THE FOOD- MOOD CONNECTION

Nutritional and Environmental Approaches
to Mental Health and Physical Wellbeing

REVISED AND EXPANDED SECOND EDITION

THE FOOD-MOOD CONNECTION

Nutritional and Environmental Approaches to Mental Health and Physical Wellbeing

REVISED AND EXPANDED SECOND EDITION

Gary Null, Ph.D.

Project Editor Amy McDonald

SEVEN STORIES PRESS
New York London Melbourne Toronto

Seven Stories Press
140 Watts Street
New York, NY 10013
http://www.sevenstories.com/

In Canada: Publishers Group Canada, 559 College Street, Toronto, ON M6G 1A9

In the UK: Turnaround Publisher Services Ltd., Unit 3, Olympia Trading Estate, Coburg Road, Wood Green, London N22 6TZ

In Australia: Palgrave Macmillan, 15–19 Claremont Street, South Yarra VIC 3141

College professors may order examination copies of Seven Stories Press titles for a free six-month trial period. To order, visit www.sevenstories.com/textbook/ or send a fax on school letterhead to 212.226.1411.

Book design by Jon Gilbert

Library of Congress Cataloging-in-Publication Data

Null, Gary.
  The food-mood connection : nutritional and environmental approaches to mental health and physical wellbeing / Gary Null. -- Rev. and expanded 2nd ed.
    p. cm.
  ISBN 978-1-58322-788-6 (pbk.)
1. Mental health--Nutritional aspects. 2. Mood (Psychology)--Nutritional aspects. 3. Food--Psychological aspects. 4. Orthomolecular therapy. I. Title.

RC455.4.N8N847 2008
616.89'16--dc22

                                        2007049987

Printed in the USA.

9 8 7 6 5 4 3 2 1

Contents

III. Disorders in Older Adults — 139

IV. Disorders in Children — 165

V. Organic Conditions Commonly Misdiagnosed as Mental Disease — 219

VI. What You Can Do: Protocols for Heart and Brain Health — 275

VII. Recipes for Natural Healing   305

VIII. Testimonials   369

Appendices   393

Author's Preface

∎∎∎

The information in this book represents nearly forty years of research and clinical experience. In seeking solutions to the complex problems of the food-mood-body connection, I have also interviewed thousands of board-certified clinicians from the fields of immunology, environmental medicine, psychiatry and psychology, as well as other behavioral sciences. From these interviews I have extracted from the clinicians' experience the information that is most relevant, and easy to understand and utilize. This provides you with the most up-to-date knowledge of the conditions you have and ways to prevent unnecessary suffering in the future.

Gary Null, Ph.D.
2007

PART ONE

Mental Health in the Twenty-first Century: Crisis or Opportunity?

Hundreds of millions of people around the world suffer from mental and behavioral health problems. Recent estimates are staggering: 154 million people with depression, 91 million with alcohol addiction, 25 million with schizophrenia, 24 million with Alzheimer's. Even more staggering is the fact that so many people endure years of chronic debility without ever receiving the help they so desperately need. Although effective treatments are available for many conditions—including a plethora of holistic nutritional and environmental therapies—mental health concerns continue to be minimized, ignored, or improperly managed by policy makers, doctors, and the general public alike.

Unfortunately, the situation has not improved over the years. "All predictions are that the future will bring dramatic increase in mental problems," says former World Health Organization (WHO) director-general Dr. Gro Harlem Brundtland, who labels mental health "a crisis of the 21st century."

According to the *World Health Organization Mental Health Atlas*, updated in 2005, global resources devoted to mental and neurological disorders remain "grossly insufficient" to address the growing burden of need. The findings "reflect the ongoing reality that the world still considers mental health care as a low priority within public health," says Dr. Benedetto Saraceno, WHO director of mental health and substance abuse. "Public health planners and decision-makers need to take the mental health needs of their populations more seriously."

Although the United States devotes more of its health expenditures to mental health than many other nations, the proportion—6 percent—is meager considering the hordes of Americans affected and the devastating consequences of these disorders. There have been advances, says Dr. Thomas R. Insel, director of the National Institute of Mental Health in a 2006 statement, but "mental disorders remain unacceptably common, causing more disability in people under age 45 than any other class of non-communicable medical illness."

Dr. Gabriel Cousens believes that what we are really facing is an epidemic of biologically altered brains caused by nutritional deficiencies. "In every generation on a universally poor diet," Dr. Cousens says, "there is a successive increasing degeneration in our mental and physical state. This has been shown in animal studies and we are now finding it in human studies. We have at least eight million children on Ritalin. At least 10 percent of our children have hyperactivity. We have 500,000 children on antidepressants, particularly Prozac. One hundred thousand children are active alcoholics. It has to do with the poor nutrition of the parents, which affects the developing brain of the fetus. Then the child is raised on a very poor diet, so the brain, which may be genetically weakened, becomes even more significantly weakened. Their neurotransmitters have lower amounts, their endorphins are not working quite right and so their brain is actually altered to the point where they need to do something to feel okay. That takes us to the epidemic of addictions which are also mental health diseases."

Despite their usefulness in shedding light on a subject still considered shameful, the Surgeon General's Report, the World Health Organization alarm, and President Bush's commission fall far short of what they might have been. Nowhere do they mention the connection between mind and body, which is the starting point of all holistic medicine. Scant attention is paid to the causes of this epidemic of mental trouble—not only "depressive illness" and addictions, but rising numbers of schizophrenics, children who can't sit still long enough to learn anything in school, and ordinary people unable to focus, sleep, or think clearly. It's taken for granted that our mental capacities weaken as we get older, but that isn't necessarily true. The environmental poisons and nutritional deficiencies that obviously contribute to mental and physical trouble, disease, or deterioration are conspicuously ignored. Even worse, the progress made by orthomolecular doctors and other health professionals still called "alternative" is missing from the picture.

The national and international experts bemoaning a mental health crisis forgot to consider the good news: most mental and emotional conditions can and have been helped, if not cured, by natural means.

As Dr. James D. Gordon, clinical professor at the Georgetown University School of Medicine says, "All aspects of diet can affect all aspects of psychological and emotional functioning," and the fact that the average doctor sees no connection between nutrition and the mind is staggering. We're not used to understanding the power of food in every healing tradition in the world. Hippocrates said 'Let food be your medicine and medicine your food.' But when we think of putting something in our mouths to affect our health, the reflex is to think of drugs."

Dr. Abram Hoffer, a pioneer in the field of orthomolecular psychiatry who specializes in schizophrenia, believes his colleagues in the mental health field are "way behind general medicine, but they're going to have to start budging. We in psychiatry are at least 10 years behind the rest of medicine when it comes to the proper consideration of nutrition, nutrients and other factors in the treatment of mental illness. They're still using treatment that was considered pretty good 30 years ago, and the only treatment today for schizophrenia is one of a variety of tranquilizers. As new ones are produced, they generate tremendous excitement as if a new tranquilizer is going to do a better job. Some of them are also very dangerous."

Dr. Hoffer uses his experience with schizophrenia to illustrate. "Standard psychiatry merely gives every schizophrenic patient one or more tranquilizers in varying doses and hopes that this will bring the disease under control. If they get well, they start to get side effects, so they cut down the tranquilizer dose, and when they do that, the disease comes back, so the patients are bouncing back and forth between the street and the hospital, between high dose and low dose, between sickness and health. You can see the result. I would guess that half of all the homeless people in North America probably are schizophrenic patients who should have been treated in a hospital and kept there. Most psychiatrists want to put their patients on a tranquilizer on Wednesday, they want to see him better on Thursday, and they want to discharge him on Friday. You simply cannot get a chronic schizophrenic patient well that fast. It takes a lot of time."

Dr. Joseph Debe underlines the time needed for good care: "There are no shortcuts to health, none. You may think it is in a bottle, or a pill, or infomercial, or some other little quick technique but it's not. We deceive ourselves when we think that. You really have to look at it like you are going back to school to learn about yourself, your body, your mind, your spirit—learn all over again because a lot of the lessons you learned weren't your own and didn't apply to you. You took them as your own, you tried to match them, but at some point you woke up and you wore a size 6 shoe with a size 12 foot. You wonder why you are in such pain and discomfort and all you kept doing is try to make it work, make it fit. Well sometimes things aren't meant to work or meant to fit based on the misapplication of our energies and our attitude. We've got to realign ourselves with what is essential to us."

In fact, the mainstream health industry has been rushing in the opposite direction. Less time. Less individuality. More and more drugs. Every year, more conditions are "diagnosed" as requiring medication. I recently saw a scientific paper claiming that the disease of "imagined ugliness" should be treated with anti-depressants. The direction is toward more pills, more "quick fixes," and more profit for the pharmaceutical industry.

For many years, the experts on my radio show and I have been protesting the huge and still increasing numbers people taking drugs to treat mental disorders. According to IMS Health, a heath-care information company, the number of pre-scriptions for antidepressants reached nearly 230 million in 2006, making them the number one type of medication in the US. That number is up from 197 million in 2002. Then there's the case of Ritalin, the stimulant used for Attention Deficit Hyperactivity Disorder (ADHD). In the last decade of the twentieth century alone, Ritalin production increased seven-fold. Ninety percent of the Ritalin prescribed in the world is used in the United States. It took the revela-tion that this class 2 narcotic was being used on children as young as six to alert the public that something was going on. Only recently have the dangers and abuses of these drugs begun to provoke an outcry in the mainstream media.

Although generally dismissed as "safe," the huge numbers of prescription drugs—especially those that alter brain chemistry—being consumed by tod-dlers, adolescents, mature adults, and senior citizens do a great deal of proven harm. Dr. Parris Kidd, a cellular biologist, says that up to 10 percent of all the people diagnosed with dementia are actually suffering from drug-induced brain damage, which appears to be dementia. "When they are taken off the drug," he says, "they begin to improve." Dr. Abram Hoffer adds that antipsychotic drugs in particular induce "the tranquilizer psychosis, characterized by a decrease in the intensity of the psychotic symptoms," though "induced in its place are apathy, disinterest, poor judgment, difficulty in thinking and concentration and inability to work."

The more we learn about how the brain and the rest of the body work, the harder it is to believe that disease and deterioration are inevitable as we age. Dr. Parris Kidd has, like many others, been insisting that "the modern pattern of brain deterioration is definitely not normal." From simple irritants like forgetting where you put your glasses or keys, to forgetting names and faces, brain impairment with aging is, most of all, a product of lifestyle, environment, and nutrition. "The brain cells are our largest and most energy-demanding and most fragile cells," Dr. Kidd says. "They are particularly vulnerable to toxins like aluminum, mercury fillings, lead from car exhaust, pesticides, even monosodium glutamate and aspartame. As the years go by, cumulative toxic damage will affect function. Although there has been a great shift in emphasis toward looking for genes that cause these problems, there is no aging gene."

What biogenetic company, I wonder, investing millions of dollars in finding a genetic marker for aging and creating a drug of some kind that will affect it, would ever acknowledge the truth of Dr. Kidd's remarks? There is no money in lifestyle change or in a healthy diet. The money is in drug therapy.

In the early twenty-first century, the money is also in genetic research, based on the idea that mental illness can be found and treated in the genes. We're told that disorders such as schizophrenia and depression seem to be passed down from generation to generation, therefore it's in your genes. A lot of research talent and money is going into trying to find vaccines so that anyone with a genetic expression of a mental disease will be able to be vaccinated against it. Dr. Ty Colbert, a clinical physiologist and active member of the National Association for Rights, Protection and Advocacy, reminds us that "while there are some true genetic disorders, like Huntington's disease, with which they are making a lot of progress, there has actually been no progress made with any mental illness. No pathophysiological evidence whatsoever exists for mental illness; it's all a series of theories."

The idea that mental illness is in the genes and can, therefore, be inherited, according to Dr. Colbert, "had its roots in the turn of the last century, when there was a strong emphasis on social Darwinism or Eugenics. There was an attempt to prove that defects are passed along, that one race is superior to the other race. So a lot of inheritance studies were developed—with a lot of errors in them—that began to show that mental illness sometimes runs in families.

They didn't consider other things that run in families—religion, accents, a lot of modeling of behavior. Just because it goes from one generation to the next doesn't mean that it's inherited."

Dr. Colbert uses the example of schizophrenia to explain. "One of the statistics most quoted by supporters of a genetic theory is that the concordance rate between identical twins with schizophrenia is somewhere between 45 percent and 50 percent. That means if one twin has schizophrenia, the chances of the other one having schizophrenia is 50 percent. That figure is used to substantiate a lot of the biological approach to psychiatry. But more recent, more accurate studies show the concordance rates actually down to something like 17 to 20 percent.

"A psychiatrist was treating a man who was schizophrenic. He also had some unusual abnormalities on his face—his ear lobes were sort of joined together next to his head and he had webs between his fingers. By chance, the psychiatrist happened to be talking to her patient's mother one day and she described an uncle who had some of the same characteristics. This uncle had been diagnosed as schizophrenic too. The psychiatrist concluded that the gene that caused the physical abnormalities in those two people may be the gene that caused the schizophrenia or that the gene that causes physical abnormalities may be close to the gene for schizophrenia. If you can find a gene for the abnormalities, maybe you can find a gene for schizophrenia. They were never able to find it. What the doctors didn't consider is that somebody with those weird characteristics is often teased relentlessly by his peers and even maybe rejected by his family, so the problems both individuals had could have been emotionally based."

1

Nutritional and Environmental Influences on Mental States

■■■

Ignoring the nutritional and environmental influences on mental states is a costly and dangerous business. Both are getting worse. Eating a healthy, balanced diet is the most effective way to ensure that our bodies receive the nutrients we need. Unfortunately, the typical American diet does not meet many of the requirements for good health, and we are paying the price physically as well as mentally. Part of the problem relates to the types and proportions of foods people eat. Just as important is how the foods are grown and processed as they make their way to our grocery shelves and kitchen tables. Scores of people have allergies, sensitivities, or intolerances to foods that they often don't even know about, all of which could be sources of emotional and mental distress. In the environmental arena, exposure to heavy metals and chemicals such as pesticides also can have devastating consequences for mental health in people of all ages.

Food: Nutrition, Allergies, and Sensitivities

Not only are the foods we eat overprocessed and robbed of all nutritional value, but the usual American diet still consists of few fresh fruits and vegetables and inordinate amounts of sugar and caffeine. When I was growing up, we got eggs or hot cereal like oatmeal, whole grain toast, and juice for breakfast. Today most children start the day with a sugared snack, a cola beverage, and high levels of caffeine. And we're supposed to believe that there is no connection between that and a child bouncing off the walls an hour later in school? Then the teacher decides that the child has something emotionally wrong with him and shouldn't be in class unless he is under the influence of a medication to control himself. We have close to nine million children taking some form of psychoactive medication each day.

Mid-morning, the kid goes out to a vending machine and gets more sugared, processed foods. By lunch time, there is almost always a toxic reaction—excitotoxins in the food are in the brain. In the afternoon, the kid is bouncing off the walls again. The kid rarely has a family meal that is also a wholesome meal. It's processed, it's pasteurized, it's salted, it's sugared, it's artificial. No one is going to stop and say, "You know, maybe the child is just having a reaction to the stimulant in the food." The latest study shows that the average child does not eat one single serving of vegetables and fruits a day. Not one. The study gives French fries the benefit of being a half serving of vegetables. So how are these kids supposed to have the biochemistry to allow their bodies and brains to function?

Dr. James D. Gordon, clinical professor at the Georgetown University School of Medicine, tells his patients to start with an experiment: "Cut out the processed food, cut out the sugar, cut out the additives and in some cases, cut out certain foods that may be likely to cause food sensitivities—wheat and milk and milk products, maybe corn. See what happens. In many cases, a kid's behavior has turned around almost 180 degrees."

This needs to be a part of our collective consciousness. Dr. Gordon believes it hasn't been so because "we keep the focus on that magic bullet. The metaphor is a metaphor of attack, an inappropriate metaphor for these kinds of conditions. The question really is—what can we do for ourselves? If we begin to pose the question that way, different kinds of answers come. You can change your diet. You can change your patterns of exercise. You can teach relaxation techniques. You can work with martial arts with kids so they can use their energy in a different way. As long as we keep posing the question—what does the expert have to do to us or for us?—we're in trouble. All we're going to come up with is more drugs."

Dr. Gordon says he's still waiting to see a good study that looks at the relationship between nutrition and the mind. "Dean Ornish did that with heart disease—he showed that if you ate a different kind of diet, you could reverse heart disease. The epidemiological evidence is that certain kinds of foods are more likely to predispose you to developing cancer, although they're not the only factor. I think we would find the same kinds of thing with behavior, but there has not been a major push in that direction, partly because there is not a major economic impetus for it. Nobody is going to make money out of basically having a decent diet. You can't patent a decent diet. You can't sell it in a pill. It's something that people have to do for themselves."

What people can do for themselves is laid out very succinctly by Dr. Gordon: "Eliminate foods that are heavily processed and have been adulterated in any way—with any kind of food additive, preservative, coloring, artificial flavoring, artificial sweetener. Aspartame has been shown to cause serious brain damage in animals.

"If possible, eat food that has been raised organically. That way, you are eliminating the pesticides, herbicides, hormones and antibiotics that go into so much of the food supply, all of which have significant biological effects.

"Eat whole foods. It's crucial. Humans were meant to eat whole foods, not Pop Tarts. If you eat a whole food diet and then eat a processed food, there are significant effects on intestinal functioning. If the intestine is not functioning well, you are not going to be taking in the nutrients, even if the food is decent.

"Eliminate all of the sugar. A natural honey or rice syrup is fine, but not the nine teaspoons of sugar in every Coke and other sweet carbonated beverages. Cut out the caffeine. Watch for food sensitivities, which are not full-fledged food allergies. The most common culprits are milk and milk products, beef, yeast, wheat, citrus, corn, soy. Eliminate those and then reintroduce them one at a time. See if it clouds your thinking or makes you anxious or depressed.

"As far as supplements go, for anybody living in a society with so much pollution and stress, I recommend a high dose multivitamin, multimineral with iron if you're a menstruating woman, without iron if you're not menstruating. And at least as a baseline, I recommend using some substance with omega-3 fatty acids—large doses of fish, like salmon, or a couple of tablespoons a day of flaxseed. (Flaxseed is somewhat better than flaxseed oil. You can grind it up and put it on your food.)

"If there are significant psychological problems, check your thyroid. A lot of people are depressed because of low thyroid functioning. Sometimes, those people may show up with normal thyroid functioning on tests. So I suggest that people take their temperature for seven days, early in the morning, putting the thermometer in their armpits for 10 minutes. If the temperature is at 98 or above, that's fine, but many people have temperatures in the 96 to 97 range. They may be hypothyroid and they may need to go to a nutritionally oriented physician or a naturopath to find out about using supplemental does of thyroid."

Even an extreme mental disease like schizophrenia can be linked to food allergies and nutrient deficiency. According to Dr. Abram Hoffer, "The nutrient deficiencies are usually some of the B vitamins, especially pyridoxine and niacin or niacinamide, and the chief mineral deficiency is zinc. During World War II in England, when sugar consumption was cut in half, when only a very dark brown flour was available for bread, and when the English were forced to depend more on their own home grown products, the incidence of schizophrenia went down, in spite of the stress of the war and the bombing of London and other cities."

The late Dr. Robert Atkins decried the inaction of conventional physicians treating mental illness when it came to identifying their root causes. Depression and anxiety, he said, are both classifiable as diet-related disorders: "I have treated about 45,000 patients in my career. In just about every community around the country, psychiatrists are doing a sort of knee-jerk reaction to the problem of anxiety and depression. They never bother to ask, 'Why is my patient having a problem?' Instead, they immediately ask, 'What is the name of the problem and what's its standard orthodox treatment?' They are bypassing the most important question of all: 'Why is my patient sick?'"

It is also important to determine how a person's anxiety and depression change over time. "If something is in the diet that is actually contributing enough to these problems like anxiety and depression, we correct the diet, and the problem will disappear," Dr. Atkins explained. "The first question you have to ask is whether the symptoms change from hour to hour. Is the depression worse for an hour, and then it suddenly lifts? Does the anxiety change from hour to hour? That is the cardinal thing to look for because if the depression or anxiety are changeable, then they are almost definitely diet-related."

Diet-related disorders can be attributed to three major mechanisms. "The first—and the most important one—is blood-sugar instability," said Dr. Atkins. "The old name was hypoglycemia, but that really doesn't describe it. It's the condition in which the blood sugar is capable of rapid escalations and rapid falls, so much so that the body is putting out other hormones—particularly adrenaline—to help regulate the blood sugar. Adrenaline is called forth when the blood sugar is on a free fall, which it usually does if something made it go up very fast, like a candy bar or a sugar- and caffeine-laden cola drink. You can make your blood sugar go up very fast and if you have this problem, which, I would say, at least half the population has to some extent, then adrenaline is released and you get a panic attack. With blood-sugar instability, typically you get your reaction before a meal, if you haven't eaten, or if you have eaten sweets and nothing else, which is the classic way to get it. That is really the basis of most anxiety states. Panic attacks can turn into an absolute phobia. You get a panic attack two or three times, and then become phobic in relation to whatever it was you were doing at the time you got your panic attack."

Food allergies are the second mechanism involved in diet-related disorders. Dr. Atkins explained, "First you eat the offending food—which is often a grain, or milk, or sometimes some of the protein foods. Usually, the foods you are allergic to are whatever you eat most often, and since in our culture so many people eat bread with every meal, you have to suspect wheat. A lot of people drink milk with every meal, so dairy is a prime allergen. After eating foods you are allergic to over a long period of time, you may develop a leaky gut syndrome, and then you will develop the inability to handle the protein complexes that are characteristic of that food. So you get a reaction after you eat it.

"The third mechanism," Dr. Atkins concluded, "is yeast, specifically Candida albicans. The yeast itself is capable, through biochemical intermediaries, of making people a little 'flaky' right from the very beginning, but it also makes you more likely to have food intolerances, especially people with sugar imbalances. Very often, people with all three of the above-mentioned conditions are going to a psychiatrist who is not trained to diagnose diet-related disorders. So even though you have psychiatric symptoms, you have a good chance of being incorrectly diagnosed."

There are two basic definitions of food allergies today. The traditional, or classic, definition describes an immunological reaction, which is usually quite severe. As Dr. Kendall Gerdes explains, "There are very good data suggesting that food allergies as traditionally defined are a fairly rare phenomenon—maybe three-tenths of 1 percent in children and even less in adults." Then there is the far more common phenomenon of food intolerance or hypersensitivity, which conventional doctors tend to know very little about. Again, Dr. Gerdes: "People read about food allergies in books they find in health food stores, but then they go to a traditional physician who thinks about allergies in a classic way. So he says, 'Well, this person is talking about something that is really rare.' But in fact, food intolerance or hypersensitivity is much more common. We have to be careful when we talk about allergies, to be sure we know whether we are speaking of the classical definition or the second, more common type.

"Many people do have significant symptoms related to foods, and these are not rare foods. They are not strawberries, or tomatoes, or peanuts that might be involved in the classic, more traditionally described immunological food allergy reactions. They are instead hypersensitivities to the much more commonly eaten everyday foods, such as milk, wheat and corn. These are the kinds of foods that can get to be problems."

Food intolerance was initially studied about fifty years ago. "A physician named Herbert Rinkel was the first one to observe that a food a person ate all the time might be causing symptoms, but you couldn't see the relationship," Dr. Gerdes says. "If you took the person off that food for a week and then gave it to them, then you might get a sharp and clear reaction. He called this 'masked food allergy.'

"Dr. Theron Randolph enlarged the concept. He observed that not only did people use these foods often, but they used the foods as if they were addicted to them. They didn't merely have wheat for breakfast, they craved wheat. They loved wheat. They might have it six times a day. They might even, if they had trouble sleeping, eat wheat in the middle of the night to help them get back to sleep. And he found that when people were using certain foods in this kind of pattern, they temporarily felt better after eating the food. By using the same principles that Dr. Rinkel had used, Dr. Randolph would take the person off the food for a week and then challenge them. In that way, many times he could see the reaction that the patients themselves could not see. The critical variable was, once he began to look for the foods that people were addicted to, he found he had a much better basis from which to determine the foods to which people were allergic."

Dr. Iris Bell, a professor of psychiatry at the University of Arizona, is also doing research in this area. "She is finding that food and chemical sensitivities probably play into the endorphin system—the same system that produces a runner's high," Dr. Gerdes explains. "The endorphin system is used as a way for the brain to give a feeling of comfort. For instance, when an infant is crying or upset, the mother gives him some breast milk, and the sugar and fat in the milk probably trigger the endorphin system so that the baby then can go to sleep. That same system can be activated under some circumstances by children and adults in order to make themselves feel good. As a consequence, people find themselves having to use a particular food or a group of foods to make themselves feel better. That is part of the basis of food addiction.

"Here's a hypothetical 35-year-old woman. (I say a woman because women go to doctors more frequently than men do, for whatever the reason. Whether this is because men are being more stoic and not coming in, or whether women are more vulnerable, we don't really know.) It would not be uncommon to find a woman who has a fair amount of fatigue, with a low-grade depression that sometimes gets to the point where she almost can't cope with things. When that occurs, and it is a variable type of thing, I will look for the two, or five, or ten foods that she is using a lot and suggest that she take them out of her diet for a week. Then, at the end of that week, many times she will find that she is not so tired and doesn't have that low-grade depression; she has more motivation to do things. Then I get more specific and test one food at a time. I ask her to have a big meal of each of those foods that she has been avoiding. Many times we can find out which food or foods have been causing the low-grade depression and her other symptoms. Though this is a generic example," Dr. Gerdes concludes, "cases just like it are fairly common."

Dr. Abram Hoffer offers another case study: "I treated a young man who was both schizophrenic and alcoholic. He had been working on his Ph.D. when he became so ill that he could not continue. Eventually he came under my care. It turned out that he didn't respond too well to my program—the vitamins and the other things that I was doing—and finally I discovered from his mother, not from him, that he consumed 12 ounces of tomato juice every morning, and had since he was a child. That was one of his basic breakfast foods. And it turned out that he had a tomato allergy. Then his mother told me that she too had been allergic to tomatoes, but she hadn't touched them for at least 60 years.

"When I put the young man on a tomato-free diet, and explained to him why, his depression and his schizophrenia vanished and he became normal. He was my second case in which a food allergy was a major factor in determining the illness of a person. It can be any one food or often a combination of foods—two or even three foods—that people have to learn to avoid, and their mental condition will then improve dramatically."

Dr. Doris Rapp is one of the world's leading experts on food allergies, especially in children. It is no accident that she has focused her energies recently on the so-called "epidemic" of Attention Deficit Disorder (ADD)/Attention Deficit Hyperactivity Disorder (ADHD) and the huge numbers of prescriptions for Ritalin and other drugs that are being prescribed for it. "There are many studies, here and abroad," she says, "that clearly demonstrate that foods and environmental factors can cause ADD and ADHD. Sixty-six percent of hyperactivity is related to food allergies. Another piece of the puzzle is clearly dust, molds, pollen and chemicals. Mint-flavored Prozac is hardly the answer if a child's depression is due to something eaten, touched or smelled that can be avoided. Environmental medical specialists can turn a child's depression or hyperactivity on and off like a switch with different dilutions of routine allergy extracts. Sure, drugs are helpful, but if the causes can be eliminated, they are not needed."

Heavy Metal Toxicity

Thousands of tons of toxic industrial wastes invade our air, water, soil, and food supply annually. Included among these wastes are heavy metals such as lead, mercury, arsenic, and cadmium. Both acute and chronic low-level exposure to heavy metals have been found to cause a host of problems, such as hyperactivity, aggression, insomnia, anxiety, depression, and reduced cognitive function.

Dr. Christopher Calapai details some of the sources of exposure to heavy metal contamination and how the problem can be so damaging to mental and physical health: "We are exposed to metals from a wide variety of places. They are in our drinking water, in some of our foods, even in our work environment where we breathe in certain toxins. Lead, for example, can come into the body through exposure to metals in paints. We get cadmium from our food, air, and water; mercury from dental fillings and shellfish; and aluminum and excess iron from pots and pans. Many of the metals that are brought into the body are toxic to the brain and to central nervous system tissue. They interfere with normal metabolism by disrupting enzyme systems.

"According to the standard textbook in the field, there have been reports of increased aluminum in the bulk of brain tissue in Alzheimer's patients and, more recently, associations of aluminum with neurofibrillary tangles and neuritic plaques. Aluminum has also been associated with neurofibrillary degeneration in patients with amyotrophic lateral sclerosis and Parkinsonism type dementia. Areas of concern with regard to mercury exposure include kidney dysfunction, neurotoxicity, reduced immune function, hypersensitivity reactions, birth defects and overall changes in general health.

"The *Food Additives Handbook* reports that lead, cadmium and arsenic are put into animal feed, as are other heavy metals. They are probably placed there intentionally to remove germs. In addition, aluminum is found in baking powder, table salt, and vanilla powder. It's used as an emulsifier, and as an anti-caking agent," Dr. Calapai adds.

The diagnosis of heavy metal toxicity should include exposure history, signs and symptoms, and lab tests.

"Before treating the condition, we perform a blood test to check vitamin and mineral levels, we examine the person's diet, consider what they do for work, where they work, and what they're exposed to at work, as well as in their home environment," Dr. Calapai says. "We also do a 24-hour urine test with an intravenous chelation procedure, and test for creatinine clearance (kidney function), as well as for heavy metals."

Dr. Richard Kunin emphasizes the importance of hair tests, as opposed to the more common blood tests, in the diagnosis and prevention of heavy metal poisoning. "A beautiful son was born to me in October 1971. In about June of 1972, he had enough hair for a hair test and I did one, and found that he had roughly 80 parts per million of lead in his hair. He should have had zero. Eighty parts per million is a toxic load and could only be coming from something he was eating. It was not something that we were putting on his hair; we certainly didn't use hair sprays or dyes. So I knew that my son, before he was a year old, was already poisoned. My heart fell. I almost fainted with grief. We checked things out and found that a toy that he had been given as a gift was tainted with 6 percent lead in the paint—that's 6,000 parts per million. If we hadn't done a hair test, he would have continued to have been poisoned and would have been mentally retarded."

Hair analysis on other patients also has been very telling. Dr. Kunin says, "I once had an 18-year-old patient, a beautiful woman, who came to see me who was depressed. She graduated from college with a C average and was disappointed in herself. She had been raised on vitamins and an Adelle Davis diet by a very caring mother. But they had lived overseas, where they had bought native pottery, and as a baby she was already lead-poisoned. I know this because I did a hair analysis of the child's hair samples that her mother had saved at various ages. At one and a half, her hair was 180 parts per million of lead. At five, it was down to 80. At age 12 it was down to practically nothing, and at age 18 we couldn't find it. As she grew, this load of lead that she had picked up as a baby was being absorbed into her tissues and being diluted. But it left behind its damage on her. Her teachers would write on her report card, 'Jennifer could have done so much better if she had really tried.' The teachers couldn't understand it. The girl had an attention deficit based on an early-life toxicity that went undiagnosed because nobody looked."

"In an enlightened society, Dr. Kunin says, "all children should be tested for lead. But their hair and not their blood should be tested. The government is spending millions of dollars to test children by taking a blood sample for lead, which is absolutely ridiculous. Lead will be filtered out of the blood in a week. If you are exposed to lead this week, by next week it will be gone, but it will remain in your hair for six months. When a hair test is done once a year, you are going to find lead contamination if it is present."

Hair analysis can be a good indicator of exposure to other heavy metals as well. "Hair analysis, for a reasonable price, gives you 30 or more real facts about the levels of mercury, arsenic, cadmium, lead, nickel, aluminum, and fluoride that have built up in your body. Everyone should know what toxic substances and physiologic minerals—chromium, selenium, boron—they're accumulating or are deficient in. We have very few tools that give us this kind of perspective," Dr. Kunin concludes. "The contamination level can be minute and still show up on the test, whose accuracy is quite high."

Treatment of heavy metal toxicity is a combination of oral vitamins and minerals to maximize immune function, exercise, and chelation therapy to remove the metals. Dr. Calapai explains, "The vitamins and minerals that we recommend are based upon the individual's particular needs. We check to see if the patient is deficient in different nutrients or if they're not absorbing certain nutrients present in their diet. The ranges are individually different and depend on the result of the physical exam."

Chelation therapy is an easily administered alternative to drugs and surgery that involves the infusion into the bloodstream of the amino acid EDTA, which moves through blood vessels and removes toxic metals. "Chelation therapy is a treatment that has been around for many years," says Dr. Calapai. "It involves using an intravenous application or induction of a protein substance that helps to bind heavy metals, to drag them out and throw them out of the body through the urine. The treatment takes about three hours to perform. It also has been shown to produce significant changes in plaque deposition in the lining of blood vessels, so it can help to open up and improve blood circulation in the body. You can detect how well the metals are being removed by means of a repeat 24-hour urine test. Chelation therapy for people who have heavy metal toxicity may be done once or twice a week for 15 weeks."

Patient Story: A Single Dental Filling

A Russian immigrant who had no fillings got a single filling when she was 20. She came to me at 22 with a shopping bag full of medicine. She didn't know what was wrong. She couldn't think. She was nauseated and sick all the time. When I asked her when it started, she said two years before. I looked into her mouth, and saw the single filling. I asked which had come first, the filling or the illness. And she said, "Oh my God. It was three months after the filling was put in that I got sick." She was a very skeptical woman who didn't trust American medicine. I told her she had to have it taken out. She was so desperate that she said, "I don't believe a word you are saying, but I'm going to have it taken out because I'm afraid that I will die if I don't."

She had the filling removed. In 17 days, she was able to start eating some foods that she couldn't eat before. It took about three months before she saw substantial results and she came back and said, "I believe it." Now that was a problem caused by a single filling.

—Dr. Alfred Zamm

Dr. Alfred Zamm explains that "mercury poisoning is like a ghost. You don't know it's there. It comes and goes, wearing masks. Some years ago, I wrote an article listing as many as 50 symptoms associated with mercury poisoning. The top three were fatigue, inappropriate coldness and sugar intolerance. These patients crave sugar and eat sweet things, and may or may not know that they will get sick. They may eat sweets on Monday and get sick on Tuesday. They may have all sorts of bizarre symptoms—muscle aches and pains, fatigue, headaches, personality changes. You don't have to have all of the symptoms; you can have one, and it may come and go."

Other common symptoms of mercury poisoning are headaches, difficulty concentrating, difficulty with reading comprehension, forgetfulness, depression, and skin changes. "It is very difficult," Dr. Zamm adds, "to prove mercury poisoning, except after the fact, when the mercury is out and the patient feels better. Taking a whole group of fillings out is not a minor matter, so I have devised some tests to assess whether or not it is worth proceeding in this direction.

"If you crave sugar and sugar makes you sick," Dr. Zamm says, "and you are already suspicious about that, then take this test. Try taking selenium, which is a mineral that binds with mercury, cadmium, and arsenic. If you feel better after taking selenium, it is a clue, not a diagnosis. About 20 years ago, when I started to investigate selenium, I realized that there was a paradox. Some people got better right away, some people took about three months, and some people got worse. I finally figured out that the patients who got worse were those who were most sensitive. They were the ones who were really sick—the ones who needed it the most but because of a peculiar intolerance to everything, including the things they needed, couldn't deal with the selenium. To overcome this, I had the very sensitive patients dilute chemically pure selenium down to very small dilutions. By starting with very small dilutions and gradually building up the dosage over a period of three months, these very sick patients started to get better."

The benefits of selenium are many-fold. "Selenium is an atom that fits into a molecule called glutathionperoxidase, which helps to destroy dangerous, foreign chemicals that just don't belong in our bodies, such as petrochemicals, floor wax and insecticides," Dr. Zamm explains. "So when you take selenium, you're not only knocking out mercury, cadmium and arsenic, you are also helping to produce more glutathionperoxidase, which protects you from environmental contaminants. So if you feel better, it is not an absolute diagnosis of mercury poisoning.

"Within pyruvate dehydrogenase complex, there are three enzymes. The first one uses thiamine, vitamin B1. If you are tired all the time, and you take 25 mg of thiamine once or twice a day, which is a low dose, and you notice you feel better, that is another clue you might have mercury poisoning. Now you have the selenium and the thiamine clue."

"The last thing is zinc. Too much cadmium and mercury in the body will replace zinc in the enzymes. Our bodies have 50 to 75 enzymes with zinc in them. So if you have mercury knocking out your zinc, then you know why it is poisoning you. It is inactivating enzymes by knocking out the zinc, which is supposed to be there, and replacing it with mercury, which doesn't work. This is cellular poisoning. You are not burning sugar, which is why you are cold and tired, and that's why you are sugar-intolerant."

Mercury does not affect everyone in the same way. Some people who have mercury in their bodies do not get sick. "We are genetically polymorphic, meaning that some people have a lot of enzymes that work very well and some people have less and what they have doesn't work very well," Dr. Zamm says. "Some of us who have mercury in our bodies are able to deal with it, while others are not able to deal with it. Those who are just getting by, who were born with a slight deficiency, will just get through. But if, at age 12 or 13, people are poisoned by having mercury fillings put in their mouths, those who have strong enzyme systems may not notice much, but those who are less strong start to manifest symptoms, although usually not right away. After a few months, a child can't concentrate at school. Maybe he or she develops allergies, and nobody connects it with the filling that was put in six months earlier."

Dr. Zamm describes how diagnosis can be difficult. "I have one patient, a young child, who had a filling the size of a pinhead and I didn't see it because it was in the back. You'd need a special dental mirror. And I said to the mother, 'I don't understand this case. This child can't tolerate sugar, he is hyperkinetic.' (Hyperkinesis, or hyperactivity, is one of the symptoms of mercury poisoning.) I said, 'This has to be a case of mercury poisoning. This child was perfectly well until he was seven. But I don't see any fillings.' She said, 'Doctor, there is a filling there.' So I got a dental mirror from a colleague of mine and looked. Sure enough, there was a filling the size of a pinhead. I couldn't believe it. I had the filling removed, and within three months the child was substantially improved. This child was genetically polymorphic in the sense that he had a very inefficient oxidation process.

"In the case of mercury poisoning, there may be enough oxygen available, but the person's body can't burn it because the burning mechanism has shut down. In every case of depression, physical deficiencies and toxic poisoning should be considered first, before resorting to therapy and psychotropic medications such as antidepressants. I have seen hundreds of these cases respond to diagnosis and treatment of the underlying physical cause."

How can mercury fillings still be considered to be safe?

"The answer," Dr. Zamm says, "is that if you did it before, it's okay to do it again. For example, lead pipes were the standard for years, so they are still okay now. Luckily, we have finally gotten around to seeing that lead pipes weren't really safe, that the lead leaching into the water causes brain damage. So we've stopped using lead in pipes. We still have tobacco from when the colonists smoked it with the Indians hundreds of years ago. You still can't convince some people that it's not healthy to smoke. We continue to sell tobacco and other poisonous substances out of habit and the profit motive.

"The same is true with mercury fillings. There is no proof that they are safe. Now, if you went out to buy a can of soup in the supermarket, it would be strange to have the clerk behind the counter say to you, 'I'd like you to prove the safety of this can.' You would say, 'What are you talking about? I'm purchasing the can. The fact that you are selling it implies that you are saying that it's safe.' But the clerk says, 'Not when it comes to soup. When it comes to soup, it is the responsibility of the purchaser to prove that it is safe or not safe. We as the sellers don't have to do anything.' That's the situation we're in with mercury fillings. No one has ever proved that mercury fillings are safe in human beings. They should prove it. But instead, the dental industry has turned it around and said, 'No, you have to prove it is unsafe.' Charlemagne said, 'If the populace knew with what idiocy they were ruled, they would revolt.' That goes for some of the things that they do in dentistry, too."

Research in recent years continues to demonstrate the devastating effects of mercury from fillings as well as other sources. Over the past decade, scientific studies have concluded that "millions of children across the world may have been mentally damaged after being exposed to low levels of mercury before they were born." Pregnant mothers with this toxicity pass it on to their unborn children, with disturbing results. In 2001, the American Academy of Pediatrics reported that the developing fetus and young children are disproportionately affected by mercury exposure. Children whose mothers ate substantial amounts of fish showed deficits in learning, attention, memory, spatial perception, and motor skills by age seven. The children performed as though they were a few months behind for their age. An Environmental Protection Agency report estimated that 85,000 US women of childbearing age have excessive exposures to mercury. The mercury in fish comes 60 percent from burning coal and oil, and 36 percent from waste incineration. The Electric Power Research Institute (EPRI) said it would cost up to $10 billion to fit power plant smoke stacks with filters to capture mercury, and that "it's just not worth it."

Dr. Ray Wunderlich offers another example of heavy metal toxicity: "A 30-year-old worker from an orange juice plant in Florida, who was a chemist and had been working there for about three years, came to me because she was depressed, irritable and anxious; she felt like her brain was in a fog. I did a chemical analysis of this patient: I looked at her blood—her red cells and her plasma—her urine and her hair. The results showed that she had excesses of five toxic metals: arsenic, cadmium, lead, aluminum and copper. Now, she had an occupational exposure to heavy metals. Many systems had gone off in the body of this relatively young woman. When she was treated for heavy metal toxicity, she progressively improved and got well. Her case is a very dramatic example of mental dysfunction and emotional problems that cleared up with the elimination of toxins.

"In the US," Dr. Wunderlich continues, "there's a lot of background exposure to heavy metals. Think about all of the auto tires on the road that are spinning off cadmium in their wheels as they wear down, all the 50,000 chemicals in the environment that weren't there 50 years ago. We are all being exposed to toxins. Dr. Davis from England has shown that these gradually and insidiously accumulate in our systems with every decade that we live. So we have to face the strong likelihood that this toxic buildup is interfering with our enzyme function."

Chemicals and Other Environmental Factors

In 2006, scientists from the Harvard School of Public Health sounded a long overdue warning: industrial chemicals are responsible for a "silent pandemic" of brain impairment in millions of children around the world. By analyzing publicly available data, they determined that at least 202 chemicals are known to have the capacity to damage the brain. However, only a few—such as lead and mercury—are regulated with regard to children. Because developing brains are significantly more vulnerable to toxicity than adult brains, children are at great risk from common chemicals used in plastics, adhesives, aluminum, paint, nylon, nail polish remover, and more. In recent years, chemical exposure has increasingly been linked to a variety of "subclinical" mental health symptoms (behavior changes, cognitive decline) as well as neurodevelopmental disorders, such as autism, attention deficit disorder (ADD), and mental retardation.

"The human brain is a precious and vulnerable organ," says Philippe Grandjean, adjunct professor at Harvard School of Public Health and the study's lead author. "And because optimal brain function depends on the integrity of the organ, even limited damage may have serious consequences. . . . We must make protection of the young brain a paramount goal of public health protection. You have only one chance to develop a brain."

Clearly, the mainstream medical and political establishment has a long way to go in recognizing and addressing the serious problem of chemical toxicity. "The government agencies and the higher-ups in the medical political structure are not even half-aware of the complexity of these environmental toxins and their effect on our health," says Dr. Richard Kunin. "They see it as very rare and therefore don't include [it] as part of a routine medical checkup. In fact, doctors have been told not to test for toxins, even though these tests are the best way to screen for poisonous metals as well as to identify how much of various substances a person is accumulating in the tissues of his or her body."

Patient Stories: Pesticides

Once at a dinner party I met a woman, and it turned out that the party was at the home of her psychoanalyst who was a transactional therapist, a psychiatrist and also an M.D. And she was a victim of a depression that would come and go. The conversation turned to what kind of therapy a doctor like myself—an orthomolecular doctor and a nutrition physician—would use. She decided to come in for a consultation to explain her depressions. In the first two months, as I went through phase one with her, which was the nutrition analysis stage, nothing came of it.

There was almost a 100-percent probability that we were going to find something chemical because the psychological inputs just didn't explain her depressions. So we went back over the whole case and hit upon something she had forgotten to tell me the first time around, which was that after she had had her third child by Cesarean, she hadn't been able to breathe for a day. Probing further, we found that the anesthesia she was administered was accompanied by a paralysis of her respiratory muscles. It's a short-term muscle relaxant that blocks the neural muscular junction and the transmitter, and you are supposed to recover in a matter of minutes. She recovered in a day. If they had not had an automatic pressure respirator there, she would have died.

She has a potentially fatal disorder. When she was measured, they found that her detoxifying enzyme, called cholinesterase, which is supposed to get rid of a chemical like this, was abnormally low on a genetic basis. She knew about this, but nobody explained to her that it put her at risk for environmental exposure to pesticides that would damage this enzyme further. The common phosphate pesticides were life-threatening to this woman. Nobody told her. Now, it turns out that she is a well-to-do woman who could afford to have an exterminator come in and spray her kitchen every month or two. And she would be disabled. The pesticide sprays are supposed to last about a week but it takes about two to three weeks to recover for an ordinary exposure, and with her low cholinesterase she would be out for a month.

She would feel depressed, weak, and shaky. She would have intestinal bloat. She would wheeze a little. She would sleep poorly, have strange dreams. Her saliva would be a little thin. In general, her autonomic nervous system was a wreck.

When she would visit her family up in Napa Valley, California, which is full of vine-yards that are sprayed, everyone else would be playing tennis, and she would be in bed with the covers over her head. Everyone thought that she was neurotic. Nobody measured her cholinesterase until I heard the story, checked and, sure enough, found she had a genetic deficiency.

In my own practice, I have come upon four cases like this, about one every two years. But in addition to these four, there have been well over 60 people I've seen in the past six or seven years who don't have the advanced or severe form, but have a milder form of environmental susceptibility.

One of these was a nurse who was in the hospital on the psychiatric ward for depression. Although her condition was improving at the hospital, she knew that this wasn't the answer. She wasn't even on medication. Just being in the ward, she was getting better, which already tells us something. She wasn't at home. She was in a new environment, and so the suspicion of environmental factors having an impact goes up.

This is an important point. If you go on a vacation and feel better, it doesn't necessarily mean that you needed a vacation. Maybe you needed to be out of your home territory where there are environmental factors that make you sick. Now in my practice I always measure cholinesterase levels. This nurse's cholinesterase were also below the normal limit. It turned out that whenever she was visiting her home territory, which was rural, she would be aware that they were spraying by airplane. From a mile away this woman would pick up drifts and her immune system was responding to the solvents and detergents that are used to disperse the sprays over a wide area. But when we measured her cholinesterase, we found that it fluctuated. When it went down—meaning it was inactivated by pesticide exposure—then she would have more symptoms, particularly depressions. When she would recover and be at her high level—meaning she was not impaired—she would feel perfectly healthy and normal and was a vivacious, dynamic person.

I call this the 'pesticide neurosis.' It's not rare and it's a very significant factor, because people are reacting to common, so-called 'safe' pesticides. These are the same pesticides that California sprayed all over the city of Los Angeles, where there were people who were having all kinds of symptoms, especially when they would spray in two adjacent areas consecutively. If you lived in the cusp between two areas, you got a double dose. In New York in 1999, the entire city was sprayed several days in a row.

—Dr. Richard Kunin

These case histories are among many in which exposure to substances was decisive, and proper diagnosis by a holistic practitioner led to a successful treatment outcome. In addition to the assessment procedures outlined above, Dr. Kunin emphasizes the importance of family history:

"Judging from the 30 or 40 cases of environmental toxicity that I could refer to from my own clinical experience, it is fairly common for a patient to have a family history," says Dr. Kunin. "You'll find out that cousin Joe had it or you'll hear that there was a suicide in the family. In fact this may have been the case with the nurse I've been describing. She came to see me looking for nutrition-related answers, and we found instead a toxin-related answer for her. She had a cousin who lived in the San Mateo area, south of San Francisco. When we had the Med Fly scare back in 1983, after the area where her cousin lived was sprayed, he went into a terrible depression and committed suicide. Of course, I can't prove that the depression was brought on by a toxic reaction to the spraying. I didn't get a blood level on him. But when you have one person with a family history of an enzyme weakness and another person with related genes who goes into a deep depression after having been exposed to a bad environmental onslaught, you have to at least consider that the two events are causally related."

These kinds of stories are a wake-up call. Today we assume everyone is so aware of and concerned about pesticides, but that is really not the case. I'm a good example myself.

For fifteen years, I didn't eat an orange or an apple because I was allergic. Then one day I was up on a farm—a friend of mine had an orchard with great beautiful-looking apples. I thought, what the heck, I know what's going to happen, I'll get red eyes, raspiness in the throat, my nose is going to run, but it's worth it. What do I care? I want an apple. So I went ahead and ate the apple and nothing happened. I thought, that's strange, maybe my fixed allergy became a cyclic allergy, so it only occurs occasionally.

I got back to town and I thought, this is great. I went to the health food store, picked up a beautiful apple, and bit into it. Within one block of walking and eating that apple, my nose was running, I had raspiness and itchiness in the back of my throat, my eyelids turned bright red, my eyes turned red. I thought, well, that's a fluke.

The next week, my buddy came to town and brought me some apples. I tried another one. Nothing happened. So then I went back to the store and asked,

"Are these certified organic?" The guy said, "Well, we think they are." I went to another store and got some that said certified organic. Nothing happened. I then got a store-bought apple that had pesticides and something did happen. I found by turning on and off my symptoms, I was allergic to the pesticide, not the apple.

I then tried the same thing with oranges and grapefruits because I'd been on vacation in Jamaica where, for breakfast, I ate papaya and pineapple and mangos and grapefruit and oranges. Nothing happened. I can eat all the oranges and apples and want, as long as they're organic. My body is sensitive to pesticides.

I told this story to Dr. Lendon Smith, who educated me further. "It may not be only the pesticide," he said. "Pesticides are disbursed in the mist of solvents and detergents, both of which are actually more allergenic than the pesticide itself. It may also be, when we say pesticide, we have to think of the whole picture. You don't get pesticide in pure form, you get it in the trade forms, whether it's kerosene or some other vehicle, and the vehicle itself may be more noxious and particularly more sensitizing than the pesticide."

Among other everyday sources of environmental toxins are paint, perfume, furniture, and carpets. Most of the fragrances on the market today do not come from natural flower scents or any natural scents; they're mostly chemicals. Some people can't go into department stores because they get violent headaches. Formaldehyde is used in inexpensive press board furniture as part of the glue. Many people get sick carpet syndrome because insecticides have been sprayed on carpets.

Patient Story: Paint Exposure

When I was injured on the job from some paint fumes, my whole life changed. I developed serious food allergies and sensitivities to everything in my environment. I became allergic to everything in my own home, I reacted to plastics of all kinds, and I couldn't breathe outdoor air. The air inside my home had to be filtered especially for me and I had to wear charcoal face masks to breathe. I was literally a captive in my home for the first year.

Also, I had depression, mood swings, and a lot of confusion and memory loss. I would go into one room and forget why I was there. I know a lot of people have that complaint from time to time, but I had it consistently throughout the day. I couldn't drive myself to the store because I wouldn't be able to find my way. I lost the ability to read normally.

Still now, two years later, I have to read things over and over in order to retain the material. I still have that deficit. I have trouble dealing with numbers.

Unfortunately, because my chemical exposure happened to me on the job, I became a workers' compensation patient. This meant that I was often sent to doctors who were unwilling to believe that there was something wrong with me or who didn't understand what the syndrome was all about. So for months at a time, because of their diagnoses, I would go without any treatment at all and I would just get worse.

Luckily I found several doctors who were able to diagnose and treat me. Dr. Wunderlich administered vitamin C drips, a vitamin supplement program, and allergy treatments, because every allergy that you can think of was triggered in my body. To this day, I cannot use any kind of lotions, cosmetics, fragrance, or hair sprays, and I doubt that I ever will be able to use them.

Very slowly, I began to get better. I still have frequent setbacks because of chemical exposures. I can't tolerate anything like gasoline fumes, new plastics, or any kind of new materials in a building. I have very restricted access to public places because of fragrances that are often used in offices, stores, or public restrooms, and because of cleaning solutions and sprays used in public places. After two years, I am still slowly making progress, but I know that I have several more years ahead of me before I can bring my immune system back to where it should be.

I like people and I have always, all my life, been around people. One of my greatest frustrations has been that now I have to dodge people because of the cosmetics, perfumes, and sprays that they use. They set off severe migraine attacks that can put me into bed for two and three days at a time.

I was forced into changing my lifestyle. I had to change my way of eating and a lot of the products that I use in my home. I've gone to a semi-vegetarian diet, mostly organic. I eat very little meat, and no flavorings. I have to be on a completely yeast-free and sugar-free diet. It is extremely restricted. But I have gotten used to it and I realize now that it's an extremely healthy diet.

My experience with doctors has made me see the need for more awareness. So many physicians saw me as a neurotic middle-aged woman because of the symptoms that I had. The symptoms that go with environmental illness are numerous and have to be taken seriously by the medical profession. It is not all in our heads.

—Betty

2

The Political and Social Dimensions of Nutrition and Mental Health

■■■

With so much expertise available and so many proven solutions, you have to wonder why Americans still suffer as much as they do. You also have to wonder why the number of people afflicted with mental trouble across the spectrum—from mild depression and lack of concentration to schizophrenia and other forms of dementia—continues to increase.

Despite the extent of mental disorders, the American medical establishment has paid little attention to causes, so intent are they on obtaining the relief of the symptoms of these conditions. Take alcoholism, for instance. There are dozens of studies showing that alcoholics are chronically deficient in certain essential nutrients. Other studies show that when these nutrients are given at optimal levels, the chemical imbalances that precipitate the craving for alcohol are diminished or eliminated, thus biochemically breaking the addictive response. One would think that the medical establishment would at least attempt to address the ramifications of these studies. Currently, many tens of billions of dollars are spent yearly on drug and alcohol treatments, the vast majority of which ignore nutrition-based approaches. Since few of the now-prevalent approaches have been shown to be successful, it is worrisome that nutrition continues to be relegated to the margins. We need to look at the fact that when biochemical imbalances are corrected and chemical sensitivities addressed, the treatments work, and with a lack of relapse. This is the kind of cause-and-prevention–oriented approach we should be encouraging for alcoholism and other problems. It is in an attempt to encourage such an approach that I put together this book.

Thousands of articles in peer-reviewed journals clearly demonstrate that nutrition affects the cause or treatment—or the prevention—of different diseases. It is estimated that up to 90 percent of all diseases could be eliminated if we understood the role that nutrition, environment, and lifestyle play. Now that we have the evidence, the question is, why haven't the medical community, the educational community, and the media advocated that we implement it?

One of the problems is that once a physician has been trained in a particular area of specialization in a particular way, for that physician to relinquish his or her mind-set and embrace a new paradigm of knowledge is not an easy process. Even with the best of intentions for their patients' wellbeing, doctors will continue to use modalities that have been outmoded, or that have been shown to be of no benefit, or that are actually harmful, for the simple reason that one uses what one knows.

Another problem is the ongoing politicization of medicine, not just in the mental health arena but throughout the field. Recent comments from Richard Carmona, US Surgeon General from 2002 to 2006, are revealing. Carmona says that during his tenure his speeches were censored by the Bush administration and he was stopped from providing accurate scientific information to the public on a variety of issues. If it doesn't "fit into the ideological, theological, or political agenda," he told a congressional committee in 2007, it "is ignored, marginalized, or simply buried."

"The job of surgeon general is to be the doctor of the nation," he lamented, "not the doctor of a political party."

The Drug Industry

According to IMS Health, a health-care information company, nearly 230 million prescriptions were filled for antidepressants in the United States in 2006, more than any other type of medication. Sales of antidepressants and antipsychotics combined totaled $25 billion. Two decades ago, sales were at $500 million. In the mental health arena, these and other drugs are the pillars of conventional treatment for many conditions. The power and influence of the pharmaceutical industry is enormous, and there's no end in sight. This comes despite recent governmental warnings about the dangers of psychiatric drugs and continuing strong evidence regarding the benefits of nutritional, psychosocial, and environmental therapies.

Even those in the medical establishment are recognizing the problem. In 2005, American Psychiatric Association President Dr. Steven S. Sharfstein issued this assessment: "The practice of psychiatry and the pharmaceutical industry have different goals and abide by different ethics. Big Pharma is a business, governed by the motive of selling products and making money. The profession of psychiatry aims to provide the highest quality of psychiatric care to persons who suffer from psychiatric conditions. There is widespread concern of the over-medicalization of mental disorders and the overuse of medications. Financial incentives and managed care have contributed to the notion of a 'quick fix' by taking a pill and reducing the emphasis on psychotherapy and psychosocial treatments. There is much evidence that there is less psychotherapy provided by psychiatrists than 10 years ago. This is true despite the strong evidence base that many psychotherapies are effective used alone or in combination with medications."

Why is the profession so devoted to the drugs? Dr. Peter Breggin, a world-renowned psychiatrist and founder of the International Center for the Study of Psychiatry and Psychology, explains: "The answer lies in maintaining psychiatric power, prestige and income. What mainly distinguishes psychiatrists from other mental health professionals, and of course from nonprofessionals, is their ability to prescribe drugs. To compete against other mental health professionals, psychiatry has wed itself to the medical model, including biological and genetic explanations, and physical treatments. It has no choice: anything else would be professional suicide. In providing psychosocial therapies, psychiatry cannot compete with less expensive, more helpful nonmedical therapists, so it must create myths that support the need for medically trained psychiatrists.

"After falling behind economically in competition with psychosocial approaches, psychiatry formed what the American Psychiatric Association admitted is a 'partnership' with the drug companies. Organized psychiatry has become wholly dependent for financial support on this unholy collaboration with the pharmaceutical industry. To deny the effectiveness of drugs or to admit their dangerousness would result in huge economic losses on every level from the individual psychiatrist who makes his or her living by prescribing medication, to the American Psychiatric Association, which thrives on drug company largesse. If neuroleptics were used to treat anyone other than mental patients, they would have been banned a long time ago. If their use wasn't supported by powerful interest groups, such as the pharmaceutical industry and organized psychiatry, they would be rarely used at all."

The medical establishment often claims that the use of psychiatric drugs helped to "empty" the US mental hospitals. "That is a myth," counters Dr. Breggin. "Psychiatric drugs were in widespread use as early as 1954 and 1955, but the hospital population did not decline until nearly ten years later, starting in 1963. That year the federal government first provided disability insurance coverage for mental disorders. The states could at last relieve themselves of the financial burden by refusing admission to new patients and by discharging old ones. The discharged patients, callously abandoned by psychiatry, received a small federal check for their support in other facilities, such as nursing or board and care homes. Some patients went home as dependents while others went onto the streets. Follow-up studies in the late 1980s and early 1990s show that very, very few patients became independent or led better lives following these new policies."

Are there any advantages to these dangerous drugs? Dr. Breggin responds, "By suppressing dopamine neurotransmission in the brain, they directly impair the function of the basal ganglia and the emotion-regulating limbic system and frontal lobes. The overall impact is a chemical lobotomy. The patient complains less and becomes more manageable. The neuroleptics mainly suppress aggression, rebelliousness, and spontaneous activity. This is why they are effective whenever and wherever social control is at a premium, such as in mental hospitals, nursing homes, prisons, institutions for persons with developmental disabilities, children's facilities and public clinics, as well as in Russian and Cuban psychiatric political prisons. They are even used in veterinary medicine to bend or subdue the will of animals. When one of our dogs was given a neuroleptic for car sickness, our daughter observed, 'He's behaving himself for the first time in his life.'"

Dr. Breggin says we need to be looking at broader issues. "How are we to understand and to show care for people who undergo emotional pain and anguish? Are we to view them as defective objects or as human beings struggling with emotional and social problems and personal conflict? Are we to drug them into oblivion, or are we to understand and empower them? Giving a drug disempowers the recipient. It says, 'You are helpless in the face of your problems. You need less feeling and energy, and less brain function.' The true aim of therapy should be to strengthen and to empower the individual. People, not pills, are the only source of real help."

Dr. Peter Braughman, a neurologist, points out that nearly twenty years ago psychiatrist Matthew Dumont suggested that the profession "give up its coquettish claims to psychotherapy and openly declare itself an arm of the drug industry." He says it need not fear an indignant response from a federal government that defines private profit as its reason for being.

Ritalin and Prozac are two cases in point. "In 1995," Dr. Braughman says, "the Drug Enforcement Administration learned of financial ties between Ciba-Geigy, the manufacturer of Ritalin, and CHADD (Children and Adults with Attention Deficit/Hyperactivity Disorder), a supposedly neutral parents' organization that was telling distraught citizens that ADHD is a disease and that Ritalin is essentially not addictive. Ciba-Geigy had given CHADD over a million dollars. The international narcotics control board expressed concern about CHADD's active lobbying for the medical use of Ritalin in children. The financial connection to a pharmaceutical company whose purpose was promoting sales of a controlled addictive substance was considered hidden advertising. Not until the spring of 2000 was a lawsuit on these matters filed. So clearly one just has to follow the money trail.

"In the 1996 elections, Eli Lilly Company, manufacturers of Prozac, made over $770,000 in soft money contributions to prominently placed politicians. By 1996, there were already over 600,000 minors on Prozac and they had a well-honed advertising campaign targeting children ready to go. There were plans for candy-coated Prozac as well."

The magic bullet theory—the idea that a single pill can cure a disease, including a mental or emotional one—not only still dominates medicine, but has become more and more prevalent. In part, this is because of the way managed care works. Judith Sachs, a professor at the College of New Jersey in Trenton, explains: "We can no longer sit in a doctor's office. The average managed care visit, whether it is for a cold or a brain tumor, is nine minutes long. In that period of time, you cannot give a full case history, you can't talk about what's going on in your life. You can talk about some symptoms, which may be somatic symptoms that come out of your stress and depression, but you can't get near the root of the problem. It's much easier for doctors to throw a prescription at it and say 'take this.'"

In the February 2000 issue of the *Journal of the American Medical Association*, Dr. Joseph T. Coyle of the Harvard Medical School says "the way mental health services are provided to children" is one cause of the increasing numbers of prescriptions for psychotropic medications being given to preschoolers. "Many state Medicaid programs now provide quite limited reimbursement for the evaluation of behavioral disorders in children and preclude more than one type of clinical evaluator per day. Thus, the multidisciplinary clinics of the past that brought together pediatric, psychiatric, behavior and family dynamic expertise for difficult cases have largely ceased to exist. As a consequence, it appears that behaviorally disturbed children are now increasingly subjected to quick and inexpensive pharmacologic fixes."

As Dr. Sherry Rogers of Sarasota, Florida, so eloquently sums up: "The drug industry clearly owns medicine. That is the bottom line. With the HMOs, medicine has clearly become a business. Every disease has become a drug deficiency. Aspirin has become a Motrin deficiency. Cardiac arrhythmia has become a calcium channel blocker deficiency. Hypertension has become a high blood pressure pill deficiency and depression has become a Prozac deficiency. All of the thought has been removed from medicine. It becomes a no-brainer. It's like a little receipt book of computerized flow sheets and the big emphasis is on labels. Label-itis is probably the number one cause of disease or death in the United States. Once you get a label, you are locked into it. Insurance companies cover certain treatments—usually drugs only—and they penalize or will not pay patients for having looked for the causes, even though they got back to work, got well, got off drugs. They will pay for several $800 MRIs, disability for being unable to work, and at least $100 a month for drugs. There is no rhyme or reason. There is no rationality. We've lost that a long time ago. So people have to take the ball in their court and find out what is wrong with them and then when they get well, to fight for their rights."

Psychiatry as Social Control

Helping people get access to the information that will actually help them get well has been my life's work. Along with others who believe in holistic healing, I have had to think long and hard about why the information doesn't get through. In part, obviously, it is blocked by vested interests.

I have been studying and speaking out against the abuses of psychiatry for a long time. One of the most important questions is, who really has the right to determine whether you are normal or not? Psychiatric terminology has always been used as a form of social control. Until the 1930s, a woman could be given a psychiatric diagnosis for just having her period. For PMS pain, she was considered insane. Before that, women were considered so emotionally imbalanced, they weren't allowed to vote. The "greatest minds" had written scholarly books on it.

In the 1930s, ice pick frontal lobotomies were done frequently and with such brutality that many patients died. But the procedure was widely accepted, and there were dozens of "scientific" articles on the importance and rightness of this procedure and who should benefit.

Electroconvulsive therapy is another case in point. Electroconvulsive therapy—shock therapy—is not a scientific procedure and does not cure depression. I have interviewed hundreds of people who have been victimized by it, generally women, and that's still going on. This treatment amounts to the destruction of brain cells by electricity. It is physician-induced brain damage.

In electroconvulsive therapy, 180 to 460 volts of electricity are fired through the brain for one-tenth of a second to six seconds. The result is a severe convulsion, a seizure of long duration, a grand mal seizure, as in an epileptic fit. As several hundred volts of electricity go through that brain, the brain becomes starved for oxygen and pulls more blood in. This causes blood vessels to break, damaging the brain. Eventually, the brain shrinks as a result of lack of oxygen and the destruction of nerves and neurons. If anyone other than a doctor did this, they would be locked up for cruel and inhumane behavior.

The usual course of treatment involves ten to twelve shocks over a period of weeks. This extreme treatment is given for depression, and it does work in the short term. A part of the brain damage is memory loss, and the patient just forgets what they were depressed about. Unfortunately, the memory loss is permanent. Permanent learning disability can be another effect of electroconvulsive therapy, not to mention emotional problems.

When the patients' underlying problems return, they're even less able to deal with them than they were before the treatment because the brain injury is so severe. The continued use of this type of medieval therapy would perhaps be understandable if it had been shown to be effective. But studies about the effects of electroconvulsive therapy directly contradict the propaganda, put forth by the manufacturers of electroconvulsive therapy devices in the United States—Somatics, Mecta, Elcot and MedCraft—upon whom physicians and the public rely for information, much as the public relies upon pharmaceutical companies for information on drugs.

The hundreds of thousands of people a year getting shock therapy generate $3 billion dollars to the psychiatric industry and the hospitals. Consider this:

there has been an ongoing campaign against the health industry in this country for well over fifty years. Every day you see advocates of the alternative position challenged as being unscientific and the purveyors of fraud. But what you have here is an industry making about one-fourth the amount of money as all the herbs and organic produce, all of the natural food stores and the vitamins and minerals that are sold, everything that we call the health movement. Electroconvulsive therapy makes that amount of money, and kills one in ten thousand people.

Here's something else to consider: 51 percent of all senior citizens in nursing homes are given antipsychotic medication and yet less than one half of 1 percent have ever been diagnosed as psychotic. The horrors continue.

It's clearly arbitrary to classify people by a term that makes them seem abnormal. I am very concerned about any group that has the sole power by such non-scientific terminology to say someone has a disease. If you send me someone who is classified with bipolar depression and I find out they have low thyroid, reactive hypoglycemia, or corrective biological imbalances and they are no longer depressed, maybe they were not depressed to begin with. Someone should be looking at why they had this diagnosis in the first place.

Many of the people I have interviewed confirm my worst fears. Dr. Paula Caplan, affiliated scholar at Brown University's Pembroke Center, worked on the *Diagnostic and Statistical Manual of Mental Disorders*, the so-called bible of mental health professionals. "The question of who puts this book together and how they do it is of fundamental importance," she says, "because a very small number of people are behind decisions about which of us are crazy and which of us are not. That book is put together by a handful of mostly American psychiatrists, mostly white men.

"According to the manual," Dr. Caplan says, "there are 374 different kinds of mental illness or mental disorders. The DSM is revised periodically; seven years earlier, it had only 297 categories of mental illness. So the whole definition of what are mental illnesses is growing by leaps and bounds. Some of the people who write this "bible" really want to help, and they think the best way is by giving people labels. Other people are very territorial; they think that the more territory this manual covers, the better it is for the mental health professionals. Some people just want to make money—if I can find a way to pathologize anybody who walks through my office door, I am set for life financially."

Dr. Caplan further explains her concerns. "We are basically psychologizing, psychiatrizing, pathologizing virtually the entire population. In the current edition, the *DSM* lists Nicotine Dependence Disorder—if you are having trouble quitting smoking, you are mentally ill. There is something called Caffeine-Induced Sleep Disorder—if you drink coffee and it keeps you up at night, you've got a mental disorder.

"Because diagnoses are not drugs, the FDA doesn't regulate them; nobody does. Nobody says 'good heavens, we're diagnosing half a million North American women as having premenstrual mental illness, doesn't that seem kind of extreme?'"

DSM diagnoses can have devastating consequences. "People are losing custody of their children because they've been given one of these labels and that fact is hauled into court," Dr. Caplan says. "They can lose their jobs, though legally you are not supposed to be fired for having a diagnosis of mental illness, but in fact, it often happens. They are being declared mentally incompetent. People are being hospitalized against their will. People are being denied various kinds of insurance. If you are given a diagnosis of a mental disorder, you often cannot get disability insurance because you are considered to have a preexisting condition or you are charged exorbitant premiums.

"There should be investigations at every level of government and by private citizen groups of the way psychiatric and mental health diagnosis is done. We need to be challenging it. Like challenges to breast implants and the Dalkon shield, where the people who produced and manufactured them and the individual doctors who used them on their patients have been held liable for the harm that was done. Diagnostic labels are in that same sense products. They are produced by the American Psychiatric Association in the *DSM* and marketed just like the Dalkon Shield, breast implants and cigarettes. The dangers are being covered up. I call the whole process Diagnosisgate because of the parallels with Watergate—the lies, the cover-up. The people who are the most unhappy, in need of help, going to therapists—these are the most vulnerable, the most likely to have these techniques and what is in this book used against them. We need to do something to protect people."

Dangers of Psychiatry

PATIENT STORY: SHOCK THERAPY

When I was a teenager, I had a baby who was born prematurely. He died eleven hours after birth. I had been taught when you are depressed, you put yourself in the hands of your doctor and I did. My mother dropped me off at the hospital on her way to work. I walked in of my own free will. I brought pretty things to dress up in because I thought it was going to be like a vacation. I was told I was going to play games like ping pong and just relax. When the psychiatrist suggested shock treatments, it didn't even cross my mind that it would damage me, so I signed for them. After they started, I had excruciating pain. I could barely remember how I got in the hospital. I was absolutely devastated. I tried to leave and they called the guards, they stopped the elevators, they dragged me down the hall, they shot me full of thorazine, strapped me down in four point restraints—that means having each wrist and each ankle bound securely so that you can't move, you can't bite and you can't get away. To say the very least, it was no way to treat a lady.

—Sandra

Not only was that no way to treat a lady, it was also the making of an activist. Years later, when Sandra Everett learned that what had happened to her was still happening, even to young children, she had to get involved. As she explains, she "became a human rights activist, knowing first hand that when an innocent, harmless person gets behid those walls under psychiatric care, nothing they say is taken seriously. Everything is considered an illness."

As founder of Citizens Rescuing Youth, Everett was one of many people organizing against Goal 2000, a law signed into effect by President Clinton. This law actually mandates that a mental health clinic be established in every school. Among her concerns were that everything was being labeled as a mental illness—"oppositional defiance disorder, attention deficit hyperactivity disorder, everything is a disease. If you are bored, that is attention deficit. If you are very active, they call that hyperactivity."

The group that benefits most greatly from this is the mental health system. In Georgia, where she lives, Everett found that the local school system receives more than $6,000 per year per child labeled with attention deficit hyperactivity disorder and put into special education. With a label of mental or emotional disorder on top of that, she says, the amount increases to more than $10,000.

"If that's not putting a bounty on the heads of our children, I don't know what is," Everett says. "If a child is labeled as having attention deficit hyperactivity disorder, they have to carry behavior cards and behavior folders everywhere they go. In one school, the labeled children are not allowed to sit with the other children at lunch. They are being made into outsiders, they are embarrassed about having to go into different classes. They are taunted for taking a pill in order to be able to sit still and concentrate. And it has no scientific validity, because there is no scientific test for this so-called disease. It was invented by the American Psychiatric Association, on the basis of behaviors alone. They did test for alpha wave changes in the brain, but alpha waves change in the brain when a person is bored and not paying attention anyway."

Many parents are being told that their children could have a chemical imbalance in the brain, and that a psychological examination is warranted. "But," Everett says, "there is no scientific test for chemical imbalance in the brain and if there is indeed a chemical imbalance in the brain, it is not an imbalance of Ritalin or Dexedrine or any of the other medications that they use. On one hand, schools are saying 'just say no to drugs' and on the other hand, the school system, infiltrated by psychiatrists and psychologists, is pushing more dangerous drugs than what the child could be getting on the street."

Dr. Braughman says that behind the overmedicating of children lies the fact that "the schools today are in disarray. They confuse psychology and psychiatry with education. While academic achievement and real world preparation for life is declining, the frequency of diagnosis of so-called learning disabilities such as dyslexia, specific mathematics disorder and ADHD is on the rise. These things serve as a ready excuse for the fact that educators have failed to educate, and that is the lure. It is much more ecstatic and romantic to be a brain diagnostician than it is simply to be one whose job is to impart the skill of reading. So we have teachers all over the country who are deputy diagnosticians, in a diagnostic orgy labeling children as brain diseased and with chemical imbalances of the brain.

"These are troubled children and the adults in their lives, both at home and in schools, are not meeting their emotional needs. Parents are seduced by the educational establishment that has already been totally seduced by mental health as education. Parents tend to believe what they are told by professionals and they're being told that there is a substitute for the real work of tough love. It's a tragic deception, part of the fraud and deception of biologic psychiatry that represents emotional pains as actual diseases when none in fact are."

An ever more egregious abuse of psychiatry is the repression of information about the disastrous side effects of commonly prescribed drugs, not only in their destruction of people's brains, but also the threat to self and society posed by the propensity to suicide and violence. Thankfully, there have been some changes in this area in recent years, but they don't go far enough. Why did we have to wait so long? And at what cost?

The Citizens Commission on Human Rights reports that a review of US school shootings from 1998 to 2007 indicates that 38 percent of the perpetrators were taking psychiatric drugs. In Columbine, Colorado, Eric Harris was on the antidepressant Luvox when he and Dylan Klebold killed twelve classmates and a teacher, wounded twenty-three others, and killed themselves. Six years later, in 2005, Jeff Weise was taking Prozac when he shot and killed nine people before committing suicide. Although the toxicology report ruled out psychiatric drugs in the body of 2007 Virginia Tech gunman Cho Seung-Hui, his roommate reportedly told the media that Cho's morning routine including taking prescription medicine. This may mean that he had been taking medication but stopped before his tragic massacre of thirty-three people on the university campus.

Unfortunately, it took the Food and Drug Administration (FDA) until 2005 to require drug companies to add black box warnings to antidepressant labels about the risk of suicidal thinking and behavior in children and adolescents, and until 2007 to extend that warning to young adults aged eighteen to twenty-four.

3

The Promise of Orthomolecular Psychiatry and Psychoimmunology

■■■

Despite the forces defending the medical status quo, change is happening. There are some physicians—albeit a relative handful out of the 700,000 in the US—who are using the therapies referred to in this book. These physicians are revolutionizing American health care. There is also a growing segment of the public becoming aware of these nontoxic therapies, many of which have been around a long time. But the impact of these forces is only just beginning to be felt in mainstream America.

Orthomolecular medicine and orthomolecular psychiatry are now some forty years old, having started with Dr. Linus Pauling's 1968 article in *Science* magazine. As Dr. Philip Hodes explains, "'Orthomolecular' means the right amount of the right nutrients. Thanks to Dr. Roger Williams's concept of 'biochemical individuality,' and Dr. Bernard Rimland's concept of 'toximolecular brains,' we found that many people with so-called mental illnesses, including schizophrenia, autism, depression and manic-depression, can be helped, in a majority of cases. They must first clean the toxins out of the brain and then provide the brain with the right amounts of the right nutrients.

"Each person is biochemically individual," Dr. Hodes continues, "so the government standards for the minimum daily requirements of various nutrients actually have little if any bearing on the specific needs of any particular human being. What seems to be a mega-amount for one person is the precise amount necessary to keep another person healthy and sane."

Psychiatrist Michael Schachter says that most psychiatrists will consider the possibility of a chemical imbalance in the brain as well as any psychosocial factors. In the former case, they then immediately resort to using some kind of drug to try to right the balance, without looking into the possibility that there could be nutritional factors contributing to the patient's psychological state. "I explore possible imbalances in the body that could be caused by nutritional and other environmental, nonpsychosocial factors that might be playing a role in the development of psychological symptoms. For instance, they don't bother inquiring how much sugar a person is eating, or how much coffee someone is drinking. They do look at alcohol consumption, especially if it's excessive, but most psychiatrists are unaware that sometimes even small amounts can be a problem."

Whenever possible, Dr. Schachter prefers nutrition-based therapies. "I use nutritional substances or substances that are natural to the body, either food substances or accessory food factors—such as vitamins or minerals or amino acids—as the treatment of choice for a person's mental disorder. Sometimes the vitamins may be megadoses because a person may be what we call vitamin-dependent on a particular nutrient. For example, some children who are hyperactive or having learning disorders will respond to one vitamin, for instance vitamin B1 (thiamine), and actually might get worse if you give them large doses of vitamin B6. So treatment really has to be individualized. I try to find what seems to be most effective for that particular child's or adult's condition."

Hand in hand with the nutrition-based approach, Dr. Schachter looks closely at the clinical ecological factors: the foods in the person's current diet, the water he or she drinks, the air he or she breathes, any imbalances in the body, as well as any daily-life habits. "For example, I check for hormonal imbalances or subtle low-thyroid conditions, which are very common in depression. If these are treated, there will often be marked mood improvement. Calcium and magnesium deficiencies are very common as precipitators for anxiety in general or even panic attacks. By correcting some of these nutrient imbalances, you can reduce tremendously the chances of a person having panic attacks. Then, if everything else is not sufficient to bring about improvement, I would use psychotropic drugs if I had to, but I would try to keep them at the lowest possible dose and I would use nutrients and other dietary supplements to minimize their side effects."

In 1955, Dr. Abram Hoffer and several colleagues published a paper in which they showed that nicotinic acid lowered cholesterol levels but that you had to give

3,000 mg per day. This was a major step forward because it proved that you sometimes needed large amounts of a vitamin for a condition not known to be a vitamin deficiency disease. High blood cholesterol was not known to be a vitamin deficiency disease. The term "orthomolecular"—first used by Dr. Linus Pauling in his paper in *Science* in 1968—was based upon his recognition that certain vitamins are effective when they are used in large quantities.

At that time, the conventional wisdom was still that you used vitamins only in tiny amounts and you only needed them for the prevention of deficiency diseases, like scurvy or beriberi. A nutritionist accepted the fact that if you had scurvy you would eat oranges or you would take small quantities of vitamin C. As Dr. Hoffer puts it, "It was unheard of to give someone 1,000 mg of vitamin C. If you suggested this they would throw up their hands in horror. The idea that you could use large quantities of vitamins to treat conditions, not just to prevent them, was a major step forward. In fact, it is considered a major paradigm change. So we are now in a paradigm in which we use vitamins as treatment, not just as prevention."

Dr. Hoffer emphasizes this development in his clinical approach. "Orthomolecular psychiatry and medicine was the first major movement to adopt this treatment paradigm. What it means is that when we have a sick patient, we correct their diet. This is vital. I don't talk to any patient until we have spent some time on their diet. We also use any drugs that have to be used. If I have a schizophrenic patient I will use tranquilizers; if I have a depressed patient I will use antidepressants; if they're epileptic I'll use anticonvulsants; if they're suffering and in a lot of pain, I'll use analgesics. But that's not all. In addition to that we use the appropriate nutrients. It can be any one of the 20 or 30 nutrients currently in use. We combine them all. When the patient begins to respond, we gradually withdraw the drugs until we are able to maintain them on the nutrients alone or on such a tiny amount that it doesn't interfere with their ability to function.

"Orthomolecular medicine is the appropriate use of molecules, nutrients, which are native to the body in the appropriate concentration at the appropriate time.

"I don't like the term 'alternative.' I think, rather, that we are going back to our historical roots. If you go back one hundred years we had no treatment except nutritional treatment. For two thousand years the best doctors in the world always emphasized good nutrition, but over the past hundred years nutrition suddenly disappeared from medicine. We're just bringing it back again."

Dr. Hoffer considers orthomolecular medicine the mainstream, "even though most doctors don't yet recognize it. My colleagues in psychiatry are still years out of date. That's because of the natural conservatism of the profession combined with the fact that they have had the least training in biochemistry and physiology of all physicians and thus they are the least likely to look upon the body as a physiological organism. They look upon psychosocial problems as primary when, in fact, in many cases they are secondary. The American psychiatric establishment—including Canada, and including the National Institute of Mental Health—has taken a very strong position against the use of vitamins in psychiatry and have yet to reverse their position, because they're slow learners."

Dr. Garry Vickar believes that "doctors have a tendency to close their minds to anything other than what they read in their literature." He suggests that there are ways to help your physician be a part of the healing process. "The name of the game is getting better. You can't make people want to treat you if you come at them and say, 'You guys are all wrong. You don't know what you're doing.' Doctors want to be helpful, but how you approach them is important.

"Medicines have not been perfect. But without medicines, things are often worse. So let's assume we have to look at the role of medications up to a point. I think you have to have a framework. I think it's important not to become so radical that you say, 'Medicines are no good; they're dangerous all the time and inherently bad.' That's not true. Medicines are not always bad any more than nutritional supplements are always good, because people can be harmed from inappropriately using nutritional supplements, especially herbs that have pharmacological effects in certain doses."

According to Dr. Richard Kunin, people tend to have ideas about health habits that are too generalized. "Before Linus Pauling and the word 'orthomolecular,' most people thought they were in the avant-garde if they took a multivitamin. These days most people are still proud of themselves if they cut down on their fat consumption and increase their complex carbohydrates and their intake of high-fiber foods. That seems to be the nutritional prescription that is our current consensus. But the orthomolecular approach that, as a doctor, I have learned to respect, goes beyond a 'one-size-fits-all' prescription and looks instead to a person's individual needs as the basis for treatment.

"I have adopted a strategy that allows people a chance to test themselves where diet is concerned in order to identify their needs," Dr. Kunin continues. "I call that test the 'Listen To Your Body Diet.' The bottom line is that people find their own particular food favorites and their own particular dietary balance, especially relative to carbohydrates. Usually, however, it's a blanket thing, like avoid sugars or increase complex carbohydrates. That leaves a lot unanswered until people go for specific tests."

Dr. Kunin goes beyond testing of vitamin levels. "We go a step further and also test the enzymes that the vitamins couple with to ultimately make the body chemistry work," he says. "We see marked deficiencies in large numbers of the people who come to see us. Remember, they are coming to the doctor because they feel something is wrong. The odds of something being wrong, therefore, are 100 percent. But we catch only about 70 to 80 percent."

There have been significant advances in toxicology, allergy, and immunology over the years. For the past four decades, Dr. Kunin has been administering a screening test for toxins called the hair test. "It is possible to screen every patient for mercury, lead, arsenic, aluminum, cadmium, nickel, and get an accurate picture of the environmental input into the individual's overall health," he explains. "The test was, unfortunately, unfairly criticized by the AMA and is not used nearly as much as it should be. Those who are nickel-afflicted are likely to be more allergic. Nickel is a free-radical generator and a sensitizer of the first rank. People with nickel-tainted hair tend to have nickel in their dental alloys or fillings. Nickel is even more sinister than the more well-publicized mercury, which is also a sensitizer. There is nickel in the braces that kids wear, and they can pick up nickel in their systems that way.

"Doctors who don't test their patients for toxicities and allergens are getting a limited view of their patients," Dr. Kunin concludes. "This can lead them to rely on treating symptoms with major tranquilizers, antihistamines, or other nonspecific therapies, rather than treating the source of an individual patient's problems."

Psychoimmunology

Psychoimmunology, also called psychoneuroimmunology, is a discipline that examines how psychological and social factors affect the functioning of the immune system. It is based on the concept that the mind and the body are intricately linked. Over the years, researchers in the field have accumulated data demonstrating that the immune system is affected by factors such as stress, negative emotions, positive affect, and supportive personal relationships. Among the conditions that have been found to have immune disregulation resulting from psychological components are infectious diseases, cancer, AIDS, arthritis, heart disease, and dementia.

PART TWO

Disorders of Mood and Behavior

4

Addictions

■■■

Patient Story: Alcoholism

I am a recovered alcoholic. It's been about seven years that I've been off alcohol. At first, I ate a lot of sugar in cakes and things like that. One of the psychological-emotional components of my behavior was that I always had a very difficult time getting started in the morning. The first thing I would think about when I got up was what I was going to eat, which usually included cereal with sugar, a pastry, and sugar-laden coffee. There has been a slow, progressive bettering of my diet, but there has still always been the sugar craving. Sometimes I would be able to get away from it for a week or two weeks, but it would always creep back in.

Recently, I completed a seven-day fast and a colonic cleansing, and I found that after that cleansing process the craving pretty much disappeared. Also, I wake up in the morning feeling rather alert, and I don't have this compulsion to eat sweets. I think that because I am staying away from sugar, I generally am having better days psychologically.

—Bob

According to a 2007 study published in the *Archives of General Psychiatry*, more than 30 percent of adults in the United States experience alcohol abuse or alcoholism during their lives. We have come a long way from the idea that addicts are morally reprehensible beings who could stop whatever it is they're doing if they only wanted to enough. The medical community, as well as the homeopathic world, now understands that addictions may be diseases, degenerative ones at that. The wisest practitioners know that addictive substances change brain chemistry in ways that persist long after a person stops taking drugs and that no single "medicine" cures any addiction. They are beginning to tease out the best means of helping all kinds of addicts by addressing the specific chemistry of their addiction and recovery, as well as acknowledging the need for mental and spiritual aid.

While we remain a nation of people where, in the new century, an estimated four out of ten can't get through a day without the "fix" of tobacco, caffeine, alcohol, or cocaine, alternative treatments are becoming increasingly sophisticated. It is now believed, for example, that women's hormonal cycles probably influence the ability to stop smoking—those who quit during the first fourteen days following menstruation seem to experience less withdrawal and depression than those who quit after the fifteenth day. For some addicts, acupuncture helps, and a few enlightened medical insurance companies are beginning to cover it. In Oregon, heroin addicts must try acupuncture before getting methadone.

The "last frontier" in recognizing how addictive a society we are comes in the attention being paid to substance abuse among the elderly. It is now estimated that 2.5 million older adults have alcohol-related problems, often missed by physicians who mistake symptoms like falling or gastritis for problems associated with aging. Elderly females have less alcoholism as a group, but more depression and more problems from prescription drugs, as well as high rates of nicotine dependence. Since the nutritional situation of most elderly people is far from optimal, I'm convinced that the approaches outlined here could go a long way toward improving the situation.

Dr. John Eades has a twenty-year history of working in the field of addiction and chemical dependencies. His concerns are social and spiritual. He defines addiction as having three components: "The first is a compulsion or craving. That is a form of a hunger. The second is loss of control. The alcoholic will try to drink two drinks and go home, but he winds up drinking 15 or 16 drinks. The gambling addict may take $100 and leave a credit card in the trunk of the car, but before the evening is over, she is probably back out to the car, getting the credit card. The third is that the consequences of the behavior are bad or negative and the individual continues doing the behavior. The alcoholic gets a DUI, which might stop a person who is just a social drinker. It doesn't stop the alcoholic. A gambler may write a bad check, have problems from that, but it will not stop the behavior.

"In our culture we have addictions to more than drugs. We have people addicted to work. They are on the airplanes all the time with their computers, working and working and working to the exclusion of having a well-rounded life. People are addicted to sexual activity, alcohol, cigarettes and gambling, a new addiction on the horizon that is going to bring tremendous problems as [local and state] governments continue to finance themselves with the revenue from gambling establishments. Another one is addiction to exercise. I have some patients who, if they cannot run on any particular day, actually go into a form of withdrawal. Even when they get injured, they still go out and exacerbate that injury by continuing to exercise."

Myths about happiness, Dr. Eades says, are at the core of the emptiness that leads to addictions. "One of the greatest and most damaging is, 'I'll be happy if I am successful.' The person is always striving, never truly arriving, always reaching, not resting. When this happens we become externally oriented, looking for things outside us to define us. I've worked with too many patients who are very wealthy, but also very discontented and very disconnected in their lives."

Linking happiness to another person or an event often causes problems. "Saying 'I will be happy if I can make another person happy in a relationship' leads again to being focused on others," Dr. Eades says. "The addict's life revolves around the drug while the co-dependent's life revolves around the addict. Or, 'I'll be happy when a certain situation occurs—when I graduate from school, when I get that job, when I get married, when we have children, when I get that new house, when the children leave home, when I can retire from that job, if I had more money, if I had planned better for my retirement, if I had more years to live.' This myth of 'I'll be happy when or if' can last an entire life.

"A lot of people need the approval of others in order to feel good about themselves. They become a system of mirrors, reflecting back what people think we should be, want us or expect us to be. I also find a lot of people feel that they have to be perfect. When a person starts to fail, as is the normal way of being human, they blame others and this promotes denial of the reality of their imperfection."

What prompts people to face their addictions? "People change when the pain of where they are becomes greater than the pain to change," Dr. Eades continues. "The alcoholic reaches a place where he says 'I can't go on this way. I'm killing myself physically. I've lost my job and so forth, but I can't live without it.' In addictive relationships, they see that person when they don't want to, they see them more than they mean to, they call them.

"Psychology is limited in its ability to help the addictive mind. William James, the great Harvard psychologist, said that for human beings to change, they must undergo some type of spiritual transformation. One of the myths that permeates our society is that psychologists have all the answers. I know for sure that I don't and I know that as I listen to other professional psychologists talk, that they don't either. We have overlooked the spiritual aspect of the human psyche. Spirituality is necessary. The people that seem the happiest are well-rounded and also have a very active spiritual life. They have been able to reach a state of solitude where they can look inward and have a better understanding of life and what's important. Some people are so addicted that no matter what we do, no matter how we analyze that person, no matter what techniques or gimmicks we use, that person probably is only going to change when they undergo some form of spiritual transformation."

Dr. Eades says he has a simple formula. "One way that people get reconnected with themselves is by being responsible in their behavior. The word responsible comes from Latin, and it means to be answerable to. Indeed we are answerable to ourselves as well as to other people. The real problems begin when a person behaves irresponsibly and still feels okay about it. At that point, the person begins to distort the world, developing a whole host of ego defense mechanisms, denying and distorting and essentially losing contact with themselves.

"I tell my patients that if they want self-esteem, they have to forgive themselves for the past, realize that their futures are spotless and that they are going to have to start being responsible. I urge them to look for internal validation. Focus inward instead of focusing outward. Stop being a victim."

Patients also have to be ready to stop lying. "I ask them not to lie to anybody about anything they are doing for the next ten days," Dr. Eades says. "Well, that is a big task for many people in recovery. When they can go through a day without lying, they are probably starting to behave responsibly. If they are behaving irresponsibly and have someone they can tell, honestly, and then move on, that helps.

"In sum, people with addictions have to start being responsible, start striving to be honest, and find a spiritual life. They need to get connected in some kind of organized way perhaps. There is power in people working together toward trying to get connected spiritually. We have to slow down and say, hey, where am I going? What am I doing with my life? Nothing changes if nothing changes then nothing changes. People expect to continue their same behaviors with their same attitudes and their same thought patterns, but it doesn't work that way. We find great power in helping other people. In AA [Alcoholics Anonymous], people can stay sober because they are helping other people. People are happiest when they lose themselves in activities that help other people with no expected payback.

"Recovery for most people is not just ceasing a behavior but making a total change. A total holistic change must occur; otherwise, the person will either go back to that drug or that behavior, find another drug or behavior, or continue behaviors that make them very manipulative in nature."

Drug and Alcohol Addiction

According to 2005 data, an estimated 22 million Americans are addicted to drugs or alcohol. Of these, 3 million are dependent on or abusing both alcohol and illicit drugs, 4 million have the problem with alcohol only, and 15 million are struggling with drugs only. Unfortunately, many people either receive no treatment at all or receive it after years of dependence. Conventional treatments that have been partially successful include twelve-step programs, psychosocial therapy, and medications. As the holistic medicine community has known for years, nutrition should also be part of this arsenal.

The late Dr. Atkins considered nutritional awareness and support a necessary component of any successful alcoholism program. He explained that alcoholism is so tied in with carbohydrate metabolism that it is fair to say they are "genetically super-imposable." In other words, it is possible to understand alcoholism in terms of carbohydrate metabolism alone. This is an extremely radical assertion, but one that lends important insight into a problem that plagues our society.

"I have seen families in which half of the members were alcoholics and the other half were sugarholics," said Dr. Atkins. "And you could switch them over. You could probably make alcoholics of the people that were addicted to sugar, and it is well known that when alcoholics go through a psychologically based program, and not a biochemically based program, they have a tendency to become sugar addicts."

In fact, it is unusual for ex-alcoholics not to become sugar addicts. More commonly, individuals replace one addiction for the other. As Dr. Atkins noted: "Unless people get the clue that there is a connection between alcoholism and sugar addiction, they will just go from one to another and will not feel any better. The phrase 'dry drunks' refers to what happens to alcoholics that start switching to sugar instead of getting on a diet in which all the simple sugars are eliminated."

Dr. Abram Hoffer also believes in the nutritional approach: "The general regimen that orthomolecular medicine uses for alcohol addiction (as with depression, schizophrenia, and a number of other mental disorders) is to pay careful attention to nutrition and the use of the right supplements," he says. "The first order of business is to make sure that the individual's basic diet is optimal. We do that by trying to take away most of the additives in food he or she eats on a daily basis. It is impossible to get them all out, but we try to do the best we can. One of the best simple rules is to put the patient on a sugar-free diet, because almost all foods that contain sugar contain a large variety of other chemicals. By avoiding sugar you will cut out most additives, by about 80 or 90 percent. Since we are all individuals, and many of us have food allergies and can't tolerate large quantities of carbohydrates or protein, for example, each one of us has to develop a diet that is optimal for ourselves."

The next step involves supplements. "We add in the supplements that are right for this particular individual," Dr. Hoffer continues. "Many of us have been so deprived of these proper supplements over our lifetime that, even with a very good diet, we cannot regain our health. That's why we need supplements. This is where the treatment differs markedly from person to person (and depending upon whether someone is being treated for alcoholism, or a mental illness such as depression or schizophrenia). So while the dietary regimen is largely the same for all—avoid sugar and any foods that make you sick—supplements are determined on a case-by-case basis."

If you are taking a substance because you're depressed, you might have some form of brain imbalance, or your depression may be physiologically induced—an underactive thyroid or a blood sugar imbalance. High blood sugar or low blood sugar manifests as depression. To get away from the chronic feeling of emptiness that frequently occurs with depression, people start to drink, which takes away the feelings and gives them the sense of being in a never-never land. The same is true of many drugs. People take drugs to get a euphoria they wouldn't have achieved on their own or that they may have had but couldn't sustain. Once you get used to that, the quick and easy route is just to stick a needle in your arm or some form of narcotic up your nose or drink it or ingest it.

None of this helps us to resolve the underlying conflict. Is the conflict biological or psychological in nature, or a combination? I have found that one of the best approaches to this problem is a systematic cleansing program, through which people actually break all physical addictions, not just to sugar, but to every other thing to which they could be allergic. Their energy comes back. Any form of addiction withdrawal creates a lack of energy, so when you substitute the energy they would be getting from the drug, and you give it to them naturally through the body's own process of metabolism, they feel better.

Then you start to rebuild the brain and the center of the brain with phosphatidyl serine, acetyl-l-carnitine, phosphatidyl choline, and herbs that are known to have an impact, like feverfew and green tea. You flood the body with flavonoids. And don't forget the juice—four to six juices a day from fresh organic vegetables. After six months to a year of this regimen, I've seen about 80 percent of addicts cleared up, staying off it, and not coming back.

I would add that if you have a problem drinker in your family, one of the things you can do is just try to see that they take some vitamins. I would start with 5,000 milligrams of vitamin C per day in five 1,000-milligram doses, as well as 1,000 micrograms of vitamin B12. The most beneficial form is methol coalobin. Hopefully, they will take them. If not, try to blend them into juices—orange juice or V-8 juice, whatever they are willing to drink.

Alcohol frequently swells the brain if you have a sensitivity to it, so you need vitamin B1—a lot. If you're an alcoholic, you need at least 100 milligrams twice a day. Normally, I suggest 10 milligrams of B1, 15 milligrams of B2, and 15 milligrams of B6, but not with an alcoholic. They need the whole B complex at a higher level. Also, the essential fatty acids have been used extensively to help people who have problems with alcohol, generally one capsule of about 100 milligrams with a meal.

There are certain amino acids that are helpful. One is glutamine. Be sure not to confuse it with glutamic acid. If you take glutamine with vitamin B6 on an empty stomach—and it's best to take it on an empty stomach—along with thiamine and vitamin B6, it will affect the brain.

Magnesium is also important in brain detoxification; I've yet to see a person who drinks regularly, even beer, who is not deficient in magnesium. I also recommend pantothenic acid, which is vitamin B5, and vitamin C, which should be taken with quercetin, the bioflavonoid. The flavonoids are very powerful oxidants and healing agents. They have antiviral properties and antiyeast properties. They are great for people with Candida, fatigue, and chronic infections. Ninety percent of the vitamin C you take is not utilized unless you take the bioflavonoids with it. I take issue on this point with Linus Pauling, whom I greatly respect. I've yet to see where vitamin C taken by itself is maximally utilized. You just don't get high bioavailability, where the tissue actually utilizes it. Generally, about 2,000 milligrams of the bioflavonoids would be sufficient.

Lecithin is crucial for helping the liver and brain functioning overall because of its choline inositol. Generally, people who consume even moderate amounts of alcohol have "lipotropic factors," fat buildup in their organs, including the liver. That adversely affects metabolism.

You should also look at niacin or niacinamide, if you want to prevent the flush. Milk thistle weed helps repair damage to the liver as does valerian root.

Clearly, alcoholism is a challenge to treat. At the Health Recovery Center in Minneapolis, founder Dr. Joan Matthews Larson realized the need to "shift our focus from alcoholism as a psychological disorder to alcoholism as a physical disease that creates cravings, depression and unstable brain functioning. Otherwise, the alcohol is removed and people take the full brunt of the damage that has been done. No matter how much they talk about their resolve, 80 percent or more have relapsed by the end of the first year. One in four deaths of alcoholics who have had formal treatment is from suicide, usually within the first year after treatment."

Dr. Larson used her own personal experience in developing her approach. She had a son in his teens. When her husband's father died of a heart attack, the boy got into a lot of drinking at school. He loved the euphoria. He drowned his sorrows in the alcohol and had a tremendous tolerance; he could drink most people under the table. But after three or four years, it was changing his brain's stability. He was becoming very depressed. Dr. Larson sought help for him in a traditional hospital treatment setting. "Now this person, a kid, who had reached the stage of real emotional instability from the effects of heavy alcohol and some pot use, sat in groups and talked about the misery of his life," Dr. Larson says. "He came home from treatment and was home a very short time, a week or two, when he took his life."

Dr. Larson's need to know what might have made a difference in her son's life led to further study. Many researchers talked about the damage that alcohol inflicts on the brain and central nervous system—depression, mental confusion, anxiety, and real cravings. She began to realize that there was no way that talk could change or repair the damage one iota. There had to be more.

She began to look at the natural chemicals the brain uses that support life and sanity. In the beginning, she concentrated on just the B vitamins, to replace the obvious losses. As she became more sophisticated, she used the amino acids, especially glucosamine, an amino acid that will halt the cravings for alcohol. "If an alcoholic just opens the capsule and lets it dissolve under the tongue," she says, "it goes right across the blood brain barrier and shuts down the cravings for alcohol."

Dr. Larson has created a detox formula that includes a number of well-researched components, all natural chemicals, no toxic drugs. She had to stop using tryptophan due to the FDA ban, now lifted. She uses a group of amino acids designed to reload the brain neurotransmitters, which are low from alcohol. The neurotransmitters are important because they create our moods, memory, and emotions.

She does a lot of lab testing and matching of individuals with treatment. Depression, she believes, can run in nationalities, like the Finnish people she sees in Minnesota, many of whom have been depressed since childhood and can't lift the depression no matter what they do. Galmanic acid is particularly useful for Scandinavians, Irish, Scots, and American Indians, all of whom seem to have less availability, less ability to get that across the brain into the prostaglandin. And the prostaglandin you want is such an antidepressant metabolite. It takes about seven days.

Dr. Larson uses a lot of calcium and magnesium. The wipe-out of magnesium in the brain causes delirium tremors in the alcoholic after as little as one drink. The loss leaves the nervous system jumpy and the brain distressed.

A good multivitamin-mineral supplement is recommended. Every one of the substances that she uses are capsules because we long ago found out that alcoholics have very little ability to break down hard-pressed pills. Their pancreas produces fewer enzymes

Dr. Larson's patients also receive melatonin, so that they can sleep, as well as a substance called GABA (gamma amino butyric acid), which is how the benzodiazepines like Librium and Valium work. They push GABA into the brain and block the re-uptake. By taking GABA, you can reload those neurotransmitters, and the firing mechanism is usually fine because of the wipe-out from the drugs and the alcohol.

People who have high histamine have minds that race, so they don't sleep well, need a small amount of sleep, and are compulsive and driven. Often, they are heavy, two-fisted drinkers. In order to intercept that raciness, they take methionine; that will block the histamine. Many marijuana users tend to be imbalanced in histamine. The marijuana mellows them out, as it does block histamine. It blocks it so well that a person who has used marijuana for a long time can lose his or her zest for life; histamine levels get extremely low. Histamine fires all the neurotransmitters in the brain, so loading them up is one thing but getting them to fire is another. To reload histamine, to raise those levels, you use B3, B12, folic acid, and histidine. Within weeks, the marijuana user may be back to feeling normal again.

Alcoholics say they have been anxious since childhood. They are really enamored of alcohol because it relieves the anxiety for awhile. If their anxiety is not relieved, they will go right back to drinking again. Often there are high tryptopyrols that are blocking the B6 and zinc, keeping them anxious. That can be totally reversed once it is identified with a urine sample and a lab test. One way to know if you might be a candidate is to look at your fingernails and to think about your dreams. Are there little white dots on all your fingernails, and can you remember the content of your dreams consistently? If the answer is, "Yes, I've got white dots, and no, I don't remember my dreams," you need to be tested for phillyrea and have that corrected.

Cocaine and heroin addicts have lost certain key chemicals that need to be replaced. The cocaine and the crack cocaine user are firing off norepinephrine like the fourth of July. That's what creates that feeling they love that is so short-lived. Of course, the neurotransmitter has to be reloaded, which is done by taking large amounts of tyrosine. Also helpful is D-phenylalanine, which makes endorphins. Now, this is not L-phenylalanine; this is D-phenylalanine and it will help replace what the cocaine user has depleted.

According to Dr. Gabriel Cousens, healing the biologically altered brain is the way to eliminate those addictive pressures that send people into sex addiction, drug addiction, alcohol addiction, violence addiction, and over-eating. He begins with a familiar program: "Detox people, get them on a live food vegetarian diet, see if there are endocrine imbalances, hypoglycemia, hyperthyroid problems. The drugs they have been on—antihypertenses, antiinflammatories, birth control pills—have altered the brain's physiology."

Dr. Cousens also assesses the pH of a person's blood. "The brain seems to work at a certain pH, which is 7.46, where it has optimal function," he explains. "This research was done by Dr. Watson in the 1950s. He discovered that people could have anxiety, depression, paranoia and even schizophrenia, if their blood pH was not at the right level. In a study of over 300 people, he used proper diet to bring the brain pH back to normal and the symptoms went away. The diet is important, then, not just because it is life-force enhancing, but because it actually alters the pH and brings it back to a normal.

"Once I have corrected all these things, I will give free amino acids and other nutrients and certain B vitamins to enhance the functioning of the brain biochemistry so that all the cells are working at their optimal state. I add meditation to calm the mind.

"Lower neurotransmitters and endorphins are partially the result of drug abuse. More men than women abuse drugs—three times more—and up to five times more are alcohol abusers. Chronic alcoholics have about a third fewer endorphins working in their brains. Some of the genetic studies show that up to 69 percent of alcoholics are missing a third of the neurotransmitters in the dopamine center. Since dopamine has to do with the pleasure centers, if you are not feeling pleasure, then you have to do something to feel good, like drink or take drugs."

Prozac and related medications are problematic. Dr. Cousens explains, "Prozac and drugs like it are stimulants; they create a hypermanic state. People who take them pay a price because the drugs alter the brain even more. They are addicting. At first, everybody thought that this was the new panacea, but within a year or two, we began having Prozac survival groups. Some people did feel better—a hypermanic state makes them feel more aggressive and gives them the competitive edge. They call Prozac a "selective serotonin enhancer," but it also stimulates the androgen systems, like amphetamines and cocaine do. It also depresses the dopamine receptive centers, which are connected to the pleasure centers.

"These drugs affect the brain in ways that people do not understand. They affect the frontal lobes, which means impaired reason and impulse control, lack of ability to make future plans and for empathy. It is really important because the lack of empathy is partly connected to all the violence that Prozac seems to stimulate. At Columbine High School, at least one of the killers was on Luvox. When you don't have empathy to connect you to human beings, it's really easy to act out with violence."

Prozac also influences other parts of the brain. "It affects the limbic system, which is the emotional system, where it creates apathy and indifference," Dr.

Cousens says. "Also, the basoganglion, which is extremely important because that creates abnormal movements, this internal pressure to move around and be active. Then it affects the temporal lobes, causing loss of short and long term memory, and then the parietal lobes and every part of their brain. There is a decrease in understanding and sensory perception and language and sense of self. In the cerebellum, there is loss of regulation of muscle tone and gait. In the hypothalamus, there is loss of temperature and appetite control. It also affects the pituitary gland, the thyroid, adrenals, and sex hormones and stress reactions."

Food Addiction

Food addictions and food cravings often mask food allergies. Dr. Hyla Cass describes her experience treating patients suffering from food addiction as follows: "Some time ago, a psychologist who specializes in eating disorders began to send her clients to me because she had heard that antidepressant medications worked for these patients. I had shifted to a more holistic way of looking at things, so I told the psychologist that before I did anything with antidepressants I would try some other things. With certain eating disorders, such as food cravings, the underlying problem is a food allergy. We often crave the very foods to which we are allergic. Typically, it's the very things we want to eat that are the most damaging, that create the symptoms. In fact, it's like an addiction to alcohol: As you abstain from the foods you're addicted to, you begin to have withdrawal symptoms and crave those foods even more.

"In order to break the cycle in cases of food addiction, just as when breaking the cycle with drinking (alcoholics are actually allergic to alcohol), you need to supply the body with the appropriate nutrients. When we correct the deficiencies and restore body balance, the food cravings and allergy symptoms will often be relieved. Rather than having to rely strictly on 'willpower,' it is possible for individuals to break addictive cycles by achieving metabolic balance, through avoiding the offending foods and supporting the body with a balanced nutritional program of vitamins, minerals, and amino acids. Often, the cravings will then simply go away. It's quite remarkable: With a good vitamin and mineral product, you can often put a stop to the food allergy and its accompanying symptoms."

Dr. Cass often orders a plasma amino acid analysis, a blood test to determine which amino acids are low. "The amino acid glutamine, in a dosage of 500–1,000 milligrams, is particularly useful for reducing cravings, including alcohol cravings," she says. "Addictions and allergies are often related to magnesium deficiency and can be corrected by supplementation. There are also techniques that can actually eliminate food allergies through the use of acupuncture and acupressure. As we can see," Dr. Cass concludes, "there are many ways, other than psychotherapy and medication, to approach what at first seems like a psychological problem."

Dr. Doris Rapp brings us more detail concerning the connection between food cravings and allergies: "In my experience, eating disorders and alcoholism can be related to allergies. Frequently, eating disorders are food addictions. When you have a food sensitivity, there is a certain phase of it that makes you really crave that food. And if you happen to be addicted to wheat or baked goods, for example, you can never get enough of them, with the result that you may become obese. To give another example, men who are addicted to corn may drink a lot of beer and they can become alcoholics. They're sensitive to and addicted to the beer, but it's the corn—or sometimes some other component— in the beer that is causing the problem. Sometimes, for those with an allergy to grains, they may feel 'drunk' after eating cereal or certain types of baked goods."

5

Anxiety Disorders

■■■

According to 2006 data from the National Institute of Mental Health, 40 million American adults are affected annually by anxiety disorders. Anxiety disorders include panic disorder, obsessive-compulsive disorder, posttraumatic stress disorder, generalized anxiety disorder and social phobia, as well as other specific phobias. They often co-occur with other mental and/or physical conditions. Although each disorder has a different set of symptoms, common to them all are excessive, irrational fear, and dread.

Conventional treatment of anxiety disorders involves medications—including antidepressants (primarily the newer selective serotonin reuptake inhibitors, or SSRIs), antianxietry drugs, and beta-blockers—as well as psychotherapy, particularly cognitive behavior therapy. In cognitive behavior therapy, the goal is to change a person's thinking pattern and the way he or she reacts to situations that provoke anxiety.

From the perspective of orthomolecular psychiatry, practically any nutritional deficiency that affects the mind—and almost all do in one way or another—can cause anxiety. Therefore, nutrition is often the starting point in treatment.

Dr. Michael Schachter emphasizes the importance of proper diet: "If you suffer from an anxiety disorder, you really need to clean up your diet. Getting off sugar and taking calcium and magnesium works. Also, balancing the stresses in your life, through meditation and other anxiety-reducing disciplines, is important."

According to Dr. Allan Spreen, "some amino acids, when given individually can be very effective in calming down the symptoms of anxiety disorders and panic attacks. . . . Some doctors use tyrosine for depression and anxiety. The 'DL' form of phenylalanine is often used on a short-term basis for depression and can be very effective if given correctly. It can lessen anxiety and depression in people by giving them more of an 'up' mood. Phenylalanine is also an appetite suppressant for many people. If they're given correctly there seems to be no toxicity associated with amino acids and they're much cheaper than antidepressants or anti-anxiety prescription medications."

Dr. Walt Stoll has a different approach: "In my clinical experience, I have found that emotional disorders are often linked to the inability to completely break down proteins, during the digestive process, into their amino acids. Just three or four amino acids still hooked together (peptides), if they get through the intestinal lining, can stimulate the immune system to make antibodies against them. Since our body is also made up of peptides, hooked together to make proteins, these antibodies can attack us. To an antibody, a peptide is a peptide. It frequently doesn't matter whether the peptide came from outside the body or is a part of the body. Many of the chronic diseases, which presently are so baffling to the allopathic disease philosophy of conventional Western medicine, are now being found to be related to autoimmune processes.

"In addition," Dr. Stoll says, "some of these peptides have been found to be identical to certain brain hormones (endorphins) that are associated with panic attacks, depression, manic depression, schizophrenia and other conditions. In these cases—with more certain to be discovered—there is no need for the immune system to be involved; the effect is direct. The two first examples to be discovered were peptides from imperfectly digested casein (milk protein) and gluten (wheat protein). Of course, these are two of the most commonly eaten foods in our culture!

"All of the mental states listed above are at least partially caused by brain chemistry abnormalities. Generally, I see patients who have already tried many different therapies. These patients come with stacks and stacks of records documenting that nothing seems to have worked in spite of every imaginable test having been done and every imaginable treatment having been tried. Psychoactive drugs have either worked poorly or have even caused the problem to worsen due to the side effects exceeding the benefits.

"Since every other conceivable cause has been ruled out by the time I get to see them, I am free to look for the things that have not been evaluated. One of the first things I look for is how well the lining of their intestinal tract protects them from their environment. I frequently find that either they don't have the normal bacterial balance in the colon or that they have gone beyond that stage to having candidiasis. Candida can only escape from our control if the normal bacteria are not in control. If Candida has converted from the normal yeast form into the disease-causing fungal form, it further damages the lining so that the leakage of peptides is much greater.

"The greater the amount of peptide leakage, the more likely it is that the brain will interpret these protein particles as being identical to the endorphins it produces during panic attacks, depression, etc. This same leakage is responsible for the increasing sensitivities we see in patients who are sensitive to environmental substances other than foods. It is much simpler, in most cases, to correct the leakage than it is to eliminate the substance. But why not do both?

"Once the reason for the leakage is corrected, the patient usually sees dramatic improvement in a very short time. The antibodies involved only last for 72 hours. Once the leakage is stopped completely, symptoms lessen substantially in just a few days; and just reduction of the leakage helps. There are many patients today that have had that kind of experience. Not everyone's mental symptoms are caused by poorly digested food playing tricks on the brain. However, in my experience, it is the most commonly missed diagnosis and one that is relatively easy to resolve."

One of the most popular herbs for treatment of less severe forms of anxiety—as well as for menopausal depression and insomnia—is kava. According to Chris Kilham, author of *Medicine Hunting in Paradise*, which recounts his work as founder of the Cowboy Medicine Expeditions, specializing in researching and creating plant-based products, kava has an exotic history. It was "brought to the Western world after Captain Cook's first voyage to the South Pacific in the late 1700s. There has been ongoing scientific interest in kava since then. It actually was a registered drug in the United States in 1950 for gonorrhea and nervousness. It was never really popular because you can't patent a plant and so drug companies can't make millions of dollars on it. Kava has been for the past several years very popular in Europe and is finally hitting the US."

As Kilham explains it, the Polynesians and the Melanesians pound the root and make a beverage out of it, which they drink on an almost daily basis as a relaxing beverage. For medicinal purposes, use extracts of the root. The root contains a group of naturally occurring compounds known as the kava lactones. They are skeletal muscle relaxants. They work in the limbic system of the brain, that area of the brain that has control over emotions, and homeostatic mechanisms like the waking and sleeping cycle, appetite, and the sexual urge. An area known as the amygdala in the brain is the seat of the emotional responses of fear and anxiety. The kava lactones in kava work in the amygdala to mitigate anxiety and they work centrally in the nervous system to relax skeletal muscles. You only require a small amount of kava. Clinical studies—which have included toxicological studies, anxiety studies, studies on depression, and studies on sleeplessness—show that kava does not impair function driving an automobile or operating heavy machinery. Toxicity occurs with very large consumption, in excess of a gallon of the beverage a day, in conjunction with malnutrition. People who are eating a reasonable diet and taking medicinal doses of kava have no cause for concern. The primary toxicity that kava exhibits when it is taken in huge amounts is a patchy skin condition.

But the form in which you take kava does matter. "There is no benefit to consuming capsules or tablets of ground up kava root," Kilham says, "it simply doesn't do anything. You couldn't swallow enough kava root to get an effect. Kava is one of those wonderful plants that actually imparts something you can feel. In that regard, it's quite rare. Clinical studies are done with standardized kava extracts; the doses needed to produce an anti-anxiety, anti-depression or sleep enhancing effect are in excess of 70 milligrams of kava lactones in one, two or three doses a day. What a customer wants to look for is a standardized kava extract with at least 70 milligrams of kava lactones per dose.

"The ultimate test is, do you feel it? I've walked into stores and seen ground up kava root capsule and I've thought, 'People are going to swallow them, nothing's going to happen,' and they'll say, 'Oh, this stuff really doesn't work.' What will work is the right quantity of a standardized extract, and if you feel it, you know you've got a good kava product on your hands."

I would add a caveat. If you're depressed, if you have hyperactive disorders, if your personality is always aggressive, if you have unexpressed anger and keep turning around and burning your own bridges, isolating yourself from people, and being short-tempered, then kava at about 100 to 150 milligrams could do you a lot of good. But almost all the companies out there who make it use the leaves. The leaves don't have the power. The bark doesn't have the power. The root is potent, the bark and the leaves are not. And it's best in a plant extract form, as Chris Kilham says, because kava lactones should be standardized, and that way you get a pure amount each time. It's been used for thousands of years and it can create a very calm, smooth, and even sense of well-being.

Dr. Ray Sahelian, a board-certified family practice physician who has written a number of books on natural health, tells us that there are several supplements and herbs that can reduce anxiety and stress. In addition to kava, these include passionflower, ashwaganda (an Ayurvedic herb), fish oils, St. John's wort, valerian, hops, and scullcap.

Certain homeopathic remedies are successful in treating anxiety. There's been a lot of work on homeopathy in children reported in the French scientific literature. One study involved "high anxiety" children needing instant gratification, who were easy to overreact, with stomachaches from the anxiety and the fears. They were given nux vomica and it worked. Another group of children had anxiety because of underlying fears—that they wouldn't succeed, wouldn't be accepted, that their parents couldn't accept them unconditionally. Ignatia proved to be beneficial. Dr. Lynne Freeman, director of the Open Doors Institute in Los Angeles, also recommends calcalcarea carbonica, essentially derived from oyster shells.

According to Dr. Freeman, "a homeopath takes a lot of things into consideration, not just your physical symptoms, your anxiety reactions, but your personality and how you think and operate in the world. If a remedy is not prescribed properly, if the energy is too strong, some people may experience heart palpitations, which can translate into more anxiety reactions, so homeopathic remedies really have to be properly prescribed." That means you should not simply get something off the shelf that has some broad-based appeal.

Music therapy and relaxation techniques have also been proven to be beneficial.

Panic Disorder

Panic disorder strikes about six million adults in the United States, and twice as many women than men. Dr. Lynne Freeman, director of the Open Doors Institute in Los Angeles, describes panic disorder as "very dramatic episodes that involve heart palpitations, sweating, feelings of disorientation, shaky limbs and the feeling that one is about to go insane or die." Panic attacks often begin in late adolescence. Many people have an attack or two in their lifetimes but do not go on to develop the repeat sudden attacks that characterize the full-blown disorder. Panic disorder can be extremely incapacitating, causing sufferers to restrict many activities of daily living as a result of their attacks and the fear of not knowing when the next one will occur.

If you have panic disorder, it's crucial to look at what is going on medically. One physical condition that often contributes to anxiety is mitral valve prolapse. This is a small heart valve that isn't functioning well, so when the blood passes through the valve, it rushes. A person can experience the quicker pace as a fluttery feeling or a palpitation. This is a pretty innocuous condition, but if you are predisposed to panic disorder or another form of anxiety, you may interpret this sensation as a heart attack, which would set off an anxiety reaction.

The same is true of gastroesophageal acid reflux, which is basically indigestion. Excess stomach acid can produce heart palpitations, arm pain, a feeling that the chest is closing—so it resembles a heart attack or an anxiety attack. Other medical conditions often interpreted as anxiety are hormonal changes involved in menopause and premenstrual syndrome, hypoglycemia, even Crohn's disease, during which the person sometimes has periods of dehydration.

Environmental allergies are also linked to or mistaken for panic disorders. A significant part of the population is allergic to aspartame, which we find even in natural vitamins. It could be mistaken for anxiety. Or perhaps you're driving and feeling anxious, not realizing that one of the things you may be responding to is the carbon monoxide fumes coming at you.

Natural treatment, in addition to that described earlier in this chapter, may involve acupuncture and massage. Both, according to Dr. Freeman, "essentially find a way to reorganize the body's natural chemistries." An acupuncturist can read your body through your pulses. They understand that different organs hold different emotions. For example, the kidney is known to hold fear, so an acupuncturist, by checking pulses and skin temperature and other things can determine that the kidneys need to be "tonified," or rebalanced. Since the kidneys produce adrenaline, which in turn produces panic reaction, you can see that acupuncture can be very effective in regulating their biochemistries.

Obsessive-Compulsive Disorder

In the movie *As Good As It Gets*, Jack Nicholson's character checks and rechecks the locks on his doors, uses a new bar of soap every time he washes his hands, and avoids stepping on sidewalk cracks at all costs. He eats the same food in the same restaurant at the same time every day, served by the same waitress. Like an estimated 2.2 million other Americans adults, this character suffers from obsessive-compulsive disorder. When his rituals are interrupted, he is gripped by a heart-palpitating, sweat-dripping anxiety attack. In the movie, love cures him. In life, there are other alternatives.

Obsessive-compulsive disorder affects both men and women, and is more common than severe mental illnesses like schizophrenia or bipolar disorders (manic-depression). It is characterized by repetitive thinking and the inability to control or put a stop to this thinking. As Dr. José Yaryura-Tobias explains, the process is "very forceful, practically taking over the mind. It doesn't allow you to think about anything else. Compulsions are urges that are so extremely demanding that they appear to have to be carried out." Some of the main compulsions are double-checking and hand washing.

Dr. Yaryura-Tobias describes some of the peculiar characteristics of obsessive-compulsive behavior: "It usually takes about seven years or so for a patient to come in for a consultation, which tells us that the condition tends to occur gradually, becoming a part of the patient's behavioral system in a very, very slow manner. Fifty percent of obsessive-compulsive patients manifest their sickness during childhood or adolescence. Later on—primarily after the age of 40—it fades away, and it becomes very rare after the age of 50."

The treatment of choice would include behavior therapy, amino acids, and medications, says Dr. Yaryura-Tobias. "We basically treat with behavioral therapy. We try to use thought-stopping, exposure (flooding) and response prevention to prevent the brain from repeating the same thought. That is difficult, so we also use cognitive therapy to explain the reasons we think the things we do, and try to modify the thought.

"Compulsions are the area where behavioral therapy is most effective. We expose the patient, either in reality or in his or her imagination, to face what he is afraid of. If you have fears of AIDS or of blood, you are exposed to blood or taken to the hospital where there might be patients with AIDS. Or you will read articles on the condition.

"If it is contamination from dirt the patient is afraid of, we teach the person how to touch objects and not to be afraid of them. Then we prevent the patient from washing their hands; in other words, they must remain unclean for awhile. I'm talking about patients who, when they are seriously ill, might completely use up one or two bars of soap per day. They might engage in rituals of washing for many hours. They may wash their hands sometimes a hundred or more times a day. Some of these patients, in addition, will clean their hands with alcohol or other substances. Sometimes their skin becomes extremely raw. I've seen cases where patients require plastic surgery.

"Overall, the treatment takes about six months. With medication there is improvement up to 60 or 70 percent of the time."

Dr. Yaryura-Tobias describes his amino acid approach. "My colleagues and I were the first to use tryptophan and with it we were able to reduce and almost eliminate completely the use of drugs for this condition, and we obtained very good results. . . . We were using between 3000 and 9000 milligrams per day.

"Then we used vitamin B6, 100 milligrams, three times a day. Vitamin B6, pyridoxine phosphate, is a vitamin that is very important for the breakdown of tryptophan into serotonin. The idea behind this was that either these patients didn't have enough serotonin in their brains, were very dependent on serotonin, or that the normal conversion of tryptophan into serotonin was not occurring.

"When we found by measuring that there was a lack of serotonin, this could be reversed by the administration of L-tryptophan with niacin and vitamin B6. Some medications also accomplish this result, but with medications we face many types of side effects.

"About 30 percent of patients do not respond to any form of therapy. But it is not a closed chapter for these patients either. An investigation has to be conducted. Now that we have brain imaging, we are able to visualize the brain. We can measure, for instance, the metabolism of sugar in the brain. We find, for instance, the frontal and temporal lobes and the basal ganglia, which are related to Parkinson's disease, disrupted. We see the metabolism of the breakdown of sugar and also images of an abnormal brain. The same can be seen with some electrophysiological measurements of brain wave tests and so forth.

"Interestingly," Dr. Yaryura-Tobias concludes, "work has been going on using pure behavioral therapy before and after measuring serotonin. With just behavioral therapy, we were able to modify the levels of serotonin in the body. In other words, we may not need medication to change or challenge the presence of a neurotransmitter such as serotonin. Simply the mere interaction of behavioral technique may have an effect."

According to the late Dr. Robert Atkins, there is some common ground between conventional Western medicine and more holistic approaches such as orthomolecular psychiatry, Both recognize that if a certain neurotransmitter is in short supply, certain syndromes will result. Dr. Atkins explained, "A classic example is that the serotonin-deficient person will often be an obsessive-compulsive. These are the people who can't get out of the house because they've got to make sure the light switches are off or the gas jet isn't on—the people who have to wash their hands 20 times a day, and whose desks have to be perfectly neat. These same people are serotonin-deficient."

The difference between the conventional and the alternative medical communities lies in how they address the problem. Dr. Atkins described the conventional approach: "Now there are drugs that block the degradation of serotonin and allow the serotonin level to lift, but these drugs do a lot of other things: They poison a lot of enzyme systems and that's why so many people got into trouble with Prozac and drugs like that." And the more enlightened alternative approach: "However, you can increase serotonin with the nutrition precursor, tryptophan.

"Dr. Russell Jaffe has done research to indicate that the best treatment for the bad tryptophan syndrome (the eosinophilia myalgic syndrome) is the use of pure unadulterated tryptophan," Dr. Atkins said. "People with obsessive-compulsive and anxiety disorders often improve on tryptophan."

Some pharmacies, according to Dr. Atkins, "will compound capsules of 5-hydroxy tryptophan. This compound is an intermediary between tryptophan and 5-hydroxy tryptamine, which is serotonin, the neurotransmitter you are trying to build up. The whole idea of supplying a precursor to build up a neurotransmitter that is in short supply is a fruitful approach to treating psychiatric disorders and should, in my opinion," concluded Dr. Atkins, "be considered before the use of nonphysiologic psychotropic drugs, which have more potential for toxicity."

Acupuncturists also have had a great deal of success with obsessive-compulsive disorder. In some situations, their treatment has proven to be more effective than medication.

6

Eating Disorders

■■■

Patient Story: Bulimia

The woman was 47 years old, a psychotherapist with a doctoral degree who had been treating patients with eating disorders for almost 15 years. She herself had bulimia—about five binge-purge episodes per day for the last 34 years. She could hardly recount a single day since she was 12 when she did not engage in bulimic activity. We gave her a small amount, about 5 or 10 milliliters, less than a tablespoon, of liquid zinc and asked her to swirl it around for a few seconds and tell us what she tasted. If people can't taste the solution, it's evidence of systemic zinc deficiency. This has to do with a zinc-dependent polypeptide known as gustine, which helps us to distinguish metallic taste, and zinc has a strong metallic taste. She couldn't taste anything. It tasted like water to her. She thought it was a placebo. She was given about 120 milliliters of this solution spaced out throughout the day at about 30, 40 milliliters each time, on an empty stomach. Four days later, she called to say she couldn't explain it, but she had no desire to binge or purge that day. That was the first day she could recall feeling good in 34 years.

—Dr. Schauss

Eating disorders, which afflict some 8 million Americans, have the highest mortality rate of any mental illness. The main types of eating disorders are anorexia nervosa and bulimia nervosa. Symptoms of anorexia include refusal to maintain a normal weight for age and height, intense fear of gaining weight or becoming "fat," body image misperceptions, and loss of menstrual periods. Bulimia is characterized by binge eating and compensation for binges using measures such as self-induced vomiting, laxatives, and excessive exercise. While the most visible sufferers of these diseases have been young women, recent research—in magazines, books, television, and school programs—indicates that men, too, struggle with them. Males with eating disorders are more likely to have alcohol-related conditions and to have had their illness overlooked by doctors, who see it as a specifically female problem.

Particularly among women, disordered body images and destructive eating behavior came "out of the closet" about thirty years ago, spurred in part by the revelation that popular singer Karen Carpenter had died of anorexia. Social critics and psychologists have looked to media pressure—and the more available surgeries for reshaping the human body—as some causes of the dissatisfaction women often feel about "normal" bodies.

Most experts agree that a spectrum of factors contributes to these diseases—individual, family, interpersonal, biological, and cultural. Treatment, often multidisciplinary, addresses both the physical and psychological components of the eating disorder. Among the interventions being used are individual and family therapy, support groups, medical treatment, and medications to treat associated depression or anxiety. Nutrition has been recognized as part of the problem and part of the cure.

Julia Ross, who has worked for years in the field of nutritional psychology, has developed a treatment model that blends nutrition and holistic medicine with traditional methods of counseling and education. In her book *The Diet Cure*, she outlines the vitamin and mineral deficiencies that can result in anorexia (including vitamin B1 and zinc) and tells how protein malnutrition can cause "brainpower outage." She explains the process by which depletion of the amino acid tryptophan, as is common in dieters, can cause serotonin levels to drop. This can result in mood disregulation, as well as obsessive thoughts and behaviors, all of which figure prominently in eating disorders.

Dr. Alexander Schauss, who provided the patient story above, has done a lot of important work in the field of eating disorders. He spearheaded the understanding of the role of zinc in diagnosis and treatment. Dr. Schauss and his staff were intrigued as to how a simple nutrient like zinc could cause a major change in the way the brain functions. "When you've done something for 34 years, whether it's cigarette smoking, biting your nails, or you're phobic about something, or engaged in bulimia, you have to wonder how it would be possible that in four or five days, such an obsessive-compulsive type behavior would just disappear. Five years later, she had not gone back to binge-purging. More important, she was provided no therapy. I never actually met her; the protocol was given to her by a staff member. We're quite convinced in this case and in hundreds of others that it was the liquid zinc that was effective rather than some tangential treatment, which of course would confound our conclusions."

In fact, five-year follow-up studies done by Dr. Schauss show a 64-percent success rate for bulimics on the liquid zinc treatment and an 85-percent recovery rate in anorexic patients. These are extraordinarily high recovery rates for a condition considered quite difficult to treat and quite insidious.

"We've known since at least the 1930s," he says, "that when animals were experimentally placed on diets deficient in zinc, they developed anorexia. By 1958, Professor Kung in China—who became a victim of the Cultural Revolution and we lost track of him—was the first to recognize that zinc was essential in humans. A paper he wrote in Chinese unfortunately never got published in English. About four years later, an American researcher from Wayne State University, working in Egypt, discovered that zinc was intimately required by the human body to develop secondary sexual characteristics. His research eventually lead to the National Academy of Sciences' establishing zinc as an essential nutrient.

"Zinc is pervasive, found in every tissue cell, organ and fluid in the human body, and involved in over 200 enzyme reactions in the brain. That is why we've taken a great interest in what zinc does in the brain that might be of therapeutic value to people with various kinds of neurological psychiatric conditions. We've learned that when humans are placed on zinc-deficient diets, they develop eating disorders."

People who are obese have been found to have lower zinc levels than nonobese people. Dr. Schauss explains, "In morbid obesity—when people are so significantly overweight that it could shorten their lifespan or increase their risk of disease—there is an inverse relationship between the level of obesity and the level of zinc. The more obese they are, the less zinc they have in their body. We don't know yet whether this is cause and effect, but it's a very important observation because at the other end of the continuum, with anorexia nervosa, self-induced starvation, people are always zinc deficient. There is strong evidence today from studies done at the University of Kentucky School of Medicine, at Stanford University, and the University of California at Davis, in addition to our research institute's work, that the lower the zinc status is, the more likely it is that the patient will be able to recover from anorexia."

Dr. Schauss explains that "the liquid zinc is absorbed directly in the stomach much like water and alcohol, which then goes into portal blood and into the liver. The treatment doesn't cause any favorable response for three to four days because in order for zinc to get into the brain or any other tissue that requires it, it needs a metal carrier, a type of protein that carries metals. That protein is metallothionein. We need to have enough of the protein carrier to help move the zinc to where it's needed in the body. It usually takes several days for the body's extra levels of zinc to facilitate the production of higher amounts of metallothionein. As you continue the treatment, eventually you have a considerable amount of this protein carrier to help move the zinc to where it is required.

"I've had cases where it's taken almost three weeks before the zinc finally starts to saturate brain tissue, which then influences the person's perception of themselves, and that begins to disturb the underlying mechanism that contributes to the eating disorder."

In times of psychological stress, people actually lose zinc. "You can, in fact, measure a two to three fold increase in the amount of zinc in the urine under conditions of psychological stress," Dr. Schauss says. "Most nutrients are lost at higher levels under physiological stress, such as wounds, surgery, injury, burns, physical trauma. But we lose more zinc if the person's internal, mental ideations place them under constant stress. They may actually be losing zinc at a higher rate than they can replace it through the diet. Combine that with binge-purge activity, where a person is losing a lot of the calories and nutrients in the purge cycle, or with anorexia, where they don't consume enough calories to sustain a balanced level of minerals and vitamins . . . you begin to understand this problem."

The zinc connection also may help explain the predominance of eating disorders in females as opposed to males. "We finally realized that zinc is highly concentrated in the male prostate, providing a mineral essential for sperm development," Dr. Schauss says. "If a male is under psychological stress, he has storages of zinc in the prostate. Since women don't have prostates, they catabolize the zinc from other tissue. The richest tissue in the human body for zinc is the muscle tissue. In anorexia, a common feature is muscle wasting. They're actually eating their own muscle tissue as a way of releasing nutrients that they need to survive.

"It is very, very important to realize that one of the reasons we use zinc is to stop that muscle wasting because the last muscle, one that only contains about 1 percent of zinc, is the heart muscle. Twenty-nine percent of the zinc in the human body is in skeletal muscle; only 1 percent is in heart muscle tissue. But when, unfortunately, the body starts to scavenge zinc out of heart muscle tissue, it starts to damage the heart. A weakened heart can result in bradycardia, tachycardia, arrhythmias and eventual heart failure. It is particularly dangerous in patients who are recovering from anorexia—the muscle tissue in their hearts has been damaged and taking on weight puts extra pressure on the heart. That is how the singer Karen Carpenter died.

"After the first studies, which were just case reports, showed remarkable rates of recovery for anorexics and bulimics, we started to do control trials. One of the first was to see whether in fact there was a difference in taste perception between those who are deficient in zinc and those who are not. We wrote a paper that was presented at the American College of Nutrition in 1986 and published in *Nutrients and Brain Function* in 1987, demonstrating that in fact patients who have zinc deficiency are unable to taste the zinc solution. So we provided relatively strong evidence, based on double blind placebo controlled studies, that this simple noninvasive procedure could be very effective."

Dr. Schauss's research findings were confirmed by the National Institutes of Health-funded studies at the University of Kentucky Medical Center and several California universities. "Giving them liquid zinc could be highly therapeutic, they found, confirming our earlier clinical observations," he says. "But they also found that a diet rich in zinc actually made the patients worse. We still do not understand why. A few years ago, I heard the head of the eating disorders program at the Gutenberg University in Sweden tell a radio audience that she believed that up to 100 percent of patients with eating disorders, including morbid obesity, were zinc deficient. She felt it was imperative that any program that treated patients with an eating disorder use zinc as an adjunct in treatment."

Dr. Schauss says that the zinc research helps provide an explanation of how non-zinc related therapies also work. "Remember, you lose zinc under psychological stress. If you send a patient who is stressed to a supportive, warm, nurturing environment, as many of the eating residential treatment facilities are, after several weeks much of their stress is alleviated. Suddenly the amount of zinc that the body is losing has been decreased, and we believe that that's partially why various treatment modalities have been helping people."

The cost for zinc treatment is minimal compared with that of traditional interventions for eating disorders. Unfortunately, that poses a problem for some treatment centers. Dr. Schauss explains, "I might be invited to a hospital that has an eating disorder unit. I present the data to the staff, they are enthusiastic and usually they've tried it out on a few patients and seen the benefits, but then the business manager steps in and talks about how much money the hospital will lose if it engages in what is basically an outpatient treatment program. That happened at a local hospital here in Washington state, and I got so mad that money was more important than health that I went to every support group for bulimic and anorexics I could find in the area and showed them how they could use this on their own. Within a year, that eating disorder unit closed down because it didn't have enough patients to sustain it. The trustee who had invited me to the hospital resigned his position. But it didn't really solve the problem, which is how do patients get this information?"

Dr. José Yaryura-Tobias strongly believes that any nutritional approach must be preceded by a program of cognitive therapy. "Anorexia nervosa, from our perspective, is an obsessive-compulsive disorder that is related to self-image, the way that we perceive ourselves. Basically, anorexia nervosa is the process by which a human being self-starves. Thirty percent of the population who self-starve eventually die.

"From the biochemical viewpoint, in the vast majority of cases when patients come for a consultation, they are already very emaciated. The chemistry we can measure is very altered. We know that there is a groove that is related to an area of the brain called the limbic system. This is the hypothalamic area, which regulates sugar, thirst, appetite and so forth. This information can help us classify some of these patients, but does not tell us how to manage and eventually cure the problem. The rest of the problem, we feel, has to do with body image perception, the way that these patients see their own bodies. They feel too fat, too slim. They have different perspectives than the rest of us."

Dr. Yaryura-Tobias says that cognitive therapy is needed to educate patients about their problems and the way they think about themselves. We need "to discuss with them how many false beliefs they have about who they are, why they think this way, why their body looks the way it does, and so forth. So false-belief modification is an important part of treatment."

Psychologist Lynne Freeman treats patients with eating disorders from a different point of view. "There's clearly a relationship between anorexia and anxiety. In fact,

38 percent of anorexics have reported a history of having anxiety. At some point, an anorexic may recognize that if she doesn't eat, she will die. But she has been avoiding food for so long—much as the agoraphobic has been avoiding leaving home—that she has developed an actual food phobia. She can sit there with a plate of food, knowing that she needs to eat and completely unable to eat, no longer in that place of intentionally withholding. She really wants to eat, and can't. This is one of the reasons doctors are using a lot of antidepressant medications on anorexia just as they would for someone with an anxiety disorder, hoping that they can somehow break that food phobia. Unfortunately it hasn't been very successful.

"Bulimia is a slightly different situation because it does involve the compulsion to eat as opposed to the avoidance of eating. Certainly the dehydration and the physical symptoms do eventually erupt in a bulimic, and so they can experience anxiety as well."

Laura Norman is a registered, certified reflexologist and a New York state-licensed massage practitioner in private practice for twenty-five years. She defines reflexology as "a science and an art that deals with the principle that there are reflex areas in your feet that correspond to all parts of the body. When we stimulate these areas, it helps to bring about homeostasis, balance in the body, without side affects. It deeply relaxes, which helps to reduce vascular constriction, so your blood and nerve supply can flow more freely. Improving circulation can help to eliminate toxins in the body and break up congestion or blockages resulting from the accumulation of excess mucus, uric acid, lactic acid, calcium deposits. It enhances the flow of blood, helps to relieve pain and discomfort, and activates the release of endorphins. It's a natural opiate, like substances normally produced in the brain that alter and regulate moods. Mainly, it helps to promote a sense of inner peace, tranquility and well being."

"There are more than 7,000 nerves in each foot," Norman says. "When we stimulate a reflex area, there is a response to this stimulus; that is why we called it reflexology. A well trained reflexologist can apply specific pressure to reflex areas using their fingers and thumbs. Anorexia and bulimia are mostly stress induced. The main thing the reflexology will do is help the person relax. For all eating disorders, anorexia, bulimia, or even people who are just plain overweight, we focus on the same organs and glands to help balance the eating disorder."

The first and most common technique is called thumb walking. Using the thumb, the reflexologist moves in a forward motion, inching along "like a caterpillar" on the sole and sides of the foot. The second technique is known as finger walking. The pointer finger, bent at the first joint, travels forward motion on the top of the foot. The third technique is called rotation on a point. The reflexologist presses a little deeper into the point using the thumb, while the other hand holds the foot and rotates it.

According to Norman, "for eating disorders, the points are these:

■ the pituitary gland (to coordinate activity of all the other glands and to stimulate and regulate the hormonal secretions);

■ the brain, to enhance circulation of blood to the brain and to promote normal brain wave activity);

■ the solar plexus (to orchestrate and increase circulation to the abdominal organs and help relax the person overall);

■ the spine (to soothe the nerves and enhance transmission of impulses to all the parts of the body);

■ the thyroid (to regulate metabolism and to modify activity of the nervous system);

■ the parathyroid (to promote metabolism of calcium and phosphorus, to enhance nerve transmission, and for muscle tone);

■ the adrenal gland (to release hormones to regulate metabolism, rejuvenate hyperactivity in response to stress, and stimulate energy);

■ the kidneys (to maintain water balance, balance blood pressure, and filter toxins and waste from the blood);

■ the stomach area (to help soothe the muscles and nerves and increase blood circulation into the stomach);

■ the pancreas (to control balance of blood sugar and aid in digestion of food and nutrient extraction);

■ the liver (to filter toxins from the blood and regulate nutrient absorption);

■ the gallbladder (to release bile to encourage peristalsis and promote absorption of fat and soluble vitamins); and

■ the intestines (to promote peristalsis and increase blood circulation and nutrient absorption, and to stimulate elimination of solid wastes).

"For bulimia," she adds, "I would also work on the mouth, teeth, gums and the esophagus."

7

Depression

■■■

Patient Stories: Depression

I could not connect with people. I felt distant. I was dissatisfied with my job. Depression was exhausting. I could not handle more physical and emotional trauma. I entered a support group, just in case I could learn something. I learned the theory behind detoxifying the body and mind. After a short time juicing, eating vegan, eliminating food allergies, my energy picked up. I no longer have PMS [premenstrual syndrome] symptoms or feel cysts in my breasts. Depression lifted within six weeks. Eye floaters lessened. I notice new hairs on my head growing in darker. As my body eliminated and uncluttered, so did my relationships. I slowly allow new friends in my life and accepted a job I enjoy at a higher wage.

—Athena

I can't remember when I first felt depressed—it was always with me. I began seeing psychiatrists at the age of 16, and began taking various medications at age 18. I was hospitalized at the age of 20. At the time, the inference was that I should be very ashamed of myself. I was on lithium and antidepressants for 18 years and I developed chronic fatigue as a result of the side effects of all the medications. The whole time I was on drugs, I was suicidal every other month. When I first got off my drugs, I had to spend a lot of time taking care of myself. After being told all my life that the best I could do was to take drugs, talk about my childhood forever and shut up to the rest of the world about it, I want to offer hope that it is possible to overcome depression.

—Catherine

Depression is a great leveler. It affects one in four Americans and doesn't differentiate between rich and poor, although it does appear to afflict women more than it does men. It is a serious disorder, often related to—some even think it is a contributing cause of—other illnesses like heart disease, arthritis, allergies, and cancer. Recent estimates are that half the people diagnosed as suffering from depression could obtain relief simply by having an underlying physical disease identified and treated. Among the conditions I have discovered are underactive thyroid, low blood sugar, cerebral allergy, a nutritionally induced or environmentally induced allergy, a nutrient deficiency, or simply a life issue that could have been dealt with in a nontoxic way. There are many practitioners within the orthomolecular movement who see things this way, yet most people continue to go right off to the psychiatrist or psychologist and get into standard therapeutic models. I have a great deal of concern about this, because of the dangers of Prozac and other psychiatric drugs, as discussed in Chapter 2.

Catherine Carrigan, whose self-healing from crippling depression and the books she has written about it have inspired many other people, believes the disease has mental, physical, and spiritual causes and solutions. She recommends checking for physical health problems first, particularly since "studies show that if you go to a psychiatrist alone, the chances of medical, nonmental factors being discovered are less than one in ten." In addition to those mentioned above, physical health problems that may contribute to depression include Candida or yeast infection, amino acid deficiencies, electrolyte imbalances, toxic exposure to heavy metals or chemicals, cardiopulmonary obstructive disease, brain tumors, Alzheimer's, stroke, seizure, hypertension, viral infections, diabetes, insulin resistance, and difficulty metabolizing carbohydrates.

There are different degrees of depression, and its treatment has varied considerably according to trends in psychiatry, psychology, and psychopharmacology in recent decades. Some people use the term "depression" when they are struck by feelings of mild sadness, the kind that affects nearly everyone from time to time, often for no obvious reason. Certain times of the year are associated with mood lows, particularly at the beginning and end of winter, for example. Commonly, when someone close to us moves away or dies, or if we lose a job or have some other major disappointment, there's apt to be an even stronger mood reaction. There will be some sadness, perhaps some grief. Usually such periods of sadness or grief are of a limited duration. When they drag on for a longer period of time, or become much more profound, we may begin to speak of clinical depression.

The causes of depression may include genetic factors. As Dr. William Goldwag explains, "These may be related to changes in the brain metabolism and the nervous system. We know about genetic factors through the action of certain drugs. We see what chemical changes take place. Obviously our individual chemistry is to a great extent determined by our genes. There are genes presently under investigation that are believed to be responsible for manic-depression type illnesses, in which one fluctuates from hyperactivity to depression or limited activity. Every day another gene is being found that is responsible for some of these illnesses. The gene expresses itself through a change in chemistry."

It is common for depressed people to have a family history of depression. In addition to the genetic factor, such family histories may also be due to common environmental factors, shared experiences in depressed families, and poor eating habits that are passed on from one generation to another. "Just being exposed to depressed people can be an influence," Dr. William Goldwag says, "since children learn how to behave by imitation. Also, family members are eating the same food, and if, for instance, the mother is depressed and cooking and serving her family, that food is apt to be sparse in nutrients since she is interested in just getting the meal over with and has difficulty finding enough energy to prepare it."

Dr. Doris Rapp explains that mood disorders often lead to abuse of family members and intimates. "Husbands batter wives, wives batter husbands, they both batter the children. Mother battering, I might add, is very common. Many of the children I treat beat, kick, bruise, bite and pinch their mothers. When some individuals have typical allergies and environmental illnesses, if they have a mood problem, they can become nasty and irritable and angry. All I ask is, 'What did you eat, touch and smell?' To help find the cause I try to discover whether the change in behavior occurs inside or outside, after eating, or after smelling a chemical. It might be a food, dust, mold, pollen or chemical, which not only affects the brain [as a whole], but discrete areas of the brain. As a result, the allergen or food or chemical exposure might make you tired or, if it affects the frontal lobes, it might make you behave in an inappropriate way. It could affect the speech center of the brain so that you speak too rapidly, or unclearly, or stutter, or don't speak intelligently. It's just potluck as to what area of the brain or body will be affected when you are exposed to something to which you are allergic."

Symptoms of depression may include reduction in appetite, reduction in sleep ability, fatigue, lack of energy, agitation or retardation in motor activity, loss of interest in usual activities, loss of interest in sex, feelings of worthlessness or guilt, slowed thinking, inability to concentrate, and recurring thoughts of suicide, or suicide attempts. Everyone from time to time has one or more of these symptoms. "Generally these should be present for at least two weeks and represent a change from a previous state," Dr. Goldwag says. "But when approximately four or five of these are present for a long period of time, and when this represents a departure from a person's usual personality, the possibility of depression should be considered."

Several types of antidepressant medications are used to treat depression, including the newer selective serotonin reuptake inhibitors (SSRIs), the tricyclics, and the monoamine oxidase inhibitors (MAOIs). Dr. Goldwag briefly describes the history: "The first drugs ever used for treating depression were amphetamines. In their time, before they got such a bad reputation, they were considered helpful. In the old days, amphetamines were used for weight control. They did diminish the appetite, and they also made a person feel good, alert, and more energetic. People who went on diets and took amphetamines felt great."

Problems arose, however, when the medications were stopped. "People would go into a depression," Dr. Goldwag says. "For that reason amphetamines were recognized to be very habit-forming. In order to feel good a person had to keep on taking them. For many people that still seemed okay, at least for a while. For a fair percentage though, the dose became inadequate as the person started feeling like he or she needed more and more of the drug. This created all kinds of problems with the body's chemistry.

"There are still some medications on the market that act a little bit like the amphetamines, although they are not anywhere near as powerful. These are mild sympathetic nervous system stimulants that are sold over the counter, such as those people use to keep awake when they have to drive. In some instances I'm sure there are people who take them as a way of counteracting depression."

After amphetamines, the tricyclic antidepressants were introduced. Dr. Goldwag explains, "They're called tricyclic because of their chemical structure, which is a triple cycle. There are a whole bunch of them now on the market. The newer group of medications are those that inhibit the enzymes that break down serotonin. They are designed to try to raise the serotonin level in the brain. In that way they counteract depression.

"They are all to varying degrees effective, but they all have side effects. Some of the side effects are severe; some are mild. They usually take days or weeks before they are effective, and in this way they are different than the amphetamines, because those would work in a matter of minutes or hours."

As mentioned in Chapter 2, the dangers and abuses of these drugs have provoked well-deserved outcry in recent years. This has come in the form of research studies, newspaper articles, legal actions, and congressional investigations. There is increasing concern about the repression of information on the side effects of commonly prescribed drugs. Among the actions have been a 2004 lawsuit against the makers of Paxil for concealing information about the antidepressant's safety and efficacy in children, and a 2006 study published in the *New England Journal of Medicine* which determined that women taking SSRIs during the second half of pregnancy were more likely to deliver children with birth defects. In addition, there is the FDA's 2005 requirement for drug companies to add black box warnings to antidepressant labels about the risk of suicidal thinking and behavior in children and adolescents, as well as its 2007 extension of that warning to young adults.

According to Dr. Goldwag, "There are many, many things that individuals with depression can do to help themselves. What we want to ask is, what can we do nutritionally and in other ways? What lifestyle factors are under our own control that we can manipulate in order to alleviate symptoms of depression or prevent them?"

It is surprising how often diet and nutrition are factors in depression, and how effective enhanced or improved nutrition can be in helping someone to improve their mood. As Dr. Goldwag says, "Often the quality of the diet suffers in depressed people. If the depression is profound, the individual doesn't even feel like eating. Depressed people who live alone or who are major providers or cooks in the house may not feel like preparing meals or even shopping. They're apt to restrict their nutrition to fast food or just anything to get eating over with." In many cases, weight loss is a symptom of severe depression. In other cases, there is substantial weight gain.

As Dr. Goldwag notes, significant weight loss is likely to bring about "marked deprivation of the essential nutrients, including the amino acids needed to manufacture the proper proteins, as well as a deficiency in many vitamins and minerals. That in itself can then aggravate the depression."

There are many straightforward solutions to at least some of the challenges associated with depression. Dr. Goldwag suggests preparing food in advance. "I recommend preparing a raw salad once a week. Certain fresh vegetables can be stored for quite a period in a refrigerator and will keep quite well. There are a whole variety to choose from: carrots, celery, radishes, cauliflower, broccoli, peppers, red cabbage, green onions, snow peas, string beans. These can all be cut up and mixed together. They can be stored in a plastic bag or sealed container. When mealtime comes, a person can take a handful of these vegetables and then perhaps add some other ones that don't keep as well, such as tomatoes or sprouts. You then have a fresh salad that is already prepared with a lot of important nutrients. This is just one way of having food prepared in advance. It's good for people who are depressed and don't have the energy to make a whole meal."

The B complex vitamins are especially important. Dr. Goldwag explains, "Years and years ago, when people suffered from severe vitamin deficiencies, some of the resultant diseases like pellagra and so forth were characterized by accompanying psychotic reactions. That is, the thinking process was the most obvious one to be affected by the vitamin deficiency. Simply providing the proper vitamin, in this case vitamin B3 or niacin, was the treatment. It cleared up the psychosis.

"Niacin is often used in much higher doses than the others in order to accomplish some of these changes. Niacin is a ubiquitous vitamin. It is being used greatly to help reduce cholesterol levels, to improve the good cholesterol and reduce the bad. The dosages being used are much greater than those used to simply overcome a deficiency.

You have to be a little bit careful of niacin because over long periods of time, in high doses, there can be some effects on the liver. The doses of niacin that have been used, mostly by Dr. Hoffer, have been in the ranges of 1 to 3 grams a day. That's thousands of milligrams a day, whereas the requirements for avoiding a deficiency are measured in just 10 or 20 milligrams."

Among the other B vitamins that can affect mental processes are B1 or thiamine, riboflavin, B6 or pyridoxine, and B12.

Researcher Sid Baumel says that "the most often studied vitamin connection to depression has been the B vitamins, which are the most closely associated with the normal maintenance of mood and the brain." If you have a really significant B vitamin deficiency, the kind that gives you bleeding gums and obvious skin problems, depression is one of the other symptoms you'd be likely to have. People who are clinically depressed don't routinely get their blood levels of B vitamins measured, but it has been proven that depressed people have lower levels of the B vitamin folic acid. There have been a number of studies looking into blood levels of folic acid and the prevention of relapse in people who have recovered from depression. These studies found that people with high levels of folic acid—whether because of their diets or because they are taking a supplement—were less likely to suffer a relapse. People low in folic acid have been given supplements and reported to have a very good clinical response.

More recently, there have been studies of a natural derivative of folic acid called methyl folate, showing it to be as effective as the antidepressant drug to which it was being compared. This supports the claim that nutritionally oriented doctors including orthomolecular psychiatrists have been making for many years now: folic acid prescribed in megadoses appears to be a stimulating antidepressant for some patients.

The amino acid tryptophan can be another key substance in the treatment of depression. According to Dr. Goldwag, tryptophan helps to raise the levels of serotonin, a naturally occurring chemical in the brain that has been found to be abnormally low in depressed people. "We learned about serotonin from experiments in which certain drugs that preserve it from being destroyed in the brain seem to work as antidepressants. The theory is that whatever can supply or aid the serotonin factor will help depression. Some foods that contain tryptophan can act as antidepressants. It is found most abundantly in milk and turkey."

Tryptophan is a precursor to Prozac and other drugs like it, drugs that amplify the activity of serotonin in the brain. Tryptophan, the substance from which the brain manufacturers its own serotonin, does the same kind of thing when it is taken as a supplement. In controlled studies, it was found consistently to be as effective as the antidepressant drugs that were available. Five hydroxytryptophan (5-HTP) is another natural compound, which is a little bit closer to serotonin. It seems to be even more effective than tryptophan.

The late Dr. Robert Atkins distinguishes between two types of depression, each with its respective type of therapeutic approach. "Clinically, you can divide depressions into two different categories: the apathetic depression where you just can't get interested in or enjoy anything, and the agitated or anxious depression, where basically you are depressed and nervous. The latter is responsive to increasing serotonin levels and is best treated with tryptophan. Tryptophan is extremely valuable in cases of agitated depression. Apathetic depression is best treated with tyrosine or what we now call acetyl tyrosine, and a product called Noraval."

Public sale of tryptophan was banned in the United States from 1990 until 2005. Dr. Goldwag explains that the FDA took it off the market because there were some serious blood problems in people who took it. "This was later tracked down to a contaminant; the problem was not due to the tryptophan itself."

While milk and turkey, as well as kiwi fruit, figs, and dates are good sources of the tryptophan, there are plenty of foods that should be avoided. Fast foods can affect mental symptoms by causing blood sugar abnormalities. People who tend to hypoglycemia or low blood sugar patterns should avoid eating too many simple carbohydrates, such as candy bars, which are converted very rapidly to sugar in the blood. As Dr. Goldwag says, "Simple carbohydrate foods temporarily raise the blood sugar, but then they drop it to a very low level several hours later, resulting in depression. This encourages the individual to repeat the cycle of taking sugar or some simple carbohydrate that's converted to sugar in order to feel that high again. This constant seesaw from high to low mood can account for many episodes of depression in individuals."

Catherine Carrigan recommends investigating amino acid imbalance. "Researchers have discovered that the bodies of people with mood disorders have difficulty producing a specific amino acid called GABA, gamma amino butyric acid. In fact, this is the closest thing scientists have ever come to a blood test for predisposition to mood disorders. GABA is supposed to synthesize in the body from other amino acids. Even 4 years after they are no longer depressed, people with mood disorders still have trouble making GABA. GABA helps you to relax."

Dr. Michael Schachter reports that "sometimes depression is caused by a deficiency of the neurotransmitter for norepinephrine. In such a case the amino acid L-tyrosine, or the amino acid DL-phenylalanine, may be helpful. DL-phenylalanine consists of two forms of phenylalanine, namely D-phenylalanine and L-phenylalanine. L-phenylalanine is used by the body to make proteins. D-phenylalanine is a precursor of the brain substance D-phenylethylamine, which is frequently deficient in people who are suffering from depression. I also recommend the mineral magnesium, and vitamin B1 (thiamine) for depression. But the course of treatment really has to be individualized."

Dr. Jonathan Zeuss, who has no doubt that depression is "to a very large degree, a nutritionally caused disease," touts the benefits of omega-3 fatty acids. "They are absolutely crucial," he says. "There is a huge amount of evidence now linking omega-3 deficiency and depression. Around a quarter of the dry weight of our brains is made up of omega-3s and if you are deficient in them, the cells in your brain malfunction and you are much more likely to become depressed."

Omega-3s are known as essential fatty acids. "Your body can't make them itself, so it's essential that you get them in your diet," Dr. Zeuss says. "Omega-3 is found in fish and green leafy plants like spinach and in supplements you can buy like flaxseed oil and fish oil. You can't get them any other way. Most Americans do not eat enough fish and greens. If you look at other countries, you can predict the prevalence of depression in the population just by knowing the average annual fish consumption. In Germany, the average person eats just 20 pounds of fish per year and they have a very high rate of depression there. In Japan, fish is a staple of the diet, the average person eats about 150 pounds of it per year and they have an incredibly low rate of depression. The US is about in the middle between those two extremes.

"We already know that fish oil is quite effective for treating manic depression or bipolar disorder and schizophrenia. Fish oil capsules have two different types of omega-3s in them called EPA and DHA. It usually comes in 1000 milligram capsules and you need to take quite a lot of it. I recommend a total of about 10 grams per day of EPA and DHA divided into two doses. That usually works out to about 20 capsules per day. You should also increase the amount of fish and greens in your diet. If you have a bleeding disorder or if you are on aspirin or Coumadin or other drugs affecting your clotting, you should really only take fish oil under the close monitoring of a physician because fish oils do thin the blood. It takes several weeks to alter the fatty acid composition of the cell membranes in your brain, but some people feel the depression lift before that. Take vitamin E along with the fish oils to protect yourself from any peroxidized oils in the capsules."

Both alcoholics and chronic dieters often have depressive tendencies. Alcoholics often suffer from symptoms of low mood. Although alcohol may appear at first as a stimulant and mood enhancer, it is in fact a depressant and substantially decreases the ability of the body to extract nutrients from the food we eat. Dieters tend to eat very few B-complex-containing foods, and they often suffer from depression as well.

Dr. Richard Kunin believes that "most of the problems that we would identify as fatigue and depression up to the moderate level—depression that makes life an effort but not impossible—are environmental problems based on nutrition, environmental pollution, toxins in the environment, sensitization due to chemicals that stick to our cell membranes and alter them and make them allergy causing. These are the things that cause people to feel miserable, and to feel miserable for long enough so that when you add to it the slings and arrows part of life, it's not hard to understand this thing called depression. Psychotic depression is different; it's a distinct minority of cases."

Dr. Lendon Smith agrees: "A poor immune system as the result of bad diet, and pesticides on top of some genetic deficiency are leading to a lot of sickness now. A balanced chemistry will lead to a reasonably normal life. We are just bags of chemicals. People who have allergies are usually too alkaline and they need some vinegar, ammonium chloride or some acidifier and that will balance their chemistry, so their allergies are under control. We can balance their chemistry to handle the ordinary pesticides. Why doesn't everybody who is exposed to pesticides get sick? Well, maybe they don't have enough of some nutrients, but there are other ways to improve this and we know that naturopathic methods work. We've got to get people to be more aware of the alternate methods of care."

Patient Story: Tobacco Allergy

A high school teacher and principal developed a severe depression. In fact, I believe he was misdiagnosed as a schizophrenic. He exhibited what we call a straightforward, deep-seated, endogenous depression. He was in a mental hospital for about a year or two, and then discharged. He was so depressed that no one could live with him. His wife divorced him and eventually he was living with his aunt, who looked after him as if he were a child. As a last resort, he was referred to me.

When he came to see me, which was many years ago, I had just started looking into the question of allergies. At that time, I wasn't very familiar with food allergies, but I thought he was a very interesting case and I said to myself, 'He is a classic case of a depression, maybe schizophrenic. He'd be the last person in the world who would respond to this antiallergy approach.' At that time I was using—and I still do—a four-day water fast. This is a way of determining whether or not these allergies are present. He agreed that he would do the fast, which also involved refraining from any smoking or consum-

ing of alcohol; he had to drink about eight glasses of water a day and nothing else. His aunt said she would help make sure he complied. When he came back to see me two weeks later, he and his aunt explained that, at the end of the four-day fast, he was normal. All of the depression was gone.

This same man then began to get tested for food allergies and he found that not a single food made him sick. But now he began to smoke again. Within a day after he resumed smoking, he was back in his deep depression. The ironic thing was that he had a brother who was a tobacco company executive, who kept sending him free cartons of cigarettes. Now when we made the connection to his cigarette smoking, he stopped smoking. Thirty days later, after he had been depressed for four years and hadn't been able to work, he was back in school teaching. And I remember this clearly because the insurance company that was then paying his monthly pension was so astounded at this dramatic response that they sent one of their agents to see me, to find out what the magic wand was that I had waved to get this patient off their rolls. This is a classic case of an allergy to tobacco that was causing this man's depression.

—Dr. Abram Hoffer

Dr. Smith addresses some of the more baffling aspects of depression in today's society. "The more we hear about the rising tide of suicides in adolescents and even in children as young as 8, 9 and 10, it seems astounding that such a thing should overwhelm substantial numbers of children in what is supposed to be the happiest time of life. I evaluate children and adults who are depressed. For some of them there is no apparent reason for their overwhelming sadness. They've got good relationships with other people. Their social organization is intact. They've had a good upbringing. They have a good self-image. They have good school or work performance and they're getting nice accolades from relatives and friends. Why are they depressed? It just doesn't seem right."

Blood tests often reveal nutrient deficiencies. "In the particular program I'm doing," Dr. Smith said, "we go by the deviation from the mean. If, for instance, calcium's range is 8.5 to 10.5, then 9.5 is the mean. If they're down to 9 or 8.6, the doctor will say, 'Everything is okay.' Still, if there are enough of those scores below the mean, these people don't have enough wherewithal, enough nutrients, to satisfy all their enzyme requirements."

Patient Story: Nutrient Deficiency

Fifteen years ago, a 20-year-old woman came to see me who was depressed for no apparent reason. She came from a good family, and had a nice boyfriend and a good job. Everything seemed fine but she would still get depressed every once in a while. At that time I was experimenting with vitamins. I thought it would be quite safe to give her a shot of the mixed B complex vitamins. I included a cc of everything from B1 to folic acid and B12. I would give about 50 milligrams of each one of these vitamins and 50 micrograms of the B12 intramuscularly every day.

After two or three of these shots this patient told me that the treatment wasn't working very well for her. She asked, 'Couldn't you give them as separate vitamins?' I started giving her injections of isolated vitamins. I gave her a shot of 100 milligrams of B1 on Monday and B2 on Tuesday. I gave her separate shots of B3, B6, B12 and folic acid.

She reported feeling terrible after receiving B1, thiamine. She asked me never to do that again. I thought that seemed odd. After the B2 she came back and said that it was okay but nothing special. She said the same thing after receiving the B3. But after B6 she came back and said, 'I think you're onto something.' She also really liked the B12 and the folic acid.

These three vitamins were the important ones for her. I mixed them up and gave them to her every week or two. With that combination, she was apparently satisfied.

—Dr. Lendon Smith

Chocolate cravings also may be indicative of depression. "It usually means that people need magnesium, because there's magnesium in chocolate," Dr. Smith said. "Women, the day before their menstrual period, often find themselves searching through the cupboards for chocolate. They find a big canister of Hershey's and drink it down before feeling better from the magnesium. I often had the delightful experience of giving an intravenous mixture of vitamin C, calcium, magnesium and B vitamins. Usually it has more magnesium than calcium. Afterwards I asked patients whether they would like some chocolate and they told me they didn't need it. It really is connected.

"Women in the sixth month of pregnancy will often send their husbands out for ice cream because the baby is starting to grow fast. The woman has a conscious need for dairy products because she knows they will bring her the calcium she needs, but she also says, 'Don't forget the pickles.' She knows, somehow, that she needs to acidify that calcium source for the baby. She will not get much out of it and she will suffer from leg cramps.

"Magnesium is one of the first minerals to disappear from food when it's been processed. Magnesium is also one of the first minerals to leave the body when there is stress, which accounts for how many women behave a day or so before their periods. They feel stressed because they're losing their magnesium.

"We need to supply magnesium to these people. We can determine who needs it by the blood test and by the sense of smell. If people smell a bottle of pure magnesium salt—magnesium chloride is a good one—if it smells good or if there's no smell, then the person needs it. The blood test we usually use is the 24 chem. screen, the standard blood test.

"Many symptoms of depression, hyperactivity, headaches, loss of weight, and other conditions are related to genetic tendencies. If there is a tendency to be depressed in the family, a magnesium deficiency will allow that tendency to show up. If there's alcoholism, diabetes, obesity in the family, then low magnesium may allow those things to show up in a person. There are reasons to explain all these things and nutrition is basic to this. The patients don't have an antidepressant pill deficiency; they usually have a magnesium deficiency."

Dr. Sherry Rogers is even more emphatic. "In 27 years of medical practice, the one nutrient I have been very impressed with is magnesium. In treating people with panic disorders, anxiety, insomnia, fatigue and depression, just by merely correcting their magnesium—something so simple, so inexpensive, so relatively harmless—has made a dramatic difference."

The first thing Dr. Smith did was ask people what they're eating. "If I find that they're eating a lot of dairy products, and that as a child they had their tonsils taken out, and that they had a lot of strep throat and ear infections, then I know they're allergic to milk and they're looking for calcium. Sure enough, the blood tests will show this. That's the first thing they have to stop. Whatever they love is probably causing the trouble because food sensitivities can cause low blood sugar."

Dr. Goldwag adds that people "have to supply their bodies with proper nutrients and eliminate excesses or chronic addictions to alcohol, drugs, or food (including sweets and sugar). Inevitably, I find that if someone gets away from an addiction to sugar, they function much better. The old term hypoglycemia is very appropriate for their condition, particularly for people with chronic depression, chronic fatigue syndrome, and chronic immune system dysfunction. These people find that when they modify their diets and get off sugars, their mental functioning improves considerably."

Recent years have seen remarkable breakthroughs in the use of natural substances to fight depression. For Dr. Rogers, "phosphatidyl choline in its pure form has made a dramatic difference for many people with severe depression. It should, because the cell membranes are where the "happy hormones" or the neurotransmitters have to hook into the cell. In order for them to insert into these cell membranes, the receptors have to be healthy. Healthy receptors in the membrane are made out of the constituents that make up cell membrane. Phosphatidyl choline is one of those. People just don't get enough of it any more because they don't eat beans, which are rich in phosphatidyl choline. It is considered a peasant food because you have to soak them and cook them a long time and people are into fast foods. They don't eat eggs because they are trying to lower their cholesterol—but you do need cholesterol for the brain. In fact, one of the reasons many people on certain cholesterol lowering drugs have high suicide rates is because they got depressed when their cholesterol got too low. They didn't have enough cholesterol in the hormone receptors in the brain and died by suicide."

Phosphatidyl serine is another brain nutrient that has been found to decrease depression and stress. Found in all cells but highly concentrated in those of the brain, phoshatidyl serine stimulates release of the mood-regulator dopamine, releases levels of the stress hormone cortisol, and increases brain glucose metabolism.

The most popular natural supplements for mild to moderate depression are St. John's wort and SAM-e. Dr. Jonathan Zeuss calls St. John's wort (Hypericum perforatum) his "first choice for antidepressant treatment for most people," although he is emphatically against using anything, including natural supplements, as "magic bullets" for a disease as complex as depression. "Rather than just recommending a different kind of pill for them to take," his holistic approach includes treatment for "the levels of thought and the spiritual level, which might encompass psychotherapy, spiritual practices like prayer and meditation, and lifestyle interventions like light therapy and exercise.

"The raw material of St. John's wort is very inexpensive. It's basically a weed that grows everywhere. Manufacturers are less likely to try to thin it out by using fillers. It is pretty unique among antidepressants because it appears to work in many different ways at once. It works on reuptake of serotonin, norepinephrine and dopamine and also through a few other types of receptors. It also has immune-enhancing effects, which probably add to the overall antidepressant effect. The side effects are minimal. Don't mix St. John's wort with any other medication, except fish oils, which should be safe.

"St. John's wort comes in a number of different forms, mostly tablets and liquid extracts. The liquid is the least processed form. There are probably more than a dozen active ingredients in St. John's wort and they all contribute to its effect. Sustained released tablets have come out, naturally, they're more expensive, but it's really just a marketing gimmick. There is no need for sustained released form because St. John's wort has a long enough half-life in your body. Virtually everyone I've prescribed St. John's wort for takes a non-sustained released form twice a day and there is no problem with that at all."

SAMe (S-adenosyl-l-methionine) is a naturally occurring compound that has been available for use against depression in Europe for more than thirty years, and in the United States since the 1990s. In 2002, clinical trials revealed that SAMe was as effective as the tricyclics with fewer reported side effects.

Letha Hadady, herbalist and certified acupuncturist, has a different approach. She uses certain Asian herbs because "when we take serotonin drugs, we lose our connection with our own body and our own healing powers. Simply breathing in the light and sending out love opens up all our possibilities for self healing. There are other sources of serotonin—sunshine, bananas, the ions from the seashore—but herbs also can give us the natural warmth and grounding and centering."

She starts by focusing on digestion "because when we have better metabolism and better digestion we have fewer toxins in the body that can interfere with our processing; our emotional center is also our digestive center. By clearing the problems of digestion, we can also digest our thoughts and our problems better. There is a very good Chinese remedy for this called Xiao Yao Wan. Several very important herbs that you can find easily are in that remedy to balance and strengthen our digestive center. This morning for breakfast, I had ginger, which is one of them. I had green tea, which I drink all day. Radish has anti-congestion energy that clears our senses and helps us think better and I wanted to add a sour taste to balance the hot, pungent and bitter. Lately I have been eating a lot of star fruit, which is slightly sour, but other people might want to have lemon. So we have green tea, ginger, radish, and something sour, like lemon. This helps balance and strengthen the digestion.

"The link between digestion and depression is very clear. When our digestion is weak, we can't process our foods, but neither can we process our emotions and our sadness. We feel overcome; everything is too heavy for us to deal with and we give in to an addiction, like ice cream—milk and cheese and cream—which makes it all worse, which makes our digestion weaker and sets us up for major problems. Barley soup helps clear away the kind of congestion that makes us feel heavy. Sometimes feeling loaded down with problems is really water retention and excess phlegm. Barley soup helps. You might want to chop in some garlic and ginger and cardamom. Cardamom is very spicy and delicious and it speeds and strengthens the heart and strengthens the heart, but it is also sharp and piercing and cuts through phlegm. Another herb that is good for that too is hawthorn."

Several herbs are important for improving circulation clarifying a person's thinking. "Sometimes we get depressed because we don't have good circulation from our hearts," Hadady says. "When our energy cannot nourish the brain, we have problems like speediness and heart palpitations. There are remedies in the Chinese medical tradition, such as cerebral tonic pills, which help ease the heart action so we don't wake up with panic attacks at night or become so maniac because we are depressed, we cannot sleep. Asian remedies do not sedate our brain in the hopes of trying to rid us of our problems. We don't put our brains to sleep, but we clarify our thinking and clarify our senses so that we can actually deal with our problems better.

"Some people just don't have the energy to get up out of their chair and do what they need to do. Or they have abused their energy with stimulants like coffee and cocaine so they don't have the energy for strong sexuality or for concentration. They need a tonic, something to pick their energy up. One that is used a lot is ginseng tonic pills. It's ginseng with other ingredients that help nourish the brain. A number of good stimulants use ginseng and fo-ti. Fo-ti nourishes the brain and the brain cells and the moisture in the body, and ginseng balances and speeds our metabolism. So we need both, the hot and the cold, the yin and yang.

"People sometimes feel chilled and weak and have sexual weakness, which can lead to depression. They also have frequent urination. They feel weak from the waist down. This kind of depression happens after jet lag, after childbirth, with chronic asthma or chronic diarrhea. There are a couple of wonderful things you can take for that. One is a Chinese remedy called sexoton, it comes in pills, you can take ten pills three times a day if you need it. Clove can have the same effect, giving you a deeper breath and more courage. When we breathe in deeply and our adrenal glands are strong, we have the fortitude and the vitality to go out there and do our work and get it done. Clove clears our congestion and strengthens the adrenal glands in our lungs so that we can take in that deep breath."

According to a 2007 study reported in the *American Journal of Psychiatry*, people who seek treatment for depression are less likely to attempt suicide. The study, involving more than 100,000 patients, found that the act of seeking help—not the type of help received—was the determining factor. Clearly, as this research shows, it's so crucial to take that first step.

Catherine Carrigan says it is important to "do what you can to lower your stress level because when you get stressed out, your cortisol level goes up. Cortisol is a hormone secreted by the adrenal gland. When your cortisol level is high, you get depressed. Stress equals high cortisol, high cortisol equals depression. Cortisol balances in the body with insulin, so to recover from depression, you need to lower your stress level and balance your blood sugar.

"If you tend to be a negative thinker, studies prove that even antidepressants won't help you. Five minutes of pure anger raises your cortisol level for up to six hours. On the other hand, five minutes caring about other people, such as praying, raises your immune system for up to six hours. If you are depressed, you need to understand that there is a direct chemical connection between how you choose to think and your body chemistry and how you end up feeling.

Detoxification is a powerful treatment for depression. "There are forty chemicals proven to depress the nervous system," Dr. Goldwag says. "Detoxing could include taking special supplements to remove heavy metals, improve your digestion, clear your liver, etc. Detoxification has been proven to be a short cut to recovery for numerous mental and physical diseases."

Aromatherapy also has been found to be beneficial in people with depression. This practice depends on the therapeutic powers of essential oils, which are generally inhaled or applied to the skin. Among the essential oils with known antidepressant properties are ylang ylang, geramium, jasmine, orange, sandlewood, lemon, and mandarin.

Spirituality is an important lifestyle factor that can affect the course of depression. Dr. Goldwag emphasizes, "Don't overlook the spiritual connection. What have you learned? Ask yourself what depression has to teach you. For myself, depression was all about learning faith because anyone can have a lot of faith when the sun is shining and everything is going great but it takes a special kind of person who can have faith when they feel terrible.

"The next step may involve doing some volunteer work, getting out and doing things for other people. This is very important in trying to get the depressed person's mind off himself or herself. Depressed people are continually negative. They have dark thoughts, guilt, sad feelings, grief, regrets. Such negative thoughts are characteristic of depression. You can't talk the depressed individual out of them or try to convince them otherwise, but you can distract them. Physical activity is one distraction. Doing things for other people is another. So getting the person involved in someone else's problems can be a very effective way of dealing with depression."

Dr. Goldwag insists on the importance of those changes which can be made by the patient himself or herself. "When we have patients who are depressed and we can get them moving, the depression is greatly alleviated. Of course, drugs have changed the whole treatment of depression greatly, but the impact exercise can have on depression has often been overlooked, and it needs to be re-emphasized. People who are on antidepressants may improve, but the way for them to really get back to functioning well—back in touch with their environment, back to work, back in relationships with their family—is to get them moving. And there's no better way to get people moving than through exercise, whose healing potential has no limits.

"Those of us who exercise regularly have had days when we just didn't feel like it. That's the way depressed people feel about everything. They just don't feel like it. They don't have the energy, the motivation, the stimulation to go and do even the ordinary things. When it's severe, the person may not even have the will or desire to get out of bed in the morning."

An exercise program can be simple and gradually build on itself. "The exercise may consist of very, very simple things, like just getting out and walking, getting up and doing some simple movements, some mild calisthenics, any kind of physical movement that gets the body in action," Dr. Goldwag says. "For some people just getting out of bed and getting dressed is a big accomplishment. That may be the first step.

"It is important for depressed people to get up and get dressed. They should not walk around in pajamas or nightgowns because this maintains that connection to the bed and the bed means inactivity. That's the thing you're trying to overcome. Exercise may take the form of walking, walking the dog perhaps, or going outside to do some simple gardening. These are all very important for overcoming that feeling of lassitude that is so characteristic of depression.

"Another benefit of exercise is a feeling of accomplishment. Even doing a little bit of exercise will make you feel more energized later on. Finishing an exercise routine, even one that's fatiguing, after a brief period of rest, will give you a feeling of revitalization, of energy, and a psychological feeling of accomplishment. It gives a feeling of, 'I've done it. It's completed.' For the depressed individual, the boost to self-esteem that this can give is important."

An exercise program must be tailored to the individual. "There is no one exercise that is good for everybody," says Dr. Goldwag. "Some people can just do a little bit; some can push themselves much further. Ask anybody who has gone from a relatively sedentary life to an exercise program and they will all report the same thing: more energy, more interest in what is going on, a clearer mind and less stress. Being active, therefore, is an integral part of any kind of medical program, particularly for people who are having mental disturbances."

Dr. Judith Sachs agrees that exercise "triggers all of these brain stimulants that make us feel good, these natural opiates. This is another system we have in the brain that takes away pain and gives us pleasure. A lot of people who run say, 'well it feels so good when I stop,' but even people who are not crazy about that kind of exercise are finding that they feel better. They feel efficient, like the body is not just this house that they happen to live in, but has actually become an integral part of their mind, their spirit, the whole way that they approach themselves and other people. That can really turn around a lack of self confidence, a lack of self esteem. When you've said 'all I could do was to walk down to the mailbox to get my mail' and suddenly you are able to run up five flights of stairs or run a mini-marathon—that can make you feel very effective as a person.

"I suggest to people who are feeling kind of low and blue that they set themselves some kind of exercise goal. Something that they enjoy doing, whether it is rollerblading, dancing (maybe they enter a dance competition with a partner) or taking a class in something they have never done before. It can make you feel effective and part of things, especially if you do a team sport that involves a group where people rely on you, you count. It's not whether you have made that home run but how you have helped other people to get to that home run. Exercise actually works the body, but it also revitalizes our sense of spirit and I think that is really important. It can also help to motivate us to stick with a good diet, a good helpful diet. I don't mean a weight loss diet.

"After paying attention to exercise and nutrition, you need to be aware of the stresses of your own lifestyle, your own patterns of behavior, how they are manifested, and how they may be altered by more healthy ways of thinking. For example, if you frequently get upset by dwelling on the past, then you need to try not to think so much about what took place in the past or what is going to happen in the future. Your emotional work is to learn how to focus on the present reality, what's going on now, by putting the body in a mode where it is accepting what's happening now, so you're ready for anything that may happen, instead of reliving crises over and over again."

Qi gong is an ancient Chinese practice that uses aerobic exercise, meditation, relaxation techniques and isometrics to control the vital energy of the body in the most efficient way. Like many Chinese therapies, it emphasizes the unity of mind, spirit and world. According to a 2006 study, Qi gong was found to reduce the symptoms of depression after eight weeks of practice.

8

Bipolar Disorder (Manic Depression)

■■■

Bipolar disorder, also known as manic depression, affects 5.7 million American adults annually. It manifests as serious cycles of depression and mania. In the depressed phase, the person may be sluggish, sad, hopeless, and withdrawn. In the manic phase, the person swings to the opposite extreme: hyperactive, energetic, impatient, easily distracted, and "too busy" to sleep. Bipolar disorder usually develops in late adolescence or early adulthood. It is a chronic, recurrent condition that often goes undiagnosed or misdiagnosed for years.

Today it is uncommon to see people whose illness is so out of control that they become truly manic. "More often," says psychiatrist Dr. Garry Vickar, "you will see individuals who are manic-depressive becoming excessively elevated in their moods. They become more expansive. They might go on spending sprees and spend money they don't have, or get involved in activities that they truly are not qualified for. They may run up charge cards, or get involved in gambling, financial affairs, extramarital affairs, alcohol or drug abuse that they would not otherwise be doing. It becomes almost the reverse of the depression spectrum—they need less sleep, they need less food, and everything is very intense. It can become rather horrific because people can become exhausted. They're sleeping two or three hours a day, if that. They may be getting by on a cup of coffee and a soda and cigarettes. At the same time they have this overwhelming sense of omnipotence about themselves and their abilities. So it can be a very, very dangerous period of time."

Another manifestation may be that the person becomes overly suspicious and paranoid. "Sometimes," Dr. Vickar explains, "the grandiose patient grows irritable, angry, and upset at other people who are getting in the way of the wonderful achievements he or she has to offer the world."

Some people with bipolar disorder become suicidal. The risk of suicide is greater in the beginning stages of the illness.

Conventional treatment of bipolar disorder involves mood-stabilizers and anticonvulsants, such as lithium and valproate, and psychosocial therapy. Some doctors use antidepressants as well, but even mainstream medicine has realized that adding more drugs to the mix is not the answer. According to a 2007 study published in the *New England Journal of Medicine*, the antidepressants bupro-prion (Wellbutrin) and paroxetine (Paxil) were no more effective than placebos when taken in combination with mood stabilizers.

Newer antipsychotic medications are also being used. Unfortunately, as we are becoming all too aware by the growing number of lawsuits, governmental warnings, and media attention, these medications often end up causing more harm than good. Zyprexa is just one case in point. Approved in 1996 by the FDA to treat bipolar disorder and schizophrenia, it has been associated with increased risk of hyperglycemia and diabetes to such an extent that its manufacturer Eli Lilly agreed in 2005 to pay nearly $700 million to settle thousands of claims.

When treating patients with bipolar disorder, Dr. Vickar recommends tryp-tophan or lithium. "I don't use other amino acids but I certainly use lithium," he says. "Now we're discovering that some of the other antiseizure medications may work in patients with lithium intolerance. Lithium is a naturally occurring substance so I prefer it over the other antiseizure medications which are, of course, man-made. In fact, lithium is a perfect example of a naturally occurring substance being used by traditional psychiatrists to treat biochemical diseases. Sometimes you use lithium in schizophrenic patients who also have secondary depressions of their moods. You want to be cautious, however.

"If a patient is manic and having psychotic symptoms, I tend to use a formu-lation similar to that given to psychotic patients. Lithium is certainly added in large part. If the patient's mood is low and he or she is depressed, lithium is sometimes of value, but not always. In addition to traditional antidepressants, I make sure they have enough B complex vitamins. There are some people who use phenylalanine or tyrosine, and these substances can be purchased, but it is often difficult for patients to get them. Not every hospital will stock them for you either. Also, sometimes the quality of the product is hard to verify."

In a 2001 article in the *Journal of Clinical Psychiatry*, Dr. Charles Popper described his experience with the Hardy-Stephan nutrient supplement, a combination of minerals and vitamins, amino acids, and antioxidants. Other researchers had already determined that this supplement could reduce symptoms and enable patients to decrease their doses of psychiatric medications. After finding it could eliminate severe temper tantrums in one of his ten-year-old patients with bipolar disorder, Dr. Popper used the supplement in twenty-two additional patients, nineteen of whom had a positive response. Acknowledging that more research must be done to assess safety and efficacy, Dr. Popper commented, "Psychiatrists do not normally think of vitamins or minerals as modifiers of the effects of psychiatric medications, but the early anecdotal evidence with this nutrient supplement suggests that there may be strong micronutrient-medication interactions. This mineral-vitamin supplement seems to generally potentiate the clinical properties of psychiatric drugs."

Other nutritional remedies that have been shown to be beneficial in treating mood disorders include omega-3 fatty acids, phenylalanine, triiodothyronine, l-cysteine, folic acid, inositol, vitamin B12, and vitamin C.

Patient Story: Bipolar Disorder

I treated a patient who, for 40 years, exhibited a history that was very clearly that of a manic depressive: He was erratic, impulsive, had marital problems, and was in and out of jobs. His response came when I added lithium to the vitamins, and nothing else. In over 40 years, nobody had ever taken a look at the possibility that he had a biochemical abnormality. They just thought he was immature, or impulsive, or perhaps a bit anti-social. I see him once a year, and he takes lithium and vitamins and nothing else. Lithium is a naturally occurring substance that manic-depressives need in higher doses than the rest of us. So here is a case of somebody who, for the better part of a lifetime of illness, hadn't been diagnosed at all.

—Dr. Garry Vickar

9

Schizophrenia

■■■

Patient Story: Schizophrenia

I was seeing about three different psychiatrists and they were unable to help me. One psychiatrist thought I was manic-depressive. I wasn't being treated for schizophrenia, which is what I have. Now I am on a regimen of vitamins and antipsychotic drugs. The vitamins, I am told, enhance the good effects of the drugs so that I don't have to take high doses of the drugs in order to remain normal or stable. Before I got on this regimen I had not been taking any vitamins. Using the orthomolecular approach to help treat my schizophrenia, I basically feel normal and have my life back again.

—Howard

Schizophrenia is a severe, chronic mental disorder that affects approximately 1 percent of the American population. It may be characterized by hallucinations, delusions, abnormal thought processes, abnormal movements, disrupted speech, social withdrawal, emotional distress, lack of motivation, and cognitive decline. Subtypes include catatonic, paranoid, disorganized, and undifferentiated schizophrenia. Psychotic symptoms generally begin in adolescence or early to mid-adulthood. Schizophrenia is associated with a higher rate of substance abuse and suicide than that which occurs in the general population. Although the causes of schizophrenia remain unknown, it is believed to result from a combination of genetic and environmental factors.

According to psychiatrist Dr. Garry Vickar, "schizophrenic illnesses as a group are among the most serious biochemical disorders there are; it can be said that schizophrenia is to psychiatry what cancers are to general medicine. The bulk of the lost revenue to society, the bulk of psychiatric expense, and the sheer horror to the families, which is not easily quantifiable, are unfortunately all consequences associated with the diagnosis of schizophrenia."

Dr. Vickar says that abnormal thought is the most disturbing part of schizophrenia. "These are patients who may have vague symptoms, who go through periods of what German psychiatrists used to call 'stage fright,' and then something happens and they start to believe that their disordered perceptions represent true events. Their strong belief in these disordered perceptions transforms them into delusions, which are simply fixed, false beliefs. Patients will start to believe their delusions and then start to believe their misinterpretation of a perceptual nature. They may hear a voice and believe that the voice is real and represents some real event or real person. They'll act on that. An example would be, if I hear somebody calling my name, if I don't think it's my thought anymore but that there really is somebody calling my name, I will act accordingly. If I think that people are looking at me and making faces, I might think there is something very wrong with me and feel bad or upset about it. If I'm eating my meal and there's a piece of moldy cheese, I might think I've been poisoned and that someone did it to me purposefully. The process starts to escalate and snowball."

Then there's the loss of insight. "The most diabolical part of the illness is the loss of insight, loss of the ability to reality-test," Dr. Vickar says. "For instance, if you're driving down the street at night and it's dark and hard to see, and you see something at the side of the road, you might slow down to be cautious, thinking that somebody is going to cross the street. Then you get close enough and see that it's really just shrubs or a mailbox or just part of the normal landscape, and you say, I'm glad I was cautious. If instead, however, you start to distort the original perception and really believe that there's someone who might jump out on the road or that somebody is trying to hurt you and can get in the way of your vehicle, you might take evasive action. In the process, you could have an accident or cause somebody else to have one. You start to distort things without realizing that you are distorting them. That's similar to what happens when the really disastrous part of the illness takes over. . . . Such paranoid delusions can become all-consuming and unfortunately very painful."

Conventional treatment of schizophrenia involves antipsychotic medications and psychosocial intervention. According to the National Institute of Mental Health in a 2007 update on schizophrenia, the medications alleviate symptoms but do not cure the disorder. In addition, side effects can be serious and patients must be monitored very closely. Among the older antipsychotics are Thorazine, Haldol, and Prolixin. These have been associated with muscle spasms, tremors, and rigidity. In the 1990s, the atypical antipsychotic clozapine (Clozaril) was introduced. Although not associated with the extrapyramidal side effects of the earlier drugs, it has been associated with agranulocytosis, a loss of infection-fighting white blood cells. Other second-generation drugs that came on the scene after clozapine—including Risperdal, Zyprexa, and Seroquel—bypass the already mentioned side effects but pose a whole new dilemma: weight gain and metabolic changes linked to an increased risk of high cholesterol and diabetes.

Beyond the known side effects, there is question about the relative effectiveness of these drugs. According to a 2006 study published in the *Archives of General Psychology*, there was no reported clinical advantage to the more expensive and highly touted second-generation antipsychotics when compared with the first. In a commentary in the same issue, Dr. Jeffrey A. Lieberman, chairman of psychiatry at Columbia University, stated that the lack of difference in effectiveness between first- and second-generation antipsychotics in nonrefractory patients is "a conclusion that runs counter to the impressions of many clinicians and previous studies suggesting marked superiority of the second-generation antipsychotics and that belies the huge advantage in market share enjoyed by the second-generation antipsychotics in the United States and other parts of the world."

Nutritional treatment of schizophrenia has a decades-long history. Dr. Philip Hodes sketches an overview: "In the field of schizophrenia, in the 1950s there were three pioneers in orthomolecular psychiatry: Dr. Abram Hoffer, Dr. Humphry Osmond, and Dr. John Smythies. They used large amounts of niacinamide, vitamin C and some of the other B vitamins to help their schizophrenic patients recover. In the 1970s, Dr. Alan Cott went to Russia and brought back the practice of fasting, and helped to detoxify many of the brains of schizophrenics who had not responded to any other kind of treatment. He helped them clear their brains so that they became rational and normal."

Orthomolecular doctors realized that something must be done to counter the effects of environmental pollution. "There are over 90,000 chemicals in the external environment that we ingest through what we eat, drink and breathe," Dr. Hodes says. "Contaminants are in the soil, water, air, and food supply. The particles that are toxic penetrate and leak through the blood-brain barrier over time and get into the brain. This process also happens with several of the heavy toxic metals, such as lead, cadmium, copper, iron, arsenic, mercury and aluminum. These chemicals and heavy metals, by affecting brain chemistry, affect the mind and behavior, so they must be removed. They need to be chelated out. . . . People can develop bizarre behavior and distorted thinking, along with warped perceptions, as a result of these toxic metals. Add to this toxic stew all the insecticides, pesticides, and herbicides that we ingest daily.

"The late Dr. Henry (Hank) Newbold demonstrated that many of his schizophrenic psychiatric patients were suffering from a vitamin B12 'dependency' and that they needed large amounts in order to feel well and sane again. Then as the years went by, orthomolecular doctors discovered that the essential minerals—macro minerals such as calcium and magnesium, as well as the trace mineral elements zinc, manganese, chromium, and selenium—also helped balance the cerebral chemistry of schizophrenics. Dr. Priscilla Slagle published her research in a book, *Up From Depression*, showing the important role of amino acids in the brain, including L-tyrasine, 5 L-hydroxytryptophan, as well as dehydroepiandrosterone, and in the treatment of manic depressives and schizophrenics."

Researcher Eva Edelman adds that a low state of histamine is sometimes associated with schizophrenia and that this, too, can be environmentally related. "Perhaps 40 to 50 percent of individuals diagnosed as schizophrenic are low histamines. They typically have a pear shaped body, low metabolism, and a tendency to dental cavities. They may have upper body pain, and tend to be young looking and resistant to shock—because histamine plays an important role in producing shock reactions in the body. They also tend to have food and chemical sensitivity.

"This condition produces the most typical mental symptoms of schizophrenia, the kind conventional psychiatry would readily identify. Low histamine is often caused by an excess of copper in the body. While copper is a very important nutrient for most people, it's very easy to get an excess because copper is prevalent in our diets and in good herbs; it's often in the pipes that conduct water to our houses. Also in vitamin pills—a lot of companies provide what would be a maximum dose for many people. Blood type A can create a tendency to accumulate copper. Copper depletes histamine levels and it also depletes vitamin B3 and C, which are needed to support mental functioning in low histamine individuals."

Dr. Abram Hoffer, who has researched and published extensively in the field, tells how the early treatment efforts influenced today's thinking: "The orthomolecular treatment of schizophrenia was started in Saskatchewan in 1951 when we ran the first double-blind controlled experiments in North American medicine and also the first in worldwide psychiatry. On the basis of these experiments, where we compared the effect of vitamin B3 against a placebo, we found that the addition of the vitamin to the standard treatment of that day, which was only electroconvulsant therapy, doubled the two-year recovery rate from 35 percent to 70 percent. That was the beginning.

"After that we ran another three double-blind controlled experiments. Since that time we have accumulated massive clinical experience; I myself have seen many thousands of schizophrenic patients. The treatment for the schizophrenic patient is really relatively simple. It's a combination of the best of modern psychiatry, which includes the proper use of tranquilizers, antidepressants or other drugs, with proper attention to diet and the use of nutrients.

Vitamin B3 is the main nutrient used in treatment. It is given in large doses. "It's not enough to give the tiny amount present in food," Dr. Hoffer says. "One will have to give many thousands of times as much in the standard dose. For the patients I work with, I give 3000 milligrams per day of either nicotinic acid or nicotinamide, which are both forms of vitamin B3."

Other nutrients include vitamin C, vitamin B6, and manganese. "I also use vitamin C at the same dose level and sometimes a lot more because vitamin C is a very good water-soluble antioxidant," Dr. Hoffer explains. "It is considered the foremost, the most active water-soluble antioxidant present in the human body. That's extremely important."

Manganese is used to protect against tardive dyskinesia. Dr. Hoffer says, "This is a condition which afflicts chronic schizophrenic patients who are placed upon large quantities of tranquilizers. According to Dr. Richard Kunin from San Francisco, when you take tranquilizers for a long period of time you take manganese out of the body, which is the reason patients develop tardive dyskinesia. When you give them back the manganese this condition may go away."

Of course, it's important to pay attention to diet. "I put my patients on a diet that is junk-free," he says. "I exclude any of the prepared foods that contain additives, including sugar. I also pay attention to patients' allergies, because 50 or 60 percent of all schizophrenics have major food allergies. If these are not detected and eliminated, the patients are not going to get any better."

Dr. Hoffer provides this review to illustrate his treatment successes: "I have re-examined 27 of my chronic schizophrenic patients who have been working with me for at least 10 years. They had been sick an average of 7 years before they came to see me. They had all failed to respond to any of the standard treatments. They had not been given any vitamins. I did a survey of what happened to them after being with me for 10 years. Of the 27 really chronic patients, 17 today are normal. They really are well. They're paying taxes."

One of the patients, a man from eastern Canada, was a very paranoid schizophrenic. He was in and out of the Ontario mental hospital system. He was so sick that his wife divorced him and his family disowned him. He moved out west to Victoria and was living as a homeless person there for awhile. He came under Dr. Hoffer's care and remained on the vitamins, to the doctor's surprise. Three or four years ago he got his degree at the local university in Toronto and the last time Dr. Hoffer saw him he was looking for a job. He thinks this is quite an accomplishment for someone who had been a very sick patient.

"Another patient," Dr. Hoffer says, "was a woman who, in a psychotic frenzy, burned down her house. She now runs her own business and supervises 12 people. These are examples of some of the recoveries we've had.

"The other ten are not well yet. Some may never be well because they've been sick for too long, but they're certainly an awful lot better than they were when we found them. They're now comfortable. They're able to live with any hallucinations or delusions they still have. This is a very chronic group of patients, the kind that normally don't respond. The important thing—going back to the view that you have to expect slow, progressive improvement rather than any sudden cure—is that it took 5 to 7 years of continuous treatment before they reached their current stage of improvement.

Dr. Garry Vickar emphasizes the holistic foundation of the treatment approach he prefers. "I think in any chronic illness, such as schizophrenia, you have to maximize the person's whole functioning. You want to make them as healthy as possible. You don't want to have an imbalance where your left arm is really maximally in shape because you're a pitcher but the rest of you is flab. You have to have the whole organism as healthy as possible.

"If, in fact, people have abnormal thinking because of deficiencies of B12, maybe they have a lack of an enzyme in their stomach that doesn't carry out the necessary conversion of B12 into what the body needs. These people have a disease called pernicious anemia that can result in their becoming paranoid. Once in a while you'll find a person who lacks this thing called intrinsic factor. You have to give B12 supplements to prevent them from becoming paranoid and from developing nervous system signs and symptoms and gait disturbances. With B12 they get better. So there are simple things like that which can be done and which, in this modern age, can get overlooked by conventional physicians."

Dr. Vickar says he checks for magnesium levels in all of his patients, "especially adolescents who drink a lot of soda pop. I also do zinc, copper, and manganese levels because there is some evidence that low manganese is implicated in tardive dyskinesia. A low magnesium level is implicated in irritability, nervousness, even nerve conduction problems and seizures. The worst-case scenario is a premenopausal woman who just had a baby, was on birth control pills prior to her pregnancy, is on prenatal vitamins, and goes back on the pill after the baby is born. She'll have sky-high copper levels, almost toxic relative to zinc.

"With the schizophrenic patient I use niacinamide or niacin (more frequently niacinamide because most patients won't tolerate niacin). I tend to use much of what Abram Hoffer has come up with. I look for a minimum of 3000 milligrams of niacinamide a day with an equal amount of vitamin C. I recommend a B complex with 50 to 150 milligrams of the entire B complex, mineral balance, depending upon zinc and copper levels. We try to titrate a dose until we reach a level of improvement with the least amount of medicine and the amount of vitamin and mineral supplements that the patient can tolerate."

Dr. Vickar continues, expressing the broad philosophy of his treatment of schizophrenic patients: "I have patients who have been diagnosed as having schizophrenia, and while I don't argue with the diagnosis, it hasn't captured the whole essence of what is going on with that patient. I prefer to see it as an incomplete diagnosis, rather than as a misdiagnosis. Very often the goal, in the schizophrenic diagnosis, is just to subdue behavior. When people are in such states of distress that their behavior is inappropriate, or agitated, or out of control, the goal is primarily to treat that behavior. I think that there is more we can do. We have to try to understand why the patient is doing what he or she is doing—not necessarily psychologically, but in some way biochemically.

"We don't know what the ultimate causes of schizophrenia are. Each new drug that comes along throws the current theory into such disarray that it doesn't apply anymore, because the new drug doesn't work the way that those preceding it did. So I don't think that anybody knows the causes, but there is one thing that we are sure of: We can make a big difference in how a schizophrenic is doing by applying two basic principles, as Dr. Hoffer has indicated: good sound nutrition and vitamin supplements.

"These are not synonymous. Nutrition has to be the floor upon which the treatment is built. Then, after that, you have to start looking at other factors—whether it be smoking, co-existing alcohol-related problems, dietary disturbances or absorption difficulties. Also, the patient may not be doing well because what they have been given is, in fact, creating more problems. So we have to be sensitive to such reactions to treatment and continue to modify the treatment all the way along. And again, the approach I find to be most useful is that schizophrenia is not so much a missed diagnosis as it is an incomplete one."

Dr. Peter Breggin points out that "studies have shown that patients diagnosed with acute schizophrenia improve better without medication in small home-like settings run by nonprofessional staff who know how to listen and to care. The patients become more independent, and do so at no greater financial cost, because nonprofessional salaries are so much lower. As an enormous added benefit, the drug-free patients do not get tardive dyskinesia or tardive dementia, as well as other drug-induced and sometimes life-threatening disorders.

"But isn't schizophrenia a biochemical and genetic disease? In reality, there's no convincing evidence that schizophrenia is a biochemical disorder. While there are a host of conjectures about biochemical imbalances, the only ones we know of in the brains of mental patients are those produced by the drugs. Similarly, no substantial evidence exists for a genetic basis of schizophrenia. The frequently cited Scandinavian genetic studies of the mid-1970s actually confirm an environmental factor while disproving a genetic one. But even if schizophrenia were a brain disease, it would not make sense to add further brain damage and dysfunction by administering neuroleptics."

At the Pfeiffer Treatment Center in Illinois, named after the late Dr. Carl Pfeiffer, who worked with thousands of schizophrenic patients, practitioners individualize all therapies. After determining a patient's biochemical subtype, the following supplements may be administered in varying doses: omega-3 fatty acids, zinc, manganese, vitamin C, glycine, tryptophan, histidine, and tyrosine.

Patients are tested for allergies to wheat, dairy, tobacco, and gluten, as some researchers have found that "cerebral allergies" may affect 10 percent to as many as 50 percent of people with schizophrenia.

Dr. Abram Hoffer estimates that about 10 percent of all schizophrenic patients are also alcoholic. "It's not a big figure," he adds, "if you remember that 10 percent of all adults in North America are probably alcoholic. In other words, the same proportion is present in schizophrenics. If you start the other way, a certain percentage of alcoholics are, in fact, also schizophrenic. There is an overlap.

"It has been acknowledged for many years that this particular group that has both problems is very tough to treat. The first person to really show that you can help them was Dr. David Hawkins, who was then practicing on Long Island. He found that when he placed his alcoholic schizophrenic patients on the proper vitamin treatment, including mostly niacin and vitamin C, he began to see a fantastic number of recoveries. I have seen some recoveries, but not as many as he has.

"I think that whether or not they are alcoholic they have to be treated the same way. If they're alcoholic, it's vital that they stop drinking. The best way to achieve that is to try to get them to join Alcoholics Anonymous."

10

Insomnia

■ ■ ■

Although we spend roughly a third of our lives sleeping, the essential nature of sleep still isn't fully understood. Brain longevity expert Dr. Dharma Singh Khalsa tells us that "recent studies have shown that you don't need to sleep as much as you think. In the last two hours, you have weird dreams and the rapid eye movement sleep is very intense. This raises cortisol levels and can actually cause you to awaken with stress and anxiety, which can lead to memory loss and other illnesses. In fact, people who have heart attacks have them most often in the morning. Ancient and modern thinkers recommend that you don't get up, take a shower, or have your coffee first thing. Take a little time for yourself—this has been scientifically shown to be one of the most important things you can do to put on a suit of armor against stress and have a great day."

Many people wake up tense because they have been unable to sleep. Insomnia is common problem, affecting one-third of all adults and accompanying many of the disorders discussed elsewhere in this book, ranging from anxiety to schizophrenia and various other mood disorders. Typically, anxiety makes it more difficult to go to sleep, and depression can cause early waking. Insomnia can also result directly from physical symptoms such as pain or indigestion, or as a side effect of drug medication. People with chronic fatigue have serious sleep disturbance, are usually unable to fall asleep, wake up frequently, and don't feel restored.

Norman Ford, a health reporter and a researcher with nearly forty years of experience, says "tossing and turning and laying awake at night is not a reliable indication of insomnia. If you wake up each morning feeling fresh and recharged and you function efficiently during the day both physically and mentally, you probably do not have bonafide insomnia. The symptoms of true insomnia are feeling drowsy and uncomfortable during the day with a definite impairment in cre-

activity, memory recall, cognitive ability, and mood, or falling asleep when you should be awake. Even though you believe you're getting adequate sleep, if all these happen together, you may have true insomnia."

Ford describes six types of insomnia: subjective insomnia, which is when you think you have insomnia, but you really don't; initial insomnia, which occurs when it takes thirty to sixty minutes or more to fall asleep; sleep maintenance insomnia, which occurs when you lie awake between sleep cycles during the night; delayed sleep phase insomnia, which is when you can't fall sleep before 2:00 to 3:00 a.m.; unfinished sleep insomnia, which occurs when you suddenly awake at 5:00 a.m. and can't go back to sleep; and disturbed sleep insomnia, which is when you are suddenly awakened by nightmares.

"The best way to improve your sleep," Ford says, "is to cut out all daytime napping and consolidate your sleep into a single nighttime unit. Get up at the same time every morning and don't sleep in on weekends. Go to bed only when you feel drowsy and tired, not when you think it's bedtime. Tire the body and mind by using both actively during the day. Watching TV is the most passive, inactive thing you can do, probably the greatest thief of sleep in existence. Instead, try to exercise abundantly every day and use the mind actively by studying, learning or playing mind taxing games like chess or anything else that makes you think, like creative writing or even surfing the Internet.

"Once you're in bed, relax in a comfortable position, take several slow, deep belly breaths, and then briefly review all the good, pleasant things that have happened that day. If they didn't happen today, they could have happened the previous day, so review them anyway. If you're not asleep within 10 minutes, get up, go to another room, and do something monotonous and repetitive. Write letters, pay bills, water indoor plants or practice deep relaxation. Return to bed only when you feel drowsy and ready to sleep. If you don't fall asleep again within 10 minutes, get up and go back to the same room and repeat the whole routine. Keep repeating it until you do fall asleep."

Sleep needs are not the same for everybody. "The fact is," Ford says, "if you really need sleep, you will sleep, but many of us go to bed too early and we spend biologically inappropriate time in bed for the demands of our lifestyle. If our lifestyle activity demands that we only need six and a half hours of sleep and we spend eight hours in bed, we'll toss and turn for one and a half hours, it's just as simple as that. The answer, of course, is to lead a more active lifestyle so that you do need eight hours of sleep.

"Many people just worry about the fact that they can't sleep because we're conditioned to believe we need eight hours a night. The more we worry about not being able to sleep, the less we sleep and the more we worry. A good technique to overcome this is called paradoxical intent. It's based on the principle of the harder you try to fall asleep, the longer you remain awake. Paradoxical intent forces you to do the opposite—try as hard as you can to stay awake. The result is, you usually fall asleep. During a study at Temple University, for example, a group of chronic worriers, people who normally took 60 to 90 minutes to fall asleep, were able to drop off in six to seven minutes. Every night millions of people lay awake worrying about how they will perform on the job next day. So one of the best ways to fall asleep is to try as hard as you can not to, and it frequently works."

People often assume that sleep needs change with age. "One person in three age 65 and older complains of poor sleep, but the explanation is that as they grow older, most men and women use their minds and muscles increasingly less and less," Ford says. "When we function like an old, sedentary, unhealthy person, we get the sleep of an older, sedentary person, regardless of chronological age. A man of 70 who walks five brisk miles each day and spends several hours studying and learning will have approximately the same sleep needs as when he was age 25. Sleep needs decrease as we become less active physically and mentally."

"People over 40 complain that they wake up in the middle of the night and can't get back to sleep for 30 to 60 minutes. The reason is that every 90 minutes during the night, most adults wake briefly as one sleep cycle ends and the next begins. Each sleep cycle lasts 90 minutes. But after 40, inactive people may remain awake for 30 minutes at the end of a sleep cycle before they can drift back to sleep and into the next sleep cycle. This is actually a bonafide form of insomnia, called sleep maintenance insomnia, and it's caused by failing to exercise and tire the body by bedtime. It's also caused by failing to spend at least 30 minutes outdoors in the daytime. It's caused by eating a large, high fat, meat-centered meal late in the evening. It could be caused by consuming alcohol after 7:00 p.m. or going to bed feeling hungry or by daytime napping."

Relaxation is key when problems arise. Ford explains, "If you do wake up after a sleep cycle in the middle of the night, the solution is to relax the muscles with deep relaxation and relax the mind with abdominal breathing—breathe deeply, use deep belly breaths, take several deep belly breaths slowly in and out.

That will tame a racing mind. As the body slows, it slows the mind, and as the mind slows, it relaxes the body. In just a couple of minutes, these combined steps will turn on the relaxation response. The mind enters a calm reverie-like state, your brain wave frequency drops and you're on the brink of sleep."

Dr. Samuel Dunkell is a psychiatrist and sleep clinician working in an insomnia outpatient clinic, and former director of the American Sleep Disorders Association. His work concerning the position of the body in sleep is intriguing. He says, "The way we sleep at night reflects the positions that we take in our daily lives. Our general approach is reflected in terms of body language. Different types of people show different configurations.

"The person who sleeps on the back is a person who is ready to receive, who is used to being given everything; the world shares their products and wealth with them. A person who sleeps on the side sleeps between the face-down and the back position, so is flexible. This position is characteristic of the majority of Americans. Sixty percent, I would say, sleep in the side position with the knees slightly bent, a semi-fetal position. Another group, quite large in number, sleeps face down. These people like to know where they are at all times. They like to be in touch with their world and to a certain extent, in control. Such people tend to be short sleepers, not to dream too much, to go to bed early and to arise early. They are somewhat compulsive, driven or active; their lives are geared for success in our society, which rewards that type of behavior. If we don't assume these positions we are restless, we can't fall asleep, we might even have insomnia."

Although sleep research focuses on the individual with the problem, most adults share beds for most of their lives. "This has not been studied too extensively because laboratory instruments used to study sleep are geared to an individual," Dr. Dunkell says. "I've seen that the way couples relate at night in terms of the configurations that they assume on the bed reflect not only their individual positions, but the relationship between them and their attitudes toward one another. Most people who have a new bed relationship, like newly marrieds who go to bed regularly with one another, sleep in the 'spoon' position. Both lie on their sides, facing the same direction, with one person behind the other. The person who generally takes the rear position has their arms over the partner. This is the person who sets the tone, the pace and is generally the nurturer in the relationship.

"My studies found that after three to five years of an ongoing relationship, gradually the couples disengage from one another in bed. They go into their individual personal sleep positions, knowing that their partner is there for them and ready to give them the security, love and contact that they need at night. During the night, from time to time, they assume that original 'spoon' configuration temporarily.

"Sometimes, people have trouble sleeping because one person encroaches on the other too much and one of them feels hemmed in. If that partner has a problem with intimacy, they may want to pull away. They will try to do things to try to discourage the partner from assuming too close contact and that's bad for intimacy. We'd rather have the couple share their life together at night as well as during the day. Whenever there are instances of discord and attempts to diminish intimacy, these should be recognized and discussed and dealt with."

There are differences between men and women when it comes to sleep problems. "Pregnant women, whose abdomens have become extended during childbirth, can't fall into their usual sleep positions or have their usual contact with their bed mates," Dr. Dunkell says. "There is also an increase in insomnia caused by the pregnancy toward the end of the pregnancy period. Postpartum, women often have difficulty falling asleep for a number of days or weeks. Men generally have most of the insomnia that occurs before the age of 55 but in the postmenopausal period, women catch up. This may be due to the loss of sex hormones or to physical problems that easily add to the inability to fall asleep."

Like other sleep clinicians, Dr. Dunkell recommends relaxation techniques. "The main problem," he says, "is to get the mind off of the worry. The worry acts like a magnet that pulls our thoughts and when that magnet starts going, it starts the worry machine going. That keeps us aroused and awake. So the main trick is to occupy our minds with something else that's less stimulating, even somewhat boring, but that keeps us busy and away from the danger zone. I have an interest in geography, so if I have trouble sleeping or I wake during the night and can't fall back to sleep, I try to remember the names of the various states of the union or the major rivers of the US or the major rivers of Europe. I even go down the alphabet and try to name bodies of water. The same general principle can be used by others—if they are interested in sports, they can try to name teams and players and years and averages and things like that. They might try to remember the names of certain books they've read or movies they've seen or actors. Whatever is important and relevant to the individual can be drawn in. It's a very effective technique and before you know it, you're asleep.

"There is a period just prior to falling asleep when we sort of give up the world that surrounds us. Because this period of giving up the world means a kind of loss of activity and structure, it has a certain element about it that we call regressive anxiety. The presence of the bed partner whom we sleep with night after night reassures us. Being close, in touch, experiencing their breathing, their heart beat, their warmth—all this will overcome that anxiety producing phase and allow us to fall asleep much more easily.

The bedroom environment should be soothing, Dr. Dunkell says. "Loud colors, surfaces that reflect light, stimulating types of objects in the room—all distract from the ability to fall asleep."

While some people advocate the use of "white noise," Dr. Dunkell does not. "If we go to sleep with a sound going on, like a fan, the noise will grab our attention, wiping out all the other sounds we are accustomed to as part of our environment. That is called masking and when it happens, it creates anxiety. To overcome this, we try to structure the world in a way that we've found in the past has given us stability. We create a world from our past experiences that we know will help us to face the unknown. That is the masking phenomena. The world gets covered over with a mask and then we project a set of ideas or a structure formation in order to make sense of the world. It's the idea behind the so-called ink blot test. We see a kind of blob of ink and we try to make something out of it. The organizing principle each of us projects is what identifies us as individuals. The technique of unveiling the masking that I use with patients helps me find their essential approach and how they view the world."

In many cases, there is a physical cause of insomnia. For example, Dr. Dunkell says, "The amount of times a person has to get up to urinate during the night breaks up their sleep and frequently leads to insomnia. As we get older, sphincters in women weaken and men have prostate enlargements, so it's important to avoid having too much fluid before you go to sleep. Avoid types of fluid during the day that cause a tendency to urinate, like caffeine, which is not only in coffee, but most soft drinks. If you do go to the bathroom and have difficulty falling back to sleep, use some of the relaxation techniques."

Dr. James Pearl, who is a member of the Sleep Panel at the Presbyterian St. Luke Medical Center in Denver and in private practice as a psychologist, adds that many different organ system disorders can affect sleep. Foremost among them is sleep apnea. "If you or your sleeping partner experiences problems with snoring, it's important to explore whether there might be some kind of breathing disorder," Dr. Pearl says. "Sleep apnea is an episode in which your breathing is interrupted for about 10 seconds. The person will stop breathing. Ten seconds later, you hear them suddenly gasp for air once. That causes them to awaken and typically, fall right back to sleep again. A sleep apnea episode can happen as many as several hundred times a night, without the person knowing it. If you are older and overweight, if you snore and are sleepy during the day, it is important to talk to a physician about the possibility of sleep apnea."

Cardiovascular and digestive disorders also contribute to insomnia. "Angina, in which the heart muscle receives insufficient oxygen, can cause a person to awaken during the night with a choking pain," Dr. Pearl explains. "Coronary artery disease and hypertension or high blood pressure, can also influence your sleep. Medication prescribed for hypertension—usually diuretics—can cause you to awaken frequently during the night to urinate."

Among the digestive problems that affect sleep is heartburn, a relatively common condition that tends to increase with age. "It is also known as acid reflux because the sphincter that separates the esophagus from the stomach doesn't function properly and causes stomach acids to seep back up into the esophagus," Dr. Pearl says. "Lying down flat will aggravate this condition, so it is good to elevate your bed. Place blocks as high as six inches beneath the head of the bed or arrange pillows from your waist to your head so you're not lying flat on your back. It is also good to eat dinner earlier in the evening, to allow the food to be digested before bedtime."

Periodic limb movement is associated with sleep dysfunction. In this condition, the person's legs, or sometimes arms, twitch uncontrollably for a few seconds. "If you awaken in the morning with your bedcovers in disarray or if your sleeping partner says that you are kicking him or her during the night, it is very important to talk to a physician," Dr. Pearl says.

Sleeping pills, other medications, caffeine, alcohol, and tobacco are all substances that can affect a person's sleep cycle. "Both over the counter and prescription sleeping pills can improve sleep for a short period of time, but if you take sleeping medication for too long, you can build up tolerance," Dr. Pearl explains. "If you continue to take the same amount of medication, your body doesn't respond as strongly, so you need to use more and more. If you suddenly stop taking the medication, your sleep is going to become worse than it was in the first place. It's a good rule of thumb to not take sleep medications more than a few times a week or for more than about a month at a stretch."

Caffeine's effect on sleep is well known. "Most people know that caffeine can influence sleep and for most people, it's okay if you don't take caffeine within about 5 hours of bedtime," Dr. Pearl says. "But for some people, the drug is so strong that they have to stay off caffeine for about 12 hours before bedtime.

"The term 'nightcap' came about because so many people traditionally used alcohol to help them fall asleep. Alcohol is very effective to help yourself become more relaxed and drowsy and it often does help you to fall asleep. But as the alcohol is metabolized through your system during the night, if you had too much shortly before bedtime, it is likely to awaken you because of withdrawal symptoms. Your body is wanting more. Drinking alcohol also makes sleep disrupted—you awaken more often and don't sleep as deeply. Generally, it is good to avoid alcohol for at least 2 hours before bedtime. You need to see how it affects you."

Because tobacco is a stimulant, Dr. Pearl says, people who smoke should not do so in the evening. "It stays in your system and keeps your physiology aroused."

A major cause of chronic insomnia is reactive hypoglycemia. This condition is frequently exacerbated by eating late at night, especially foods with a high glucose level, such as pastries, candy, or even fruit juice. Such foods cause your blood sugar level to go up and then plummet, a fluctuation that can contribute to insomnia. Also, overindulging late at night in highly fatty foods can cause sleeplessness. That's because foods with a lot of fat take four to five times longer to empty from the stomach and be digested than simple or complex carbohydrates do.

The late Dr. Robert Atkins pointed out the efficacy of tryptophan in the treatment of insomnia. Food with high amounts of naturally occurring tryptophan, such as turkey, fish, eggs, and dairy products, may be helpful. Tryptophan in supplement form, which is no longer banned from import into the US, is "very valuable for sleep disorders because serotonin [the substance it breaks down to] is the sleep chemical. If you take it right when you are ready to go to bed, when your serotonin level is on the upswing anyway, you are really fitting in physiologically with your body's chemical rhythms."

Herbs that are nontoxic and have no contraindications can be a real help to those challenged by insomnia. Unlike sleeping pills, herbs won't leave you in a fog in the morning, or feeling like you haven't really slept. Passionflower is an important relaxant herb popular in much of Europe. Other possibilities include pheanine (at 300 milligrams, one of the best relaxants in nature), chamomile tea, hops, skullcap, and valerian root, a natural calmative used by orthomolecular psychiatrists for people who tend to be anxious. Herbalist Letha Hadady says that people who can't think clearly during the day and wake up at night sweating, with their hearts beating too fast, should consider remedies that balance the adrenal glands in the heart. "The Chinese remedy called Ding Xin Wan is very good for people under stress—if you're working against a deadline or going through a divorce and are so overwrought you can't think clearly during the day but at night, especially, your heart is pounding and you can't sleep."

Other things to try: calcium citrate and magnesium citrate—1200 milligrams of each taken any time after dinner; 50 milligrams of the B complex; and 200 milligrams of inositol. Many people use melatonin. Also, 200 micrograms of chromium in the evening will help stabilize your blood sugar level.

Dr. Pearl has additional recommendations: "If you are feeling like you are under a lot of stress and a lot of anxiety, it's important to take a look at that either with a self-help book or with a therapist to see what you can do to minimize the problems. One powerful way to improve your sleep is to maintain a regular sleep-wake schedule. Getting up at the same time every day is helpful, even on weekends. Some sleep experts say you should go to bed at the same time every night and some say go to bed only when you're sleepy. Do whatever feels right for you. But it is really good to try to get up at the same time every day.

"Sunday night insomnia is a common problem, especially for people under 40. Let's say you normally go to bed at 11:00 and get up at 7:00. On Saturday, if you sleep in an extra hour, your body rhythms are one hour behind. If you sleep an extra hour on Sunday, until 9:00, then your internal sleep-wake rhythm is two hours behind. Sunday night, if you try to go to bed at 11:00, you are not sleepy because your body clock is two hours behind. If it is really important for you to sleep in on weekends, don't go to bed that Sunday night until you feel sleepy. You might sleep one or two hours less than usual but that won't hurt you."

Light therapy can be useful. Dr. Pearl explains, "Studies show that people who spend a lot of time indoors away from windows, away from sunlight, have a disproportionate amount of insomnia. They have difficulty sleeping for the same reason that blind people do. Nine out of ten blind people have severe sleep problems because they are not getting sunlight into the retina of their eyes, into the brain to tell the brain that it is time to be awake during the day. The more light stimuli you can give your body during the day, the stronger your sleep-wake rhythm will be. I am talking about sunlight in particular. Indoor light is not going to make any difference. You need to expose yourself to bright sunlight—just your eyes. There are artificial sun boxes that are commercially available. But if you have insomnia, get outside as much as you can, during your lunch hour, during your breaks. Don't wear sunglasses, unless you've got an eye condition that requires it."

Exercising in the late afternoon or early evening may help some people with insomnia. "When you do aerobic exercise for half an hour, you raise your body temperature," Dr. Pearl says. "Five or six hours later, your body temperature drops. So working out after work or before dinner is an ideal way to get your body ready for bed. A lazy way to get that same benefit is soaking in a hot bath. It has to be really hot, at least 102 degrees. When you use passive body heating, the drop in body temperature occurs just about three hours later.

"A lot of people intuitively know that stressful experiences during the evening can disturb nighttime sleep and research has confirmed that. So it is important to think of the evening as a transition period between the day's troubles and the night's rest. Get ready to wind down. Try to leave your work at the office. If you have to bring it home, get it done early in the evening. Do stressful things like planning your schedule early in the evening or else wait until the morning."

Physical stress also can interfere with sleep. "If your muscles are tense and tight or your breathing fast and shallow, try abdominal breathing," says Dr. Pearl. "Take breaths that are increasingly deep and slow, so deep that it makes your abdomen push out. Hold it for a few seconds and let it out slowly, breathing away the tension.

"Finally, if you can't sleep despite everything you have tried, do something else. Switch on the light and read; watch a tape or clean out a drawer. A lot of people think that missing sleep is going to hurt their health, but losing sleep has very few effects. Many studies show that when people sleep less than normal, their performance the next day in most cases is just as good as when they had a good night's sleep. Highly creative tasks do sometimes become more difficult when you have lost sleep, but, for most of us, even if we go a whole night without sleep, we can get along fine the next day. Don't be afraid of insomnia. Don't lie in bed trying to sleep. Some people like to imagine sleep as a wave in the ocean and themselves as a surfer. Position yourself in this warm ocean and wait. The wave will overtake you and sweep you away."

Along the lines of positive affirmation, writing in a diary shortly before bedtime can be extraordinarily beneficial. It can be a way of really seeing what you've done that's affirmed your mental, spiritual and physical health, as well as any deeds you've done that have had positive effects on others. If a person spends some time at the end of each day reflecting on what they've done in the past twenty-four hours that's been positive, and on plans for the next day, he or she gains a sense of completeness about the day. In a sense, then, diary-writing legitimizes going to bed; it's as if you can now see that you really deserve the good night's sleep you're about to get.

11

Attention Disorders In Adults

■■■

It is my belief that, just as we have pathologized children's behavior and mental disorders, and at the same time refused to examine the role of the environment—including sugars; caffeine; artificial sweeteners; empty calorie diets; and overuse of cell phones and computers, which cause electromagnetic pulses into the brain and disturb sleep patterns, impacting a child's behavior and causing symptoms that mimic ADD or ADHD—so too have we done the same with adults. Life has consequences. We cannot always control the outcome of things. We fear loss. We go through many crises relating to relationships, jobs, aging, diseases, and finances. We now label frequently inappropriate behavior as a disease. I believe that if we had more humanistic counseling, classes in how to deal with life issues, and better support systems around these issues, we would not need the pharmaceutical-medical model that claim these are psychiatric disorders that require treatment.

Writer Peggy Ramundo is quite correct when she says that the general public usually associates Attention Deficit Hyperactivity Disorder (ADHD) with "hyperactive boys hanging from the light fixtures, running their parents and their teachers ragged." However, as she explains as coauthor of book *You Mean I'm Not Lazy, Stupid or Crazy?!*, we now know that this disorder does not simply vanish after childhood. In fact, according to 2006 data from the National Institute of Mental Health, between 30 percent and 70 percent of children with ADHD continue to exhibit symptoms as adults. Moreover, many adults with ADHD do not even know they have it. In Peggy Ramundo's case, she was diagnosed in 1990, three years after her son received his diagnosis.

The *Diagnostic and Statistical Manual of Mental Disorders (DSM-IV-TR)* defines three subtypes of ADHD: predominantly hyperactive-impulsive type, predominantly inattentive type (sometimes still called ADD), and combined type. As in children, the primary symptoms in adult ADHD are impulsivity, inattention, and hyperactivity. For adults, Ramundo's useful concept is "disregulated activity"—too much or not enough. Some of the more obvious manifestations are "chronic tardiness, argumentativeness, being unable to wait for a traffic light to change, jumping from activity to activity—having 14 projects started and none finished." It is often accompanied by substance abuse and "lots of disorganization," she says, adding, "it is not unusual to see someone hopping from one thing to another, one job to another. To those watching, this behavior looks like laziness or lack of motivation. They think of the person as hard to get along with, forgetful, irresponsible."

Educational therapist Robert Bernstein says that parents "often have a child that they bring to me and I say, 'Well, this is the problem,' and they say, 'Gee that sounds a lot like me.' Whenever I ask an adult, 'When did you realize there was a problem?' they always tell me the same thing—as long as they can remember, 'since I was four, since I was five.' It's a problem that they've been living with their entire lives and haven't been able to compensate for, which implies that it is an internal mechanism, not something that has to do with the parents or teachers.

"Recently, I saw a very successful adult who is very disorganized. His office was a total mess and he had to work sometimes all night just to kind of catch up on things that he needed to do. In the initial consultation, I gave him one of the simplest tasks you can do. It's almost embarrassing giving a 45-year-old a peg board, where he had to put the yellow pegs and the red pegs in the right places. There were five yellow pegs. He put four in perfect order. I would have bet any amount of money that he was going to put the fifth peg in, but he didn't. After he finished, I said, 'Why didn't you put this fifth peg in?' He said, 'Well, I knew it was going to happen eventually.' I asked, 'Is that the attitude you have on your job? You feel that you don't have to finish it because it's going to eventually be done?' He said, 'Yes.' So that's his process—he can control that situation and put that last peg in and finish that job.

"I saw someone else who brought problems like he cannot stand in line, he cannot be in a group. He never went out on a date. He never completed a class. His psychiatrist thought he had a learning disorder, but to me, it seemed that his problem was that he couldn't accept outside structure.

"Most people say they have learning problems. I confess I have no sense of direction. Fortunately, it didn't interfere with my academics. If it did, I would be labeled retarded. So the question for an adult is—is the problem really interfering with learning, doing a job or in a relationship? If it is, you have a problem."

Conventional treatment of adult ADHD may involve medication (stimulants or antidepressants), education, and psychotherapy.

The natural healing community has recognized the power of nutrition. Studies over the past two decades have linked attention and activity disorders to deficiencies in zinc and essential fatty acids, and consumption of caffeine, artificial flavorings, and other food additives like MSG and artificial sweeteners.

Nutritionist Marcia Zimmerman points out that the timing of what we eat has a powerful effect on the brain. "There was work done at MIT and Harvard that showed how carbohydrates raise serotonin levels in the brain. Serotonin is a neurotransmitter that is calming and tends to put children to sleep. On the other hand, protein provides the necessary amino acids that are precursors of attention-grabbing neurotransmitters, namely norepinephrine and dopamine. No wonder children who have high carbohydrate breakfasts and lunches can't concentrate at school. And adults go off to work without an adequate breakfast, then eat donuts and coffee at ten in the morning and wonder why everything is flashing past them and they're unable to concentrate or complete tasks. The timing of carbohydrates and proteins is very important."

Many people, including Peggy Ramundo, have been helped by vegetable chlorophyll green algae, a natural food that appears to stabilize the blood sugar level, provide amino acids in relatively balanced proportion and trace minerals in assimilable form, as well as concentrated sources of beta carotene and vitamin B12.

Ramundo also finds that adults are helped by exercise, "very strenuous exercise, not just your three times a week, 20 minutes of aerobics, but an hour or two hours a day. Adults say it stimulates the action in the brain sufficiently that they do not need to take medicine. They are also finding therapeutic massage useful."

For many doctors on the cutting edge of brain longevity studies, attention problems can be early signals of declining cognitive power. Dr. Richard Braverman says, "Attention deficit marks a premature aging or dysfunction of the brain. There are many different kinds. You can have attention to detail. You can have failure of consistency on attention. You can have reaction time attention disorders. You can have impulsive attention deficit disorders. You can have blanking out or almost petit mal–like attention deficit disorders. Only when a doctor distinguishes which type of attention deficit disorder you have can he say which type of treatment is going to benefit you. This is what we see in depression, anxiety, all the psychiatric conditions, bipolar, schizophrenic. These conditions are all medical disorders of the brain with varying degrees of loss of brain function, metabolism, attention and memory.

"People with severe memory deficit have recovery if they are treated effectively. That can include everything including chelation. There are books on toxic metal syndrome describing the benefits of chelation on memory and research papers suggesting that if you do chelation you will pull out the aluminum and you will end up with improvement in memory. More work needs to be done in this area, of course."

12

Tardive Dyskinesia

■■■

Tardive dyskinesia (TD) is a neurological condition caused by the long-term use of antipsychotic medication. It is characterized by abnormal, involuntary movements of the face and limbs, such as tongue protrusion, rapid eye blinking, lip smacking, and rapid arm or leg movements. The condition develops in 15 to 20 percent of people who take antipsychotic drugs for one year or more. Women and the elderly are affected more often than the rest of the population. Tardive dyskinesia is difficult to treat because symptoms often continue even after the offending medication is stopped.

Dr. Peter Breggin often testifies in court cases brought by people who have suffered these reactions to their medications. In one recent case, a Louisiana judge ordered Bristol-Myers Squibb, the company that manufactures and distributes Prolixin, to pay $2 million to a fifty-two-year-old woman who developed severe and disabling tardive dyskinesia after taking the drug for five years. Among her symptoms were muscle spasms and abnormal movements of the face, neck, shoulders, and extremities, as well as impaired speech and breathing.

More than thirty years ago, according to Dr. Breggin, whose expert testimony in Louisiana was cited by the judge's ruling, "psychiatrist George Crane gained the attention of the medical community by disclosing that many, and perhaps most, long-term patients on neuroleptic drugs were developing a largely irreversible, untreatable neurological disorder, tardive dyskinesia. The disease, even its mild forms, is often disfiguring, with involuntary movements of the face, mouth or tongue. Frequently, the patients grimace in a manner that makes them look 'crazy,' undermining their credibility with other people. In more severe cases, patients become disabled by twitches, spasms and other abnormal movements of any muscle groups, including those of the neck, shoulders, back, arms and legs, and hands and feet. The muscles of respiration and speech can also be impaired. In the worst cases, patients thrash about continually.

"Despite this tragic situation, psychiatrists too often fail to give proper warning to patients and their families. Often psychiatrists fail to notice that their patients are suffering from tardive dyskinesia, even when the symptoms are flagrant. Many or most tardive dyskinesia patients also show signs of dementia—an irreversible loss of overall higher brain and mental function."

Dr. Breggin says, "It was inevitable that these losses would occur. The basal ganglia, which are afflicted in tardive dyskinesia, are richly interconnected with the higher centers of the brain, so that their dysfunction almost inevitably leads to disturbances in cognitive processes. A multitude of studies have confirmed that long-term use is associated with both deterioration and atrophy of the brain. Growing evidence indicates that these drugs produce tardive psychoses that are irreversible and more severe than the patients' prior problems."

According to Dr. Garry Vickar, a "massive report" issued about twenty years ago concluded that orthomolecular psychiatrists who were using vitamins did not have patients with tardive dyskinesia. "The patients I've seen usually come to me after having been treated with drugs for a very long time. If they're on an antipsychotic drug and they don't in fact have a psychotic or a schizophrenic illness, they're at higher risk. For example, somebody with a mood disorder given an antipsychotic drug is at higher risk for developing tardive dyskinesia."

Patients with schizophrenia appear to be at particular risk for TD. "Typically those with tardive dyskinesia are patients who have been treated for schizophrenia over the course of many years," Dr. Vickar says. "The ravages of the illness are combined with the cumulative effects of the medicine. The older antipsychotic drugs—Thorazine, chlorpromazine, Stelazine, Prolixin, Haldol—work in a certain part of the brain where the neurotransmitter function is tied in with movements.

"Attempts to remedy this have resulted in the creation of newer antipsychotic medications such as Clozaril and Risperdal. These are allegedly less likely to cause tardive dyskinesia because they work on different centers of the brain. They relieve some of the schizophrenic symptoms without the potential for tardive dyskinesia."

Dr. Vickar outlines the difficulty in treating tardive dyskinesia. "You have to walk a fine line. You have to help patients reinstitute the very medicine that is implicated in causing it to relieve the dyskinesia. Sometimes I call neurologists in. They may have to use, in very interesting combinations, some of the anti-seizure medicines that have antispasmodic effects.

"We used to think, many years ago, that the crucial missing ingredient in patients with tardive dyskinesia was vitamin B6. It turns out that it is probably vitamin E that is the protective element necessary with regard to TD."

Dr. Vickar describes his treatment approach. "I treat TD patients with choline and lecithin and large doses of B vitamins. The choline and lecithin are tied in with the presumptive mechanism of action of this abnormal movement. If there's an imbalance in the different neurochemical pathways, then it is thought that the choline and lecithin will help along what is called the phosphytotyl choline pathway. You add the lecithin so you don't have to give as much choline, because choline tends to lead to a very fishy smell in the body. It is presumed that this brings a balance back, or reestablishes the proper chemical balance in the brain to relieve the abnormal movements.

"If the chemical pathways in the brain were altered by the use of Haldol and other drugs, there may have been a disturbance of the intricate balance of neurochemicals necessary to coordinate smooth movements. The presumption is that choline and lecithin will help correct the imbalance that was created by the traditional antipsychotic drugs."

A 2003 study published in the *American Journal of Psychiatry* concluded that branched-chain amino acids reduced abnormal, involuntary body movements in men with tardive dyskinesia by an average 36.5 percent when compared with a placebo. The amino acids were delivered in the form of Tarvil, a "medical food" powdered drink product.

In his article in the *International Guide to the World of Alternative Mental Health* (www.alternativementalhealth.com), Dr. Walter Lemmo, a naturopathic physician, discusses other recent studies showing the benefits of nutritional treatments. In 2001, a report in the *American Journal of Psychiatry* found "significant improvement" in patients who received 100 milligrams of vitamin B6 daily increasing weekly over four weeks in 100 milligram units to a total of 400 milligrams per day. Another 2001 study, this one in the *Archives of General Psychiatry*, found that schizophrenic patients receiving 10 milligrams per day of melatonin demonstrated a reduction in their TD symptoms. These mainstream medical reports confirm earlier papers published in orthomolecular medicine journals indicating the usefulness of these and other nutrients—including manganese, vitamin B3, vitamin C, vitamin E, tryptophan, and essential fatty acids—in treating tardive dyskinesia.

PART THREE

Disorders in Older Adults

13

Brain Aging

∎∎∎

As our population ages, cognitive decline becomes an increasing concern. An estimated 24 million people worldwide currently have dementia, with 4.6 million new cases every year. By 2040, 84 million individuals are expected to have some type of age-related cognitive impairment.

One of the most disturbing symptoms of aging is diminished brain function, which can cause everything from forgetfulness and loss of concentration to Alzheimer's and other serious diseases. Fortunately, modern research reveals that much can be done to keep the brain in top form. As evidenced by recent articles in mainstream medical journals, including a 2006 editorial in the *Journal of the American Medical Association*, even conventional doctors are realizing that nondrug treatments such as nutrition, supplements, exercise, and memory training can yield safe and effective results.

Dr. Dharma Singh Khalsa, founder of the American Academy of Anti-Aging Medicine, has written numerous articles and several books on brain longevity. "When we talk about the brain, there is almost a schism in the way it's looked at these days. Many people in the medical establishment still look at the brain like it's a computer with certain files. I consider that very 20th century. In the 21st century, the brain is going to be considered more like a symphony, an orchestration that is constantly changing and vibrating and moving and having deep rich colors.

"The brain, as a flesh and blood organ, is dependent on blood flow. The brain is dependent on oxygen. Of course blood brings the oxygen. We need that. We have to have adequate nutrients like glucose. The brain thrives on glucose, so we have to have a good diet, not refined carbohydrates or sugars that do more harm than good. We have free radicals, these little products of metabolism that cause scarring of the brain. We have energy in the brain in the form of the power plant and the mitochondria. We have the synapse, a very important juncture where the electrical chemical energy is transferred from one cell to another to create the memory, to help us produce other memories, to draw up old memories, restore new memories and the emotions and all that."

In his lifestyle approach to the brain, Dr. Khalsa compares the brain to the heart. "The brain is an organ, like the heart, and I like to say that what works for the heart works for the head. When we think of the brain, we must think of lifestyle because there are things that we can do—exercise, nutrition, supplements, stress reduction, hormone replacement therapy. Don't forget the glands in the brain—the hypothalamus, pituitary, the pineal glands, so important for creating a healing environment in the body so we can regenerate ourselves, have more energy and vitality, even as we get older, rather than going in a spiral of degeneration and waiting for Big Brother to say, 'Hey, take this protease inhibitor.'

"The endocrine system is primarily the hypothalamus, which is the brain's brain. The gland in your brain that controls just about everything, including aging, is not even the size of your pinky fingernail. It sends a whole bunch of hormones—called 'releasing hormones' or 'factors'—down to the pituitary gland, which is the master gland of the brain. This orchestrates secretions from all the glands in your body—the thyroid, the adrenal, the gonads (the testicles or ovaries). When you are young, it's responsible for growth and development, and as we get older, it's responsible for reproductive functions, and then, after a certain age, these hormones decline. The pituitary gland, in response to the hypothalamus, produces human growth hormone, one of the most important, if not the most important hormone to keep in good shape as we get older. But unfortunately, all these hormones peak at age 30, start to decline a little around 40 and at about 50, start to plateau down."

Dr. Khalsa recommends a low-fat diet. Vitamin and mineral supplements provide "an all-purpose insurance policy." Other beneficial substances include ginkgo, which enhances circulation to the micro capillaries, oxygenating the tissues in the brain; coenzyme Q10, "a very energetic cofactor that works in the brain's power plant, the mitochondria"; and old-style phosphatidyl serine (PS) from bovine brains, as well as newer types of PS synthesized from soybeans.

"Everything I've talked about is regenerating or protective, not stimulating," Dr. Khalsa says. "I stay away from compounds like DMAE and acetyl carotene because I think they are not good for everybody. They are way too stimulating. There is a compound called huperzene A that, in combination with vitamin E, can be very effective in blocking the enzyme that destroys the memory. It can be taken in capsule form, 50 to 100 micrograms twice a day. I don't think it should be taken by everybody because most normal people have enough of this memory compound.

"Anybody who does not have a regular stress management program that is proactive, something like a daily or almost a daily practice of meditation, does not have to worry because they won't enjoy good health. If you don't have some type of stress management tool to reduce the nasty chemicals, such as cortisol, that come from the chronic unbalanced stress we're all feeling in the new millennium, you can count on having early degenerative disease. Cortisol attacks the memory center of the brain. It's like battery acid. Stress doses of cortisol come from chronic, unbalanced stress, not the acute stress of walking across the street and almost getting hit by a car. We are talking about daily stress over years, unresolved conflicts, anger, difficulty in the work place, difficulty at home—these all have an effect on your brain."

Exercise is critical for taking care of your brain. "If you exercise on a regular basis," Dr. Khalsa says, "you don't have to be Mr. Universe or run a marathon. You can do brisk walking, or jogging, or play tennis, or go on a treadmill, or go to the gym, work in your garden, do anything you want as long as you're getting your heart rate up and sweating three or four times a week. This has a very positive, healthy effect on the brain. It increases blood to the brain, it increases oxygen to the brain, it dilates blood vessels up there. It lets in everything that you need—because what good are nutrients if they don't get to the brain? There are many studies showing that growth factors injected into the brain can be very restorative, but you don't have to get them injected. You can produce your own growth factors just by going out and getting some exercise on a regular basis."

Physical and mental exercise should be connected. Dr. Khalsa explains, "Combine physical exercise with mental stimulation like reading a book, listening to a book on tape, or listening to an informative show and then discussing it with someone else. Combine mental and physical exercise sometimes—riding. Ride on a stationary bike and read the newspaper or listen to a book on tape. You can actually make new connections in your brain this way. I saw a video the other day showing the neurons stretching out, looking for connections. Our brains are just hungry for connections, hungry to communicate, hungry to reach out and make new neuronal connections so that we can maintain our intelligence.

At his institute in Tucson, Arizona, Dr. Khalsa offers the Brain Longevity program, which consists of four pillars:

1. Nutritional modification, including a 15 to 20 percent fat diet. Adding breast of chicken, fish, and nonanimal protein products such as tofu is helpful. Certain fish are especially good for the brain. These fish include salmon, tuna, trout, mackerel, and sardines.

2. Stress management. Meditation decreases cortisol and enhances many aspects of mental function. Massage and guided mental imagery have also been shown to lower cortisol levels in the blood.

3. Exercise. Like ancient Gaul, there are three parts: mental exercise, physical exercise, and mind/body exercise. Dr. Kalsa notes, "Aerobic reconditioning enhances mental function by 20 to 30 percent. The ancient art of brain regeneration, and innovative mind/body exercises derived from my 20 year practice of advanced yoga and meditation, are important in enhancing global brain energy."

4. The final phase comes from the forefront of anti-aging medicine. "Among pharmaceutical drugs used to help regenerate the brain cells is l-deprenyl citrate. Deprenyl has been shown to increase longevity in animals and increase important biochemicals in the brain. In recent studies of patients with moderate Alzheimer's disease, Deprenyl improved attention, memory, verbal fluency and behavior. Side effects associated with Deprenyl may include anxiety and insomnia if the dosage is too high. It may be contraindicated in patients taking antidepressants such as Prozac, and in those individuals suffering from heart disease. Deprenyl should only be prescribed and taken under the supervision of your doctor."

Hormone replacement therapy with pregnenolone, DHEA, and melatonin are also used as part of the Brain Longevity program. "Pregnenolone has been clinically shown to be useful in patients with memory loss, especially those who have difficulty finding the correct words," Dr. Khalsa says. "DHEA is currently controversial because of concerns over long-term use. When I prescribe DHEA as part of my program, I always have a blood level measured. If the patient is a male, I will also check his PSA blood test (prostate specific antigen) because of concern about the long-term effects of DHEA on the prostate. Melatonin is useful for insomnia, jet lag and renormalizing the body's biorhythms. It is my clinical observation that the generally recommended dose of 3 to 6 milligrams is too high. I prescribe 0.1 to 0.5 milligrams as a beginning dosage. Side effects with the higher dose include uncomfortably vivid dreams, morning headache and grogginess.

"While it is very true that the Brain Longevity program can help us prevent and reverse memory loss as well as develop and maintain high levels of brain power," Dr. Khalsa concludes, " it can also allow us to tap into a very special part of our being. We can enjoy discovering who we really are and exploring the true nature of life. Along the way we will be sure to create a lifetime of peak mental performance."

Dr. Ray Sahelian has evaluated leading-edge nutrients and hormones, and been actively involved in research on the use of pregnenolone. "We heard first," he says, "about DHEA, the hormone made by the adrenal gland, which is the mother of testosterone and estrogen. Pregnenolone is the mother of DHEA. The body uses pregnenolone to convert into DHEA, which in turn converts into estrogen and testosterone or other antigens. Pregnenolone can also convert into progesterone. In fact, all the hormones made by the adrenal glands start out from pregnenolone and therefore, I call pregnenolone the grandmother of all the adrenal hormones.

"We have known about pregnenolone since the early 1930s. In the 1940s, some of the research included giving it to factory workers. They found that it improved work performance. People were more energetic, there was an antifatigue factor. Later on, they tested it in pilots in simulated flights. Concentration was better, performance was better. Eventually, researchers realized that pregnenolone had anti-inflammatory abilities and testing started on rheumatoid arthritis, lupus, osteoarthritis and other autoimmune conditions. They found it had some benefits. However, about the same time, another hormone called cortisol was being evaluated. Cortisol is also made in the adrenal glands and has powerful anti-inflammatory abilities. Cortisol basically stole the limelight. Scientists doing research on pregnenolone put it aside. There are quite a few studies in the '40s, and in 1950 and 1951, then hardly anything up to 1996, 1997.

"If it weren't for the 1994 Dietary Supplement law that allowed a lot of these natural hormones and nutrients to be marketed, pregnenolone would have still been ignored. It's a shame because there is so much potential in this hormone. I was familiar with some of the studies done on mice and rats concluding that pregnenolone was one of the most potent memory enhancers. So when pregnenolone came on the market, I called up a lot of my colleagues and asked them, 'Have you ever tried this?' None of the health professionals I called had tried it. I called a lot of people in the vanguard of using new supplements and nobody seemed to know anything about it." So Dr. Sahelian decided to try it for himself.

Patient Story: Pregnenolone

I bought a bottle of 10 milligram pills and started in the morning. I took it for about a week and honestly, I didn't feel much. The year before, I had taken DHEA, also starting with 10 milligrams. I had felt a little bit of energy, a little bit of mood elevation, so I thought maybe pregnenolone didn't have the ability to cross the blood-brain barrier in the brain. Maybe it just didn't do anything to the human body.

About a week later, I increased the dosage to 20 milligrams, two pills in the morning. I thought I felt a little more energetic and alert. I could stay up a little bit later in the evening and still be active, but I still wasn't sure if that was a placebo effect. About a week after that, I went up to 30 milligrams, three pills in the morning. That day, I was really busy. I forgot that I had taken the 30 milligrams. I take a walk every evening, about four miles, so I was walking in Venice, California on the oceanfront walk, about 6:00 or 7:00 p.m., when I realized that a pleasant, harmonious, almost continuous sense of mild wellbeing had come on. It wasn't euphoria, just a mild sense of wellbeing. When I looked around, it suddenly seemed that everything was sharper, clearer. Colors were brighter. When I stopped and looked at a rose, a pink rose, it wasn't just a pink rose, there were shades of pink within it. Everything seemed like the best vision I'd ever had.

I thought this was really strange. I kept walking, noticing patterns, windows, more flowers. It seemed that my perception had increased. Instead of just going up to my normal 2 mile mark and turning around, I kept walking and walking. I did six, seven or eight miles, came home, put on some music and the music even sounded better.

The next day I didn't take any pregnenolone. I went to the library and got the research published in the '40s and '50s, all of it, read it all, word by word. I couldn't find anything about visual and auditory enhancement. One thing they did mention in the study of factory workers was that quite a number had noticed an enhanced sense of well-being.

The study of the pilots in simulated flight also mentioned an enhancement of well-being, but nothing about visual and auditory enhancements. So I wasn't sure if it was just me experiencing this.

Over the next few weeks and months, I recommended it to quite a few patients and friends. I talked to other healthcare practitioners who had heard about pregnenolone and were starting to use it. Quite a few had noticed clarity of vision on it.

It became a passion for me over the next few months to learn as much as I could. I've tried pregnenolone in dosages from 5 milligrams to 60 milligrams. I've tried it in a variety of products over the counter. I've tried it in a variety of forms. It comes in sublingual, regular pills, micronized pills, cream, all kinds of forms. It comes in combination with DHEA and other nutrients like ginkgo and phosphatidyl serine and many others.

The most significant area for using pregnenolone is as replacement therapy in our older years, our 40s, 50s and beyond. Our concept of hormone replacement is going to expand to include more than just estrogen, or testosterone. It can be used for an enhanced sense of mood, slight memory improvement, awareness, mental ability enhancement, clarity of thinking, maybe a little more creativity. A lot of aspects of our mental condition will be helped because pregnenolone is made in the human brain, like DHEA. The enzymes are available that convert cholesterol into pregnenolone within the human brain, so these neurosteroids are within the brain, they have a function there. As we age, their levels decline and it would be appropriate in our older years to take tiny doses of these things.

But until we learn more about this and DHEA and melatonin, the dosages need to be minimal. We do not know the long-term consequences of giving high doses. Generally, my dosages are between 2 milligrams and 10 milligrams. I definitely do not recommend dosages as high as 50 milligrams of pregnenolone or DHEA. I've heard of cases of heart irregularities when people took 50 or 100 milligrams of DHEA or pregnenolone. An 80-year-old woman felt palpitations in her heart the very day she took 25 milligrams of pregnenolone.

I have urged all health food stores to not sell pregnenolone in dosages greater than 10 milligrams. Many buyers are buying the 25 and 50 milligram pills and popping more than one a day. More is not necessarily better and is not a motto to live by when it comes to hormones. Besides my concern with the rare instance of heart irregularities, we have no idea how high dosages will influence tumor formation especially of the prostate gland, breast, ovary, and other tissues. You can go up to 15 or 20, but on a regular basis, stay on the very low dosages.

—*Dr. Ray Sahelian*

Dr. Sahelian continues his words of caution. About ten years ago, "I attended a natural health show where I walked around the hundreds of booths set up by vitamin companies. It was amazing how many new supplements had been introduced—stevia, pyruvate, NADH, CLA (conjugated linoleic acid), silica, chitosan, androstenedione, shark liver oil, 5-hydroxy-tryptophan, ultimate protein powders, stinging nettles, DHA (not DHEA, but docosahexaenoic acid), and others. Outlandish claims were made about a few of these supplements by some of their promoters. What were these claims based on? Nothing convincing. Sometimes a simple laboratory study done in an obscure part of the world on a small group of mice.

"Many of these nutrients, hormones, and supplements have not necessarily been proven safe before their introduction to the market. It may take months and years before any of their side effects are noticed. Often, these side effects occur when high dosages are consumed for prolonged periods."

For cell biologist Dr. Parris Kidd, the most important nutrient for good brain functioning is phosphatidyl serine (PS). He explains, "It is part of a class of nutrients that is probably as fundamental to our health as the antioxidants are because, like the antioxidants, phosphatidyl serine and its related substance phosphatidyl choline help protect our cells and tissues. They detoxify and support replacement of dead and damaged tissue, including brain cells.

"This class of nutrients used to be called lecithin, but now we have far more potent sources of PS. PS is a crucial building block for the nerve cells that make up the networks in the brain. It works particularly well because it is part of the membranes, those thin ribbons of material that are wound back and forth within the body of the cell. These enclose the cell and work inside it as surfaces on which the enzymes function to carry out metabolism, which is energy conversion. So PS is involved in the synthesis, the transport, the recycling and the functional action of all the chemical transmitters of the brain. All of these rely on the membranes working right, and nerve cell membranes rely heavily on PS to work right."

The aging brain loses its ability to make PS. "As the brain ages, it fails to make phosphatidyl serine or it substantially decreases in efficiency," Dr. Kidd says. "As we get older, we seem to need more of it. There is not very much of it in our foods except in brain and people don't eat brain very often. Brain as a food is not so safe anymore. When people in their 50s, 60s and older receive supplemental phosphatidyl serine, all of their measurable brain functions improve. Energy consumption by the brain improves, electrical currents improve, the different brain zones are better integrated functionally, the chemical transmitters go back into the normal range. Dysfunction of memory, learning, concentration and even mood and coping with stress—all seem to benefit."

"There have been more than 60 human studies on PS, of which 18 have been conducted double blind. Numerous animal studies confirm these benefits and it seems that PS works at such a profound level of function in the brain through the cell membranes that it can support just about any aspect of brain renewal. Very definitely, the human brain can renew itself. New nerve cells can be made, and existing cells can re-extend their networks and rebuild to full levels of cognitive function."

Clinical trials have demonstrated the benefits. "PS was able to turn back the clock on memory loss by 12 years," Dr. Kidd says. "That is, in matching up names and faces. People were testing at about 64 years of age and at the end of the trial, they were testing 52 years of age. So it actually turned back the clock on a measurable aspect of memory loss. It can also benefit persons who have motor problems and tremors as well as hallucinatory dysfunction. It seems to be very good for mood as well.

"The recommended dosage can be from 100 milligrams to 300 milligrams per day, depending on the severity of problems. The clinical trials used 200 to 300 milligrams in two divided doses per day with meals. In some people, doses up to 600 milligrams may be necessary and these are tolerated without any significant problems. Benefits often begin at around three or four weeks, but they continue all the time the person stays on PS. In the trials, even after being taken off PS, people sometimes continued to improve. I think they should probably stay on it because it is a very safe nutrient. It has a very good benefit-risk type of profile and is not at all incompatible with other nutrients or even pharmaceuticals. I think PS is very, very good news for the brain."

Linda Toth has a Ph.D. in communications from UCLA and was a senior staff health writer for the *Journal of Longevity Research*. Increasing memory or brain power is one of her major concerns.

"Remember," she says, "half of all the body's nerve cells are located in your head. Actually, a young baby has many more brain cells than an adult. Around age 10—we don't know why or how—the brain itself starts snipping away brain cells. We think it is so the cells don't continue growing and put pressure on the skull, which won't be enlarging too much more after the age of 10.

"The adult brain only weighs three pounds or less, about 2 percent of your total body weight, and yet 25 percent of all your body's energy is used to conduct memory activities. The brain reacts to any incoming signal in 1/30th of a second. It has about 100 billion nerve cells and each nerve cell shares information with up to 10,000 other tiny nerves in just the flick of an eye."

The brain has evolved tremendously over time. "People compare our brain to a computer," Toth says. "It really ought to be the other way around because even the computers they're developing now can't compare. Lower forms of life, like a reptile, just have a brain stem. But as the brain developed a mid brain and then the fore brain—that's where the cerebral reasoning function is—a very important center was developed deep inside the brain called the limbic system. If you were to take the brain out and spread it out, it would cover about three square feet. The brain in its evolution is like a piece of thin fabric that has been folded inside and molded into a ball to fit inside the skull. Deep inside that outer covering, what we call the gray matter, is the limbic system."

Scientists have learned a lot about the limbic system over the past two decades. Now, Toth says, "we know that the limbic system controls our emotions, it controls short-term and long-term memory, and it is a very important part of the brain to protect. . . . The hypothalamus regulates weight and temperature. It also is the place where immune function starts, signaling the bone marrow to produce killer T cells and white blood cells to fight poisons in the body. If the hypothalamus gets damaged by mercury, aluminum or other chemicals in the environment, the brain doesn't have any way to protect the body. The immune system can be entirely compromised.

"Memory usually fails today because of nutrient deficiency—high levels of salt, sugar, or processed foods are a big problem for the brain, because it needs enzymes. It's one gigantic laboratory of chemical reactions and various substances. We're not even exactly certain how many amino acids, we think it could be as many as 5,000 various amino acids in the brain, and these amino acid reactions are going on all the time. The brain is like a wheel, it never stops turning until you die."

Another major cause of memory loss is alcohol and drug abuse, including prescription drugs. Toth explains, "When you use recreational drugs like cocaine or speed, it's like putting a blow torch on your delicate brain cells. People who have chronic long-term use of these kinds of drugs tend to lose memory much faster than other people."

Cardiovascular dysfunction can cause memory loss. The blood vessels that carry oxygen and blood and food substances to the brain are stopped, either by a narrowing of those arteries or a blood clot.

"The culprit might also be free radical damage," Toth says. "Free radicals are extremely small ions that are on the loose. When they're unstable, they go looking for another ion and will actually steal an electron from a healthy cell. Free radical damage is caused by pesticides—in our foods, in the air, in the water, pesticides that we might touch. Also, by heavy metals in water, smog, air pollution. Household chemicals with chlorine, bleach or ammonia. I warn people never to mix ammonia and any kind of chlorine bleach product together, it is extremely neurotoxic."

Other factors linked to memory loss include food allergies, Candida infections, intestinal parasites, and taste enhancers. The latter are "chemicals that actually exist in the brain, glutamate, cystine, aspartic acid, but they put them in food because it excites the brain, the brain knows these amino acids, but when you get an imbalance in the brain, what happens is, it's like burning the filament out on a light bulb," Toth explains. "If you look on food packages, you'll find that these things are being hidden very cleverly. They very seldom tell you anymore, "monosodium glutamate," they say things like "natural flavoring, natural seasoning, herbs and spices, or spices." Be suspicious that that is a taste enhancer. In the mid '80s the food industry went to the FDA and got legislation passed under something called proprietary rights, which means they can hide their formula in food substances, they don't have to tell you that this is MSG."

Dr. Joseph Debe suggests a variety of special evaluative tests. One of these is an organic acid analysis. "Organic acids are metabolic intermediate compounds. They are compounds produced by the body in the course of metabolism and normally shouldn't appear in the urine in any concentration. When any particular one of these organic acids is elevated, it has a meaning. Some organic acids play a key role in producing energy, which is required to produce neurotransmitters. If we don't have adequate energy production, the neurotransmitter levels will fall. The organic acid analysis helps us get an idea as to whether serotonin levels are too low, whether dopamine or epinephrine levels are too low and then therapy can be more precise."

Organic acid analysis provides important information about the body's ability to detoxify. "It shows the possible need for specific nutrients such as individual B vitamins, alpha lipoic acid, coenzyme Q10," Dr. Debe says. "With this test, you can be sure that you need a particular nutrient rather than just using a shot-gun approach. And the organic acid analysis also measures waste products from different organisms from bacteria, yeast and parasites.

"Anyone desiring a work up for mental-emotional disturbances should have a hair analysis, which measures toxic metals and also mineral levels as well. Another important test is the adrenal stress index, a salivary test that measures levels of long-acting stress hormones, cortisol and DHEA. If you take DHEA when your body produces enough of it, it can increase the risk of imbalance of other hormones including testosterone and estrogen. That can be related to certain cancers. So it's important that you have these hormones measured before you engage in any therapy to modulate their levels."

Fatty acids should be analyzed. Dr. Debe says, "The red blood cell fatty acid analysis involves taking a blood sample and measuring the concentration of the different fatty acids. Two of these are very important for mental-emotional functioning. One is called DHA and the other one is called arachadonic acid. Probably most Americans are deficient in DHA because we are not getting it from our foods. DHA is found in highest concentration in cold water fish. But most Americans don't eat enough of it. The body can also make DHA from flaxseed oil, but there are a variety of conditions that impact the body's ability to do so, and the red blood cell fatty acid analysis can tell us whether the body is actually making that conversion or not."

Amino acid analysis also is important. "The amino acids are the building blocks, the precursors for the neurotransmitters." Dr. Debe explains. "Tryptophan is the precursor for serotonin. Tyrosine is the precursor the body uses to make dopamine and norepinephrine. These different neurotransmitters are deficient in depression, in schizophrenia, in ADHD, very common neurological conditions. With the amino acid analysis we can determine if we need to supplement for those particular compounds. And the amino acid analysis also gives us insight into nutrient deficiencies."

Herbalist Letha Hadady points us toward a couple of good memory herbs. "The simplest one is gotu kola, which helps rebuild our nervous system and our brain. Take gotu kola capsules all day for better clarity during the day and better sleep at night."

Hadady has developed a memory soup that "renourishes the brain and has a number of moistening blood building herbs."

The recipe calls for "a handful each of polygonatum, which nourishes blood vessels and bone marrow; lycium, a blood builder; cornus, a bitter dried form of cherry that strengthens adrenal glands; schizandra to keep moisture and strength in and prevents excess sweating from weakness; acornus and polygala, which work also to strengthen the adrenal glands; hawthorn and fuling, which also help in digestion.

"This soup builds blood, rebuilds bone marrow, which nourishes our brain, and keeps us from sweating too much by strengthening the adrenal glands. It's a way of building energy and holding it in so we don't lose it. That's a good approach with herbs: build energy and hold it in. With our breath and with our mind, breathe in healing energy and send out love, that will open all the doors for our self healing."

14

Alzheimer's Disease

■ ■ ■

Patient Story: Alzheimer's Disease

A patient came to my office in the Empire State Building. She could not name the building; she didn't know where she was. She could only say that she was in New York. She went on a program using NADH [nicotinamide adenine dinucleotide] and I saw her again after six months. She said, "Well, this is your office in the Empire State Building and this is a blind and this is a window." A couple of months later, her daughter went to visit her and she found a gold button on the floor. She asked her father to whom the button belonged and her mother, the Alzheimer's patient, said, "That's mine. I lost it from my jacket yesterday." She showed a constant, significant improvement of her mental activity.

—*Dr. George Birkmayer*

Alzheimer's disease is a progressive disorder marked by the gradual loss of brain cell function. It currently affects 4.5 million Americans at a cost to society of $100 billion dollars annually. By 2050, it is projected that 13 million people in the United States will have the disease. Alzheimer's usually appears after the age of sixty, perhaps tripling in numbers of cases every ten years over age sixty-five. At age eighty-five, the incidence may be as high as 50 percent. Older people with cardiovascular disease are especially prone to Alzheimer's disease, and women appear to have a higher risk, although this may only reflect that women have longer life spans than men.

People with Alzheimer's suffer a gradual decline in cognitive function. It usually starts with memory loss. First, the ability to learn new material and recent short-term memory start to go. There may be some language paucity, mild impairment in drawing or puzzles, and difficulty with higher functions such as planning and problem solving. The personality starts to change, with occasional irritable outbursts and sometimes apathy. As the disease progresses, memory problems increase and the personality may become flat. Restlessness and wandering may occur. Over time, there may be no memory, no trace of former personality, and difficulty making any sense with language. In the end, people may be unable to perform basic tasks such as eating, going to the bathroom, dressing, bathing, getting up, or walking.

There is no cure for Alzheimer's disease. Treatment is aimed at alleviating symptoms, and halting or preventing progression of the disease. Mainstream medicine emphasizes the use of medications to improve memory and thought processes, as well as other conditions that may co-occur, such as depression, anxiety, hallucinations, or delusions. The FDA has approved use of several drugs mostly for the treatment of mild to moderate symptoms of Alzheimer's disease. Although it has not approved the use of antipsychotic medications for treating associated psychosis or agitation, due to safety concerns, these drugs are often used on an off-label basis. Recently, this has prompted warnings from a variety of sources, among them the US government's National Institute of Mental Health (NIMH).

According to an NIMH position paper issued in 2006, "Although some atypical antipsychotic medications are modestly helpful for some patients, they are not effective for the majority of Alzheimer's patients with psychotic symptoms." Furthermore, it stated, "Good clinical practice requires that medical or environmental causes for Alzheimer's related agitation and aggression be ruled out and that behavioral interventions be considered before turning to antipsychotic medications." The NIMH also expressed concern about "significant limitations and risks" with regard to other types of drugs, such as antidepressants, anxiety medications, sedatives, and mood-stabilizers, in Alzheimer's patients.

Fortunately, there are a variety of natural health options for people with this debilitating disease.

Dr. Philip Hodes has developed a comprehensive approach. He says to avoid or eliminate any sources of aluminum exposure: aluminum cookware, utensils, or foil; underarm deodorants; drinking water and any juices or drinks packaged in aluminum-lined cartons. Cut out those vitamins as well as bottled water packaged in bottles with aluminum across the top.

Dr. Hodes suggests a brain and body detoxification program, which should include a supervised fast. "Now don't attempt to detoxify on your own," he warns. "You must have holistic physicians or practitioners who are knowledgeable, competent and experienced in these practices, because if you attempt it on your own you may come up with some upsetting surprises."

Raw juice therapy helps flush out the toxins and supplies enzymes as well as raw vitamins and minerals, Dr. Hodes says. Colonic irrigation will help clean out the colon of years of accumulated putrefaction and helps the body function properly. Drinking distilled water, at least in the beginning or for part of the treatment, is also beneficial, along with the use of herbal noncaffeinated teas.

Dr. Hodes also recommends that a practitioner of biological dentistry remove, in proper sequence, your silver-mercury dental amalgam fillings. Tom Warren, who wrote *Beating Alzheimer's*, emphasized the importance of this procedure.

Bio-oxidative therapies are very effective in bringing oxygen into the brain to increase the individual's ability to think. We live in an external environment with only 19 percent oxygen, when it should contain more, so we all suffer from oxygen insufficiency, Dr. Hodes says. Bio-oxidative therapies include hyperbaric oxygen chamber therapy, ozone therapy, and hydrogen peroxide therapy, among others. Also helpful are superoxide dismutase, dimethylglycine, organic-germanium-132, glutathione peroxidase, homozone, vitamin E, aerobic exercising, and deep breathing in a relatively pure environment, as well as the herbs ginkgo biloba and butcher's broom.

Antioxidants are an important part of Dr. Hodes's program. He mentions vitamin A, beta carotene, thiamine hydrochloride, riboflavin, niacinamide, pantothenic acid, pyridoxine, B12, folic acid, para-amino-benzoic acid (PABA), biotin, choline and inositol, vitamin E, vitamin C, the bioflavinoids (such as quercetin, hesperiden and pycnogenol), vitamin N, acetyl cysteine, acetyl carnitine, the sulfur-containing amino acids L-cysteine and L-methionine, and the enzymes such as coenzyme Q10, bromelain, papain, and pancreatic enzymes.

EDTA chelation therapy, performed intravenously, can be used to remove heavy toxic metals such as lead, cadmium, arsenic, nickel, copper, iron, mercury, and aluminum. A special chelating agent, desoxyferramine, works well, specifically as an aluminum-chelating agent.

Homeopathic remedies will also remove aluminum from the body and the brain, according to Dr. Hodes. "Then you have to take orthomolecular nutritional therapy, intravenously or with intramuscular shots, along with oral supplements of all the nutrients."

Dr. Hodes credits clinical ecologists with having made a major contribution in the treatment of people with Alzheimer's disease when they recognized the importance of four- to five-day diversified food-rotation diets. In a food-rotation diet, you eat a variety of foods and no one food more than once or twice a week—thus eliminating the food allergens to which you are generally "addicted." The rotation diet also lightens the load on your immune system. You should also eliminate alcohol, caffeine, tobacco, sugar, and foods that are refined, processed, or filled with chemicals and artificial colorings and dyes. Replace them with natural, organically grown, pesticide-free wholesome and whole foods.

Biomagnetic and electromagnetic pulse therapies are also valuable, Dr. Hodes says. Diapulse, magnatherm, biofeedback, acupuncture, and ear acupuncture (auricular therapy) may be tried.

Dr. Hodes notes the existence of several other, less widespread approaches that are available, involving nutrient substances that increase brain function: An Israeli egg yolk lecithin substance, AL721, which was originally used to give energy and reduce cholesterol in elderly people, and was used to combat HIV and AIDS, also helps the brain. You might try Dr. Ana Aslan's treatment called Gerovital (GH3) and live cell therapy, which are illegal in America but available in certain other countries. There is also something called super-triple-phosphatidylcholine.

"There are supplement companies which manufacture brain formulas, which are composed of various amino acids, enzymes, vitamins, minerals and herbs," Dr. Hodes says. "Niacin, or vitamin B3, is helpful because it opens up the blood vessels and brings nutrients, blood, oxygen, and other nutrients to the brain. Mineral baths, consisting of sodium, potassium, and magnesium, which seep into our bodies through the pores of the skin, are also helpful."

Among Dr. Hodes's other recommendations are herbal remedies; homeopathic remedies; developmental/behavioral optometric vision therapy for improved visualization, perception, cognition, and memory efficiency; applied kinesiology; and chiropractic and osteopathic care. Finally, he maintains: "Since the brain of an Alzheimer's patient shrinks, we have to rehydrate it with pure water, eight to ten glasses daily. It takes about six months to compensate for the shrinkage."

Dr. Dharma Singh Khalsa heads the Alzheimer's Prevention Foundation in Tucson, Arizona. His "mission" for several decades has been to make the idea of preventive medicine for the brain available to health care practitioners. He is convinced that memory loss can be prevented and reversed, and his work is critical not only for healthy people, but also for those suffering all kinds of brain deterioration, including Alzheimer's.

Dr. Khalsa's Seven Step Program combines conventional medical practices with those of alternative medicine.

1. NUTRITIONAL ENHANCEMENT. "Improved nutrition, all practitioners agree, enhances cognitive function. At a bare minimum, the diet should have low fat, moderate protein, high complex carbohydrates and a low caloric intake. Adding breast of chicken, fish and nonanimal protein products such as tofu is helpful. Certain fish is especially good for the brain. These fish include salmon, tuna, trout, mackerel, and sardines."

2. NUTRIENT SUPPLEMENTATION. "The B complex vitamins are essential for optimal neurological health. They are especially critical for neurotransmitter control and carbohydrate energy metabolism. Niacin itself (B3) has been shown to have memory-improving benefits. For this reason, a high-potency multiple vitamin/mineral package is included in each patient's program in doses above the US Recommended Dietary Allowance (RDA), but not in so-called 'orthomolecular' ranges.

"Recent dynamic research has confirmed the neuroprotective role of vitamin E. Vitamin E protects cell membranes from oxidative damage. The dose utilized in this program is 800 IU. Other antioxidants prescribed are vitamin C (3000-6000 milligrams per day) and vitamin A (25,000 IU a day). Selenium and zinc are included in the multivitamin/mineral tablet. Additional program supplements include three newer neuroactive compounds: phosphatidyl serine (PS), 300 milligrams per day; coenzyme Q10, 1000 milligrams per day; and acetyl L carnitine, 2000 milligrams to 1500 milligrams per day."

Dr. Khalsa provides more information about these newer compounds. "PS is a negatively charged phospholipid, almost exclusively located in cell membranes. It has a series of unique physiological properties that are important to neuronal functions, including stimulation of neurotransmitter release, activation of ion transport mechanisms and increase in glucose and cyclic AMP levels in the brain. In the aging brain, a decline in these functions is associated with memory impairment and deficits in cognitive abilities. PS has been found to improve short-term memory, mood, concentration and activities of daily living. Although initial studies utilized bovine PS, the concern over the risk of a slow viral infection prompted the search for an alternative plant source. A novel PS product made through byenzymatic conversion of soy lecithin has now been developed, and subsequent research has confirmed its positive effects in patients with memory loss."

Coenzyme Q10 has rapidly gained notice as a powerful agent. "It works as a dynamic antioxidant throughout the brain cell membrane and mitochondria, where it is involved in the production of high energy phosphate compounds," Dr. Khalsa explains.

"Acetyl L carnitine is a superbly versatile metabolite and plays a pivotal role in facilitating energetic pathways in brain cell mitochondria. It is a source of acetyl groups for acetyl-Co-A and facilitates release of acetylcholine and other neurotransmitters and neuropeptides. ALC also has been reported to decrease cortisol levels."

3. HERBS. "Ginkgo biloba is utilized at a dose of 120 milligrams per day. This dose increases microvascular circulation, scavenges free radicals, and helps improve concentration and short-term memory."

4. PHARMACEUTICALS. The FDA-approved drugs for Alzheimer's disease include Cognex, Aricept, Exelon, and Razadyne for mild to moderate symptoms; and Namenda for moderate to severe symptoms. As mentioned earlier in this chapter, although not approved by the FDA for Alzheimer's disease, other drugs, including antipsychotics, are being used to treat associated psychotic and behavioral symptoms. This practice has become a cause for concern by many practitioners.

5. HORMONE REPLACEMENT THERAPY. "Research on the effects of estrogen replacement therapy in the prevention of AD has been very exciting," Dr. Khalsa says. "Hippocampal plasticity and nerve growth factors are apparently estrogen-sensitive. The use of either DHEA or pregnenolone, both neurospecific hormones and precursors to estrogen, makes good clinical sense, because of the lower side effect potential. Both have proved useful in this program at doses of

50 milligrams per day. An animal study demonstrated that DHEA affects excitability in the hippocampus, thereby enhancing memory function at moderate dosages. Because the optimal dose needed to facilitate the induction of neuronal plasticity in humans is not yet certain, the dosage level used was arrived at empirically.

"Another study showed that DHEA enhances acetylcholine release from hippocampal neurons in the rat brain. DHEA has been found to be consistently low in patients with AD.

"Research in animals has proved pregnenolone to be a very powerful memory enhancer. Pregnenolone was also demonstrated to improve memory in humans. More than 50 years ago, researchers at the University of Massachusetts trained 14 subjects to operate an airplane flight simulator. Subjects who received the hormone improved significantly compared with controls. A recent study has demonstrated improved memory with pregnenolone use in older people.

"The hormone melatonin at doses of .3 milligrams to 6 milligrams is given at bedtime, when indicated, to restore circadian rhythm in place of benzodiazepines, which can depress cognitive function."

6. MENTAL TRAINING. Nowhere more than in the brain is the old adage, "Use it or lose it," more appropriate. In fact, Einstein had a fairly normal brain when it came to his neurons. However, what was extremely unusual was the structure of his brain, rich in supporting glial cells. He was the Michael Jordan of mental athletes.

We know that the risk of developing dementia decreases with the number of years of formal education. The lower the educational level, the greater the risk for Alzheimer's. This highlights research suggesting that mental activity throughout life is neuroprotective. Based on the enriched environment work of Cotman and Diamond, Dr. Khalsa's program includes cognitive stimulation, such as headline discussion, crossword puzzles, music, art, and group therapy. Mental training increases dendritic sprouting and enhances central nervous system plasticity.

"Stress management is crucial because chronic, unbalanced stress causes elevation of the hormone cortisol," Dr. Khalsa says. "Cortisol has a toxic effect on the memory center of the brain and can cause memory loss. The stress management tool of meditation decreases cortisol and enhances many aspects of mental function. Massage and guided mental imagery have also recently been shown to lower cortisol levels in the blood.

"To prevent accelerated brain aging and cognitive dysfunction, it is critical to reduce the negative physiological consequences brought about by chronic stress. For this we turn to a practice that is thousands of years old and the subject of many modern scientific research studies: meditation. Besides the awake state, the sleep state and the dream state, there is the fourth state: the transcendent or meditative. In the past three decades, numerous studies have been completed by researchers exploring the far-reaching effects of transcendental meditation, a simple mental technique. . . . The relaxation response (RR) is an innate psychophysiological mechanism first demonstrated by Walter Hess, Ph.D., in 1948, a discovery for which he was awarded the Nobel Prize in physiology. Meditation has been found to decrease serum cortisol levels and promote normalization of adaptive mechanisms. Practitioners of meditation also display lower levels of lipid peroxidase, a marker of free radical production, as well as higher levels of the hormone dehydroepiandrosterone, important for optimal brain function. Elderly meditators have been shown to enjoy greater life expectancy than nonmeditators. The use of meditation as a tool for preventing memory loss, or for reversing it in its early stages, is an avenue ripe for clinical investigation.

"Pharmacological approaches to the prevention and reversal of memory loss are likely to continue to be difficult because of the presence of multiple neurotransmitter deficits and the difficulty of replacing lost transmitter function in a way that mimics normal neuronal release. For this reason, patients are instructed in the practice of yogic kriyas: specific exercises that combine breathing, finger movement, and regenerating sound currents. The practice of these kriyas serves a dual purpose: they induce the RR and stimulate the central nervous system. Kriyas have been clinically shown to create cerebral stimulation, mental relaxation, and an increased ability to focus. A PET scan has demonstrated that kriyas enhance regional cerebral blood flow, oxygen delivery and glucose utilization."

7. AEROBIC CONDITIONING. "Finally, aerobic conditioning has been shown to improve some aspects of mental function by as much as 20 to 30 percent."

Dr. Jay Lombard focuses treatment for Alzheimer's on four areas: reducing excessive inflammation; increasing the neurotransmitter acetylcholine, which is vital to memory; reducing antioxidant activity; and boosting the mitochondria.

To raise brain acetylcholine levels, there is a natural product called huperzene A, which blocks the enzyme that breaks down the neurotransmitter. Ginkgo biloba has been shown to be effective in retarding the progression of the disease. Vitamin E and melatonin are good antioxidants. Coenzyme Q10 or an analog of it, an amino acid called acetyl-L-carnitine, is useful for increasing mitochondrial activity. Estrogen is very effective in inhibiting beta secretinase, an enzyme that is detrimental to Alzheimer's patients. Estrogen blocks that enzyme and therefore inhibits the production of these pathological proteins found in the brains of Alzheimer's patients. DHEA, a natural adrenal steroid, may also be effective.

Dr. Michael Schachter tells us that some Alzheimer's patients showing signs of senile dementia "have improved quite a bit on a program in which they received injectable B vitamins and magnesium. Some of these elderly people have difficulty absorbing vitamins and minerals simply because of long-term chronic deficiencies, so an injectable program becomes very helpful." He also uses disodium-magnesium EDTA chelation therapy to remove calcium from soft tissues, where it doesn't belong, and to try to get it back into the bone, where it does belong. The chelation process, which is an intravenous treatment, helps with soft tissue decalcification, in addition to removing heavy metals.

15

Depression and Other Mental Disorders in Older Adults

■■■

According to the American Association for Geriatric Psychiatry, nearly one-fifth of all older adults have mental disorders that are not considered a normal consequence of aging. In this population, symptoms are often overlooked, ignored, or confused with other ailments. As a result, people often are left to cope with problems that could otherwise be treated.

Eight to 20 percent of older adults living in the community and up to 37 percent in primary care settings have depressive symptoms. Left untreated, the results can be tragic. People age sixty-five and above have the highest suicide rates of any age group; although they make up only 13 percent of the population, they account for 18 percent of all suicide deaths in the United States.

Among the risk factors for depression in older adults are the presence of other illnesses including diabetes, stroke, and heart disease; recent bereavement; chronic or severe pain; fear of death; previous history of depression; and substance abuse. Many medications have side effects that can cause or exacerbate the symptoms of depression. Although it is not unusual for people to feel sad, grief-stricken, or lonely in later years, true depression is marked by persistent symptoms that interfere with the ability to function in daily life.

According to the Cleveland Clinic Health Information Center, depression in the elderly may differ from that of the general population in several ways. It is often linked with other medical conditions. It tends to last longer. In addition, it "doubles their risk of developing cardiac disease, reduces their ability to rehabilitate, and increases their risk of death from illness."

The symptoms of depression in older adults may include agitation, anxiety, memory problems, social withdrawal, decreased appetite, confusion, loss of interest in normally pleasurable activities, prolonged grief, reduced energy, and suicidal thoughts. Because these symptoms are present in many other conditions, accurate diagnosis is difficult.

Among other mental health problems in older adults are anxiety, and alcohol and substance abuse. In a given year, more than 11 percent of people aged fifty-five and older meet the criteria for an anxiety disorder. Phobias are the most common type. Three to 9 percent of people in this age group engage in heavy drinking (twelve to twenty-one drinks per week), with men four times more likely than women to abuse alcohol. Older people take prescription drugs at a rate that is three times that of the general population. They also use over-the-counter medications extensively. Problems often result from the misuse of these medications. This includes underuse, overuse, or erratic use that is contrary to label instructions.

As in the younger population, conventional treatment of mental disorders in the elderly often involves the use of antidepressant medications. The selection and dosages of medications is more complicated, however. Because many older patients take medications for other medical conditions, there is an increased risk of adverse drug interactions. Age-related physiological differences also may alter a drug's effectiveness, or cause more potential for side effects. For example, as reported in several 2007 studies in the *Archives of Internal Medicine*, elderly patients taking certain drugs, including Prozac and Paxil, had increased risk of fragile bones and fractures from falls.

A variety of effective natural therapies are available for these disorders, including diet and nutrition, nutritional supplements, meditation, exercise, and psychotherapy. These are all described in Chapter 7. Special care must be taken when providing any intervention in an older patient, particularly when there are other conditions involved.

PART FOUR

Disorders in Children

Often, those most susceptible to environmental illnesses and to misdiagnoses by conventionally trained physicians are also those who are least able to protect themselves from the dangers these problems pose. Our children live in environments we create for them, and they either benefit or suffer from the changes we make in those environments. A range of behavioral, affective, and mental disorders affects children primarily. They are discussed in the following chapters.

In many cases, the culprit is found to be environmental toxins of one type or another. Dr. Harold Buttram has been pointing out for the past two decades that "while most of our knowledge of the effect of environmental toxins comes from reports of occupational exposure in adults, there is no doubt that developing children are at even greater risk. It is a known fact that pesticides are toxic to the nervous system. Most of our knowledge in this area comes from studies of occupational exposures in adults. What is not known—and all the texts say this—is how toxic are the continual low-dose exposures that are commonly incurred from the environment, and especially, how toxic they are to children. The evidence suggests that there is sufficient toxicity, from residual pesticides in foods, air, and water, and in homes and yards, to cause neurotoxic damage—particularly to children or to the fetus during pregnancy.

"All the scientific literature emphasizes that the fetus and young children are far more vulnerable to toxic chemicals than adults are," Dr. Buttram adds. "And yet the government standards for limitations of pesticides are set by adult standards, which do not take into account the heightened susceptibility of children.

"In order to assess the damage caused by pesticides and other toxic chemicals to the nervous and immune systems in children, every educated person should read a government publication entitled *Neurotoxicity: Identifying and Controlling Poisons of the Nervous System*. It points out that behavioral problems are one of the earliest signs of chemical toxicity, which is what we are seeing in children today. In fact, researchers in the field of chemical toxicity are extremely concerned about the impact of environmental chemicals on children."

16

Aggression

■■■

Patient Story: Aggression

Just after Brittany was born, when she was about three weeks old, she started having recurring ear infections. She was always going on antibiotics—literally every two weeks—until she was about two years old. At that time a friend introduced us to an allergist in Massachusetts, who put her through allergy testing and treatment. We changed our daughter's diet after finding that there were certain foods to which she was severely allergic, such as chicken, sugar and dairy.

After a year of allergy therapy, she is doing much better. She is a relatively calm child; she can play nicely by herself and has a very good temperament. She is one of these kids that, if you have to give her an injection, she'll just sit there and maybe giggle. But when she has sugar or chicken, she turns into a little animal. She becomes extremely cranky, gets almost violent. She will want to hit you; she will cling to me and to her father.

We didn't understand what was happening until we started to see a pattern. When we found out she was allergic to these things, we started to understand that eating these foods was what caused the tantrum-like behavior. Also, her infections completely stopped during the treatment. When she went off of the allergy treatments for a little while, because our insurance would not pay for them, her ear infections immediately returned along with the other symptoms.

Before we went to the allergist, I had talked to several doctors. We had gone to the best doctors and to different children's hospitals. Their answers were operations for her ears and medication to help calm her down if necessary. After a while the doctors started to treat me like a neurotic mother, implying that I must be doing something wrong for my child to be doing this. Or else they said she was going through a phase and would grow out of it. Both those kinds of attitudes got very frustrating.

This experience has taught me to trust myself. As a mother, you absolutely know your child, and if you feel that the physician you are talking to isn't correct, then you should question it, and go with your gut instinct because chances are you're probably right. As a parent, you know your child best. Since we've been working with Dr. Buttram, Brittany is doing much better, staying on the diet and avoiding foods to which she's sensitive. The main thing I would say is, trust your instincts and keep looking until you find what works.

—Brittany's mother

Aggression in children often has an environmental root cause. Among the culprits are dust, pollen, molds, foods, and chemicals. As Dr. Doris Rapp explains, "Any of these things can turn an absolute angel into a tyrant in seconds. A frequent clue to an allergic reaction is that affected children develop red earlobes, wiggly legs, red cheeks, a red nose and sometimes a spacey look in the eyes. At times these children can be very nasty and aggressive, with a frightening demonic look in their eyes. They throw out their lower lip and their eyes are half-shut and they look as if they are going to kill you. I've seen this in three-year-old children who eat the wrong food, or if we just take one drop of an allergy extract containing a substance to which they are sensitive and prick their arm with it.

"We have videotapes documenting what we're talking about. However, insurance companies are very reluctant to pay for this kind of medical care, even though many times specialists in environmental medicine can see patients and relieve symptoms that haven't been helped by all the other medical specialists. They pay for medical care that does not help and don't pay for care that does help. We must ask why. Insurance companies say environmental medicine is experimental and anecdotal. If we take two hours taking a history and do extensive patient or parent teaching to show them how to figure out answers so they can finally detect what's causing the problem, on a long-term basis, it is time well spent. That individual stands a chance of remaining well and not needing drugs or hospitalization once the true cause has been identified and eliminated. Insurance companies should be delighted because, in the long run, this approach saves an enormous amount of their money, as well as preserving the wellbeing and preventing the heartache for so many patients and family members."

"Insurance companies are reluctant to pay the environmental specialist, but will very quickly pay the hospital. Each day in the hospital can cost $1000. The total cost for environmental treatment of a serious condition would be much less than a week in the hospital.

Dr. Rapp describes the changes she has witnessed through environmental approaches. "I have seen a number of children who have been so difficult in school that they have been singled out by school officials. First, all the usual quieting drugs were tried, and when nothing helped, they were told that they would have to be institutionalized. We have videotapes showing that these same children can be turned around. They act great, until we give them a particular food to eat or skin test them with one drop of an allergy extract solution containing the item that bothers them. Within minutes, they are absolutely uncontrollable. Four people have to hold them down. They are spitting, hitting, kicking, and then we give them the right one drop, the correct dilution of that same substance that caused the problem, and they are right back to normal. This newer, more precise, allergy detection is called provocation/neutralization allergy testing. No, we can't explain why this happens. The body is smarter than the doctors.

"I have a number of patients who were going to be institutionalized and who did not need to be. I have seen many other children who were put in classes for the learning disabled because they've been classified as learning disabled or as having conceptual understanding problems or perceptual disorders of various sorts. Many times they fall between the cracks. The school doesn't know how to classify them if, for example, they display 'autistic-like' behavior. Some (although certainly not all) of these children have responded beautifully to allergy care. Their grades go up significantly. One child's IQ changed from 57 to 125 in a period of 19 months. Some of the children have been returned to be in the classroom with their peers. Many of them can switch from home teaching to school if the parent can pay to have an air purifier put in the classroom."

An even more disturbing cause of aggression in children, as well as teenagers and adults, can be traced directly to the kinds of psychiatric drugs they have been taking. Dr. Peter Breggin, a leading critic of Ritalin and Prozac, and medical consultant in several lawsuits brought against the pharmaceutical companies that manufacture these and other drugs, calls Attention Deficit Hyperactivity Disorder "a disease of the professionals rather than of the children." The "professionals" remind him of the authorities in Aldous Huxley's *Brave New World*, except "actually, in *Brave New World* the children did not get drugs. We have reached a level of obscenity in the way we treat our kids that was not even imagined in that fantasy.

"All of these drugs can produce psychosis and violence. I went back and took a good look at the literature again. I found a controlled clinical trial at Yale in which a 12-year-old boy dropped out of school. This little boy was on Prozac and he quit because he was having nightmares of going to school and killing his classmates and being killed. These were getting worse. He was losing track of what was reality. His symptoms went away when the Prozac was stopped. In the same study, a girl who was taking Prozac developed a violent psychosis and was attacking her stuffed animals. She did not recover when the Prozac was stopped."

"Both cases were published in a major medical journal as probable Prozac reactions. Yet the experts, my colleagues in psychiatry, get on the radio, TV, newspapers, and say there is no evidence at all for this reaction when there is a great deal of evidence. Prozac, in one study, produced mania in 6 percent of the children and they had to drop out of the study. Luvox, which is another antidepressant very similar to Prozac, caused a 4 percent rate of mania in a similar study."

Dr. Breggin expresses serious concern about what this means for the general public. "These rates are occurring in little four to six week trials, where the kids are carefully monitored," he says. "When you have somebody out in the community taking these drugs and not being monitored every week, their parents are not as involved as the ones whose children are in clinical trials, so your rates of kids getting out of control are going to be even higher in the general population. We are creating thousands and thousands of episodes of manic psychosis in our children."

"My colleagues are so unwilling to face the truth. They end up saying that these kids have manic depression. So if your child gets manic on Prozac, instead of being told, 'Hey, I'm sorry, we gave your child a drug that induced mania,' the parents are going to be lied to and told that the child's disorder just happened to come out now. We won't even stop the Prozac. We may increase the Prozac, Zoloft, Celexa or the Paxil, these knock-off Prozac drugs. We'll increase it and we will give the child Lithium or Depicot or something else. In my clinical practice, I see kids on three and four drugs by the time they are 12. The doctor declares the child to have one or the other disease or disorder when it is, in fact, drug induced."

Drug-induced aggression and violence has briefly made it into the headlines as a result of recent school shootings. "A large number of the kids that have been committing incredible acts of violence have been taking psychiatric drugs," Dr. Breggin says: "Kip Kinkle, the Oregon shooter, was taking Prozac and Ritalin some time before the shooting; T. J. Solomon, who did the shooting in Georgia, on May 20, 1999, was on Ritalin. Eric Harris, the leader in the tragedy in Colorado in April, 1999, was taking the psychiatric drug Luvox at the time of the murders. Luvox is approved for children and youth with obsessive compulsive disorder, but doctors often give it for depression, since it is in the same class as Prozac, Zoloft and Paxil. While psychiatric drug use is only one of the contributing factors to the episodes of school violence, it is one of the most easily prevented factors. There is strong scientific evidence to support the view that these drugs should not be given to children and teenagers."

Dennis Clarke, chair of the Executive Advisory Board of the Citizen's Commission on Human Rights, expands our understand of drug-induced violence to include some well known mass murderers. "In Austin, Texas in 1966, Charles Whitman went up into the Texas Tower, the first school shooting in the United States. Forty-eight hours later, the FBI held a press conference and said no drugs were found in Whitman's body. This is the same report that we got on the incident at Columbine High School with Eric Harris. No drugs were found in the body. Now we learn that, in fact, Whitman had been on prescription amphetamines. He was displaying a classic amphetamine psychosis. According to the FBI, he had been eating amphetamines like popcorn while he was up on the tower shooting people. Had we learned that at the time, it would have changed the whole course of what we're doing with amphetamines and amphetamine-type drugs like Ritalin in this country.

"No one has a problem attributing increases in violence within the inner cities to the use of crack cocaine. That's 'those people over there' for the majority of the Americans. But the fact is that the rise of senseless violence among white children and young adults is directly connected to drugs, only they are legal drugs."

17

Attention Deficit Hyperactivity Disorder (ADHD)

■■■

Patient Story: ADHD

Timothy is five years old. Since his birth, I've been trying to find out what was wrong with him. It's really been a personal battle. Many people looked at me cross-eyed and said that he is a normal little boy, he is just growing, or he is immature, or it is my fault because I don't discipline him properly. I am not stern enough, they said, and I should introduce physical punishment.

Since Tim was my first child, I had nothing to compare his behavior to and since I was coming out of the corporate world, I didn't really know with whom I could share my doubts and insecurities. I felt very vulnerable exposing myself to other mothers and saying, "I can't do this. What's wrong with my child?"

By the time Tim was three, there were times when I just couldn't stand being a mother. All I did was say "No, no, no" all the time. He started doing dangerous things to his younger brother, such as pushing him down the basement stairs in a walker. And I thought, "This is not Timothy. He knows that that is not right." There was a look in his eye, and I thought, "What has possessed him to do this?" I knew something wasn't right, but I was told he was acting out because of his new brother, that this was typical, not to worry, to discipline him as necessary.

When he was four, his schoolteacher said, "I'm having a difficult time with this child. He is extremely bright, but he can't color in the pictures and he doesn't know how to socialize with other children." So I decided that it was time to go to a child behavior specialist. He said that when Tim could sit still, he demonstrated a high IQ, but he was extremely immature and needed to be observed.

By the time he turned five, his prekindergarten teacher suspected an attention deficit disorder with hyperactive tendencies and suggested medical care. We brought him to the hospital and the behavior specialist said that Ritalin would be necessary, along with counseling.

Based on our family history of chemical dependency, I felt that Ritalin was not a good option. So I started looking for other possibilities. Two weeks after the diagnosis, we had a birthday party, and I served my boy ice cream, chocolate cake and a glass of milk. He went totally off the wall. To try to control him, I had the children play school and I asked Tim to recite his ABCs. He stopped at D. Now, he had known the whole alphabet for a year and he just panicked. He looked so scared, absolutely horrified. He said, "Mommy, I don't know what to do. What comes after D, what comes after D?" I knew it was the food, and that from there, I needed to find an answer.

I happened to see Doris Rapp on a television show, and I picked up her book. I gave my son the multiple-elimination diet that she suggested and the results were unbelievable! The doctors were surprised. The chief of the pediatric staff was extremely intrigued, but because of the way he was trained, he wasn't able to offer me any medical support. But he did support my going to Dr. Buttram until he could learn more himself.

Now that I have figured out that my son's problem is food allergies as well as allergies to environmental substances such as pollens, it really bothers me that medical doctors don't have this fundamental knowledge of nutrition. Reviewing the first five years of Timothy's life, I notice a pattern. He has always been at his worst during July and August. Now I realize he is severely allergic to ragweed, to the grasses, and to dairy and corn. When he came in contact with these substances all at once, it just gave him a full-barrel effect. In the summertime we would eat fresh corn on the cob, and after, as a wonderful treat for the whole family, we'd jump in the car and go Dairy Queen, with all the ragweed blowing around. As soon as the frost hit, he was much better.

After six months under Dr. Buttram's care, Timothy is a totally changed child. The kindergarten program he will be entering next year has tested him and, in their opinion, he is a normal child and shows no evidence of an attention deficit. Plus there is no hyperactivity and has been none for at least four months.

—Timothy's mother

Attention deficit hyperactivity disorder (ADHD) is estimated to affect 3 to 5 percent of school-aged children in the United States. The term describes a wide range of learning problems. Since 1980, hyperactivity has been included in the diagnostic category instead of being treated separately, as it had been before. The list of symptoms includes short attention span, inability to concentrate, inability to sit still, difficulty following instructions, destructive behavior, tendencies to talk too much or interrupt, inability to wait one's turn, and being accident-prone.

It is a very controversial diagnosis. A child is considered to have ADHD if he or she meets certain behavioral standards, as observed by teachers. Since no teachers see a child in the same way, subjectivity is a big problem. While practitioners agree that we are in the midst of an epidemic of troubled learning and behavior among children, few assign the same kinds of cause to the problem and few are in accord about effective treatment. Opposition to the most common orthodox treatment—prescription medications including Ritalin and Adderall, as well as the newer Concerta and Strattera—has become increasingly widespread and vocal.

Dr. Harold Buttram, who helped Timothy and continues to help other children with many of these symptoms, says that the problem is reaching epidemic proportions. "I always make a point of asking patients of mine who are schoolteachers and have been teaching for 20 or 30 years whether there has been a change in the behavior of children during that time. The replies are consistently emphatic—that there has been a drastic change in children. There are more hyperactivity and attention deficit problems, more learning disorders and more behavioral problems."

On the other hand, many experts, especially over the past decade, are challenging the idea that this is a real mental disorder and objecting to the way children are being stigmatized by it. Some call ADHD a myth or a "wastebasket diagnosis" for everything else the doctors can't find another name for. Many find social and political factors at the root of the epidemic—overcrowded schools, the desire to replace family and teaching with pharmaceutical control of youngsters, and the profit motive of drug companies always in search of new markets.

Some of the children's so-called symptoms, they say, are often normal childhood behavior. Or the product of boredom in unchallenging school situations. "The fundamental problem," as Dr. Peter Braughman puts it, "is that the diagnosis is entirely subjective. Let's say the first period teacher is given a behavior checklist, the third period teacher is given a behavior checklist, so are a counselor and a playground attendant. You come up with four different views of the child.

"There is no physical marker making this a disease, so it is wholly inappropriate to talk of it having a cause or a treatment or a chemical defect or an allergic basis. As a neurologist for 35 years, it was my duty to each patient to determine whether they have a disease or not. I haven't proven that a patient has a disease until I demonstrate that they have some abnormality. That might require a brain scan to show a mass or a tumor, a chest x-ray to show a tumor, a biopsy to further define the character of the tumor, or a laboratory test to show a chemical abnormality of the blood, urine or other body fluid. When one has a patient with symptoms that persist but no abnormality can be found, one has not proven that there is disease.

"ADHD, invented in committee in 1980 at the American Psychiatric Association, has never been proven to be a disease. The whole concept of how to define 'attention' is problematic. There is no specific work to show us what it means. The main researcher in the area of attention in the 1970s, Dr. Thomas Mulholland, described a conference of the major experts in this area around the world, none of whom could come up with a satisfactory definition of attention. The methods used to diagnose attention and hyperactive disorders, then, by its very nature, are completely subjective. There is a laundry list of about 100 adjectives to describe a child with attention deficit or hyperactive disorder. Do you need three, do you need five? Is there a hierarchy, which ones are important? You just have a myth."

Dr. Braughman does not deny that many children are struggling in the classroom. "There is no question that we see children who have trouble learning in school," he says. "This is a reality and this we know is true. In my experience, these children have a very high intelligence. Their intelligence, however, is in the area of creativity, a right brain activity. In school, reading, particularly, is a left brain activity. So what we have is children who are learning with their right brain, trying to do something in an intellectual, cognitive way, and not able to do it."

Dr. Joseph Trachtman tells us that a historical link between brain defects and learning disabilities has colored our view of the problem. "In the scientific literature, starting in the early 1860s, we find a French anatomist named Broca reporting two people with lesions damaging the left side of the brain. These people had lost their speech—this came to be known as acquired aphasia, aphasia meaning loss of speech. Shortly after that, there were a number of reports about children who had trouble learning and they were labeled with 'congenital aphasia.' From those early reports of congenital aphasia, we get to the label that we have now of ADHD. It has the implied connotation of brain damage, carried over from Broca's research. In the 1970s, the same condition in children was called 'minimal brain damage,' or MBD. The physicians' handbook for screening MBD was published and supported by Ciba-Geigy, the manufacturers of Ritalin."

When there is a real learning problem, the "number one cause is poor nutrition," says nutritionist Howard Pleper, author of *The ADD Diet Book*. Again, the problem is lifestyle. Because "we believe in instant gratification, it's easy to go out and get foods with chemicals and additives, especially preservatives, so that if we decide not to eat it today, we can eat it three years from now. Also, the soil in which our food is grown is depleted of the essential nutrients, even the soil in which 'organic' fruits and vegetables are grown. There are some organic farmers who do not remineralize their soil.

"Among the environmental contaminants at play when children have learning or behavior problems are insecticide and pesticide residues in our food and water and metal contamination, especially aluminum or lead toxicity. A holistic pediatrician in Florida says the lead toxicity he finds in children comes not from paint in older homes, but from piping and solder through which lead leaks into the water itself. Indoor air pollution, food allergies and repeated use of antibiotics, which promotes the overgrowth of yeast and leads to Candida, are among the causes of this."

Dr. Joseph Debe adds that a study of children diagnosed with ADHD found "65 percent had parasites, one-third had yeast overgrowth and 75 percent had a condition called leaky gut syndrome. Leaky gut syndrome is when the intestinal lining is weakened. Normally, the intestinal lining serves two purposes: it allows for absorption of nutrients and at the same time it keeps toxins from the intestinal tract from making their way into the bloodstream. In the 75 percent of these children who had impaired intestinal barrier function, toxins were making their way into the bloodstream at greater than normal concentrations. Some of these toxins impair energy production when they become involved in biochemical reactions. One of these chemicals in particular—from yeast—has been associated with childhood autism."

As Dr. Michael Schachter notes, these conditions are frequently improved by cleaning up children's diets and removing fluoride: "Some of these children are sensitive to fluoride, which may cause headaches, hyperactivity and problems with attention. Fluoride is often present in their drinking water and toothpaste. Some children are prescribed fluoride tablets or given fluoride treatments at their dentists' offices or at school. Some of these children are benefited by removing all sources of fluoride. Additionally, vitamin and mineral supplements, such as magnesium, may be quite helpful.

"Homeopathy can also be extremely useful. I saw one little boy who suffered from recurrent ear infections and was hyperactive. When we gave him the proper homeopathic remedy, removed sugar from his diet, and gave him a little cod liver oil, the pediatricians and specialists who had been following him for his ear infections and asthma were amazed at how beautifully he did; he turned out not to require tubes in his ears, which they had recommended. Also, his attention deficit and concentration span improved."

Dr. Judyth Reichenberg-Ullman has treated hundreds of ADHD children homeopathically. She is worried, first of all, about overdiagnosis. "We hear so many stories from parents about children who have been in a classroom for just two or three weeks and they're called into a teacher's conference and the teacher says, 'Have you thought of putting your child on Ritalin?'

"Some of these are just active, normal children, and many of them are gifted. Imagine if you had an IQ of 150 or a photographic memory, you'd probably be bored to tears in some of these classes, wanting to find other things to get your attention and to keep you stimulated. It is shocking how many precocious and intelligent children are being diagnosed. Some of them are put in special education classes. One of the things that happens with homeopathic treatment is that the children get out of those classes, are back in normal classrooms, and they get their imaginative natures and their creativity back. It's very rewarding."

Of course, there are children with typical symptoms, Dr. Reichenberg-Ullman says. "We definitely do see children who are bouncing off the walls, completely unable to concentrate, legitimate examples of children with ADD. The characteristics are drifty, driven and daring. Drifty, as in, 'calling planet earth, do you read me?' Drifty means difficulty concentrating. Many children cannot understand what they read or what's being asked of them in class. They are very, very slow to comprehend and very absent minded, spacey. Their parents have to give them the same instructions four or five times, which leads to a lot of frustration. Driven is 'wired for sound,' impulsive, not thinking before a child does something. Many children grow up to be adults with these same or similar characteristics—unable to sit still, fidgety, squirmy, wandering around the room. Daring is actually being reckless. These people can put themselves and other adults or kids in danger of being hurt.

"There is no question that homeopathy can help many of these children. If parent and child stick with treatments for at least six months, we estimate about a 70 percent effectiveness rate in the hands of a experienced homeopathic practitioner."

Dr. Reichenberg-Ullman says that many studies link attention deficits with abnormalities of specific neurotransmitters. "A study at the University of California at Irvine found that children with severe ADD had a decreased sensitivity to dopamine. The homeopathic point of view would be that the neurotransmitters may indeed be found to have a correlation, but that this is a result of the imbalance in the person. Whether you talk about a neurotransmitter imbalance, or something physical like Candida, whether you talk about fibromyalgia or a strep throat, from a homeopathic point of view, these are not the causes, these are the results. Homeopathy seeks to go to the root of that energetic imbalance in a person, to address the cause. When the cause is addressed, all of these other things will fall into place.

"Sugar consumption is part of the problem. Many parents say that the day after Halloween, for example, their children are bouncing off the walls, that they notice a definite difference. However, it's not enough in the case of most ADD children to decrease the amount of sugar in the diet. We have very conscious parents in our practice and many of these parents have made these dietary changes. The same is true of allergens—from a homeopathic point of view, this is the result of an imbalance in a person, not the cause of the problem. Most of the kids that we see have seen allergists or addressed the allergies and they're still having problems.

"In homeopathy, each person is treated as a unique human being. There are over 2000 homeopathic medicines. A word of caution: it has taken me about fifteen years to really understand homeopathy to the level that I do and we do not recommend self treatment for ADD. It's one thing to self treat colds and flus, you can learn to do that, but not with ADD."

Dr. Reichenberg-Ullman provides several examples to illustrate her point. "A sixteen-year-old named Sherry was referred by her family practice physician. She had a five-year history of ADD. She had been on Ritalin since the sixth grade. Without Ritalin, she couldn't focus, she was distracted by noise, by movement, she couldn't concentrate taking tests, she stared off into space and stopped in mid-sentence. No matter how much she tried to be quiet she couldn't. She was frequently embarrassing her friends. She would be driving and would miss seeing another car because she didn't notice it. She was always fidgeting and fiddling and clicking her nails and tapping. Ritalin had given her hives. It also made her feel like she didn't know herself, that's what she said. Her tendency to procrastination wasn't affected at all by the Ritalin. She also loved pickles, ate them straight from the jar, and she loved to suck on ice. The medicine she needed was called baratrum albun. It's a plant, and for her that's what was really helpful.

"Another child was brought in because she had lots of problems in school. She was even getting an F in PE. She was getting a D in math. Her mother brought her in because she was being self destructive, mutilating herself, scratching her face, pulling out her hair. She felt that people hated her. She would lash out at her mother verbally, would kick and punch and even threatened to hurt herself with a knife. She had a very different situation and she needed a remedy called liacin, which is actually made from a very dilute preparation of rabies. So these children need all different kinds of homeopathic medicines.

"There is a medicine called stramonium, which is thorn apple, that we often give to children who, in addition to having difficulty concentrating, have a lot of fears and can be quite violent. So it depends entirely on not just the symptoms of that individual, but the states, in other words, really understanding a person in depth."

Dr. Lendon Smith summarizes some of the history of treating hyperactivity in children, and then describes his own clinical experience: "The man who discovered the paradoxical effects of stimulant drugs on hyperactive children was Charles Bradley from Portland, Oregon. In 1937 and 1938, he found that most children with 'hyperactive syndrome' came from difficult pregnancies, especially those which ended in troublesome deliveries. The hyperactive children were the second of twins or born with the cord around their neck. They were premature, or born with a collapsed lung or too much bilirubin. A number of things might have interfered with the oxygen supply to the brain. The problems had not been enough to hurt the child's intellect but just enough to hurt the part of the brain that has to do with self-control. This was Bradley's original concept.

"Then, in 1938, a mistake was made. Charles Bradley was in charge of a home for problem children when he asked a nurse to give an overly active girl some bromide. The nurse accidentally used the next bottle, Benzedrine, and the girl promptly went to sleep. The doctor commented to the nurse that the bromide sure worked well and the nurse responded by saying, 'What did you say?' The doctor asked, 'What did you give her?' It turned out that this was the first time anybody had ever used a stimulant drug on somebody who already seemed to be overstimulated. That started the seemingly paradoxical treatment approach of giving stimulants to hyperactive children."

The limbic system has been found to be the part of the brain primarily affected in hyperactive children. "Hyperactive children don't seem to have enough norepinephrine, a brain neurotransmitter, in their limbic system in the little cells that have to do with inhibitory control," Dr. Smith says. "That's why Ritalin, Dexedrine, Benzedrine, caffeine to a certain extent, and some other stimulant drugs have a calming effect on these children. They prevent the reuptake of norepinephrine at the synaptic cleft. This is something all neurologists understand.

"I was working with a lot of hyperactive children in my practice in Oregon," Dr. Smith continues. "I began to notice that these children had certain traits in common. They had short attention spans and they were unable to disregard unimportant stimuli. Everything came into their nervous system from their eyes, their ears, their skin, and their muscles with equal intensity. They were unable to selectively respond to certain stimuli and to ignore others. They couldn't just pay attention to the teacher, the board, or what was in their workbook.

"We found that many of these children would calm down after being placed on 5 or 10 milligrams of Ritalin or Dexedrine. If they responded we diagnosed them as having the hyperactive syndrome. If that didn't work, then we believed something else to be wrong.

"We had trouble ruling out psychological disorders or problems at home. You can imagine these children disrupting not only the classroom but the home environment as well, resulting in their parents either beating them or finding some other rigid disciplinary measure in their attempts to get these children to settle down and pay attention. Over a period of years I saw seven or eight thousand of these children and I noticed a pattern that interested me. I found a ratio of 5:1, boys:girls. This rules out Dr. Bradley's theory that hyperactivity was a result of a hurt to the nervous system. If he were right the ratio would have been 50:50.

Other patterns also were revealed, Dr. Smith says. "I also found these children to be fair most of the time. They were blue-eyed blondes and green-eyed redheads. We did see some African Americans but in general they were fair-headed and light-skinned. I concluded that some genetic factors were involved here. I also discovered that these hyperactive children generally were very ticklish, goosey, sensitive. When I shined a light in their ears to check their eardrums, the light would bother them as if they could hear a light and see sounds. It was incredible how sensitive they were. The stethoscope was always cold on their chest even though I warmed it up. My gentle hand on their abdomen to palpate the liver and spleen was an irritant and made them giggle and jump off the examining table. They noticed everything.

"As time went on, I started to incorporate nutritional testing and discovered that every single hyperactive child I saw had low levels of calcium and magnesium. I became interested in controlling behavior with diet after I noticed how my daughter responded to foods. If she ate sugary stuff she'd have trouble, but if she ate complex carbohydrates or protein, her level of activity was fairly even. I found that hyperactive children did well when eating five small good meals a day.

"I was hoping to discover a sugar causation and not a hurt to the nervous system. I found that about 15 percent of these children did have some hurt to the nervous system, but that most of them came from family backgrounds of alcoholism, diabetes and obesity, all sugar problems. I thought, 'Aha, I've got an answer here for hyperactivity. We should just stop the sugar.' It worked in a few cases, but not all."

Dr. Smith noticed other interesting signs. "Then I saw that most of these children had had ear infections as infants," he said. "We know that ear infections in general indicate food sensitivity, usually to dairy products. I discovered that their present diets were usually laced with milk, cheese, ice cream, and lots of other dairy foods. Stopping all dairy helped some of these hyperactive children but it still wasn't the whole answer. It showed that some of these children had trouble absorbing calcium from dairy products because they were allergic to them. Almost all these children had circles under their eyes and had had their tonsils taken out. They had retracted eardrums and would constantly clear their throats. That indicated a sensitivity to dairy products. Their intestinal tracts prevented the uptake of calcium from the milk they were drinking. Their blood and hair levels of calcium and magnesium were very low. Also, they weren't getting the calcium and magnesium they needed. We all know that calcium and magnesium have a calming effect on people.

"After many years of investigation, I had learned that hyperactive children are often ticklish, goosey and sensitive. They come from a family that has diabetes, obesity, or alcoholism. Generally, they're boys. Their teachers say they're in trouble. An especially important point is that they are usually okay one to one with their mother or father at home alone, but in a class of 30 other kids they cannot function. These children do better in small groups or one-on-one situations. That is ideal for them.

"Drug therapy helps them disregard unimportant stimuli. I found I could produce the same effect in most hyperactive children by giving them the right dose of calcium, usually 100 milligrams a day, and the right dose of magnesium, usually 500 milligrams a day. After receiving these minerals, usually 60 to 80 percent could manage without drug medication. It all seemed to fit. There was good evidence to indicate that hyperactive syndrome is related to food allergies, sensitivity to sugar, and not having enough calcium and magnesium.

"The next thing I noticed was that parents and teachers would report that many of these children were off and on, like Jekyll and Hyde. The parents would latch on to that little phrase as being almost diagnostic. That to me meant that it was not a psychiatric condition but a blood sugar fluctuation. It could come from eating sugar or from eating foods to which they were sensitive. We know that if people are sensitive to dairy products, for instance, the blood sugar will rise and get up to maybe 180 mg after eating a dairy food and then drop precipitously down to 60 mg. Then they crave these same dairy products again. They go up and down, up and down.

"If a teacher reports that a child is fine on Monday morning, doing his work and sitting still and then for no good reason on Monday afternoon he is all over the place, falling asleep or being disruptive, we can have a good idea that his behavior is related to something he ate for lunch. We have to carefully monitor the meals he eats and make sure the child doesn't get any particular food he is sensitive to. Along with milk the usual offenders are corn, wheat, soy and eggs."

Dr. Smith describes the diet he advocated. "The diet we recommend incorporates good foods as much as possible. Too much fruit may be detrimental due to the sugar. We recommend whole grain foods. We eliminate white bread, white rice, and empty-calorie foods. We don't have candy bars around. We don't have white soda crackers. We don't offer desserts to these children. We suggest good foods, complex carbohydrates, and vegetables, cooked as little as possible. Nibble, nibble, nibble is the rule we emphasize for hyperactive children. The whole family has to change their way of eating. Many of the parents find that they feel better on this diet as well.

"Once people change the diet of the hyperactive children, they find they can get off drugs, the Ritalin, Dexedrine or whatever else they are on, or reduce the dosage, or take it only on tough exam days. My results showed that 80 percent of these hyperactive children were made 60 to 100 percent better. Most of the children and their parents would notice a change for the better but still feel that something was missing.

"Then I found, as I got more into a nutritional approach, that I needed to incorporate more vitamins. I was missing vitamin B6, pyridoxine. I found that 50 to100 milligrams of pyridoxine was very helpful, especially if the child had trouble with dream recall. This is also good for children who can't seem to concentrate."

Two clues were critical, Dr. Smith says. "I would ask teachers or parents of these children, 'Is he goosey, ticklish, sensitive?' If they were, I would know it had something to do with calcium and magnesium. If they said, 'He has a Jekyll-and-Hyde personality. He's on and off, good and bad,' then I knew the problem was related to diet. As I became more nutritionally aware, I found out that many of these children had trouble with their intestinal tracts. I gave them vitamin shots. They sting. If it really stung and really made them hyper, that was because they weren't absorbing enough calcium. That was another clue. If you have enough calcium in your muscles then the stingy shots aren't so painful.

"Many parents said the vitamin shots were very important and that they really made a difference to the child, but I had no way to figure out how much B12 and B6 to give. It was helpful to me to find out that that could make some difference."

Dr. Smith worked with a chemist from Spokane named John Kitkoski, who discovered that most people in North America were somewhat alkaline. "This may be the key as to why this condition had become more common in the past couple of decades. The earth is aging and has become more alkaline. The increased incidence of this condition, even though obstetrical management has gotten better, is because our foods have gotten worse and more processed.

"This alkalinity, from which many of us are suffering, is often the key to this problem. If people are somewhat alkaline, the minerals, like calcium and magnesium, are less soluble. It's more difficult for the minerals to work with the enzymes to do all the things that they're supposed to do for the body if the minerals—especially the calcium and the magnesium—are not soluble enough to be usable.

"This is why many people have found that becoming vegetarian has made a difference for them. Vegetarianism tends to make people more acidic because vinegar is produced. Most vegetarians don't have trouble with high blood pressure.

"We can sometimes spot these people. Say a child of 9 or 10 is somewhat hyperactive. He has circles under his eyes and he's got a nose full of junk. He's got a nasal sound. We look at his jaw and it's narrow. His front teeth are crowded. We know that this child probably was not breastfed and that he probably is alkaline and probably drinking cow's milk, to which he is sensitive. Therefore, he's not getting the calcium/magnesium he needs. He's probably craving calcium and magnesium because he knows somehow that he needs it. He doesn't know, however, that he won't be able to absorb it."

Dr. Smith says it's imperative to consider all of the factors that could be causing a child's hyperactivity. "It's never just one thing. We were trained in medical school to make a diagnosis and to treat with a drug. The drug Ritalin is a standard for this. If it works that's a clue to me. If a stimulant has a calming effect then something is wrong with this person's ability to manufacture the right amount of norepinephrine for his limbic system. Therefore I can work on the diet and at the same time slow down the use of the Ritalin, which has side effects, such as leading to shortened stature. As this child grows up he is going to have to face the fact that he has got to change his diet."

Dr. Allan Spreen's position is very much in line with that of Dr. Smith. "My approach to hyperactivity is to try to get the individual biochemically in the best nutritional shape, and we usually get really nice results. Some people can have a very slightly sluggish thyroid that might not show up on blood tests. But with very low doses of thyroid, they feel so much better, even though their blood levels still remain normal on blood testing. Their whole emotional make-up improves. Their concentration gets better, and their energy level improves."

The late Dr. William Crook agreed with those who believe the disorder belongs to the modern world. "One of the advantages of having treated two generations of children is that I can say quite clearly that we did not see these children in the 1950s and early 1960s. Children now eat more fast foods, they drink more sodas, they spend more time looking at television than they spend in school, 28 hours per week. Television promotes junk food, television promotes violence. Children are indoors, not exercising, playing kick the can or riding bicycles. They're not getting full spectrum light that they get from sunlight; they're sitting in shaded rooms.

"Children need one-on-one attention. They need to be held, looked at and listened to. In our rushed world today, many parents struggle to do this, but they can't give their children the bed time stories, the hugging, the rocking to sleep, a lot of the things that I grew up with."

Increased use of antibiotic drugs is another major factor. "We were taught in the 1950s, parents and professionals, that antibiotics were wonder drugs," Dr. Crook said. "Parents would come in: 'My child has a fever, has an earache, give me an antibiotic,' and most doctors gave them antibiotics, which knocked out some enemy germs, but also knocked out friendly germs, disturbing the normal balance of bacteria in the intestinal tract. This leads to the overgrowths of a number of unfriendly organisms, including not only the common yeast, but other bad bacteria.

"This also creates what is called a leaky gut, so these children absorb food allergens that they would not ordinarily absorb. Food allergens are clearly related to ADHD. There are reports going back in the peer reviewed literature 70 years ago, and double blind studies in the 1990s, proving that children with ADHD are clearly sensitive to dietary ingredients. These included not only food but also the food coloring and additives. Also, pesticides in the food."

Dr. Crook believed that discipline is appropriate for misbehavior in hyperactive children. "The term discipline, from the Greek, comes from disciple and it really means teaching," he explained. "You've got to teach the child and there are clear scientific studies to show that rewarding good behavior, even with a smile or a pat, is much better than punishing a behavior that you disapprove of. Some children are difficult and hard to raise and you have to learn that the two to three year old is always getting into things and you don't punish him for doing the things that two to three year olds do. You have to think about what the child is saying, what the behavior means, and then you will be less apt to feel like you have to punish."

One of the main hazards of prescribing drugs, Dr. Crook said, is that you do not get to the cause of the problem. "Suppose someone has a headache. You can relieve it with aspirin or Tylenol, but suppose this person has a slow-growing brain tumor that is not recognized after you mask the pain? The second danger is that the child who takes long term Ritalin is apt to become a juvenile delinquent, to be put in jail. There was a study in the *Journal of Child and Adolescent Psychiatry* with two groups of Caucasian middle and upper class boys. One group received only Ritalin, the second group, multi-modality therapy, including psychological and educational counseling. Over a number of years, 22 percent of those that received only Ritalin ended up in a mental hospital or a jail. None of the others were institutionalized. There was, I should note, no difference in the two groups in terms of vandalism, marijuana use, alcohol use or petty crime.

"There are many, many nutrients, minerals and vitamins that are useful in treatment. Recent scientific studies support use of omega-3 fatty acids, found in flaxseed oil. We know about zinc. Studies of the effect of magnesium go back to at least 1922, when McCollum at Johns Hopkins put some rats on a low magnesium diet and those who did not get enough magnesium were irritable, had convulsions and some of them died. Much has been publicized for all of us about our needs for calcium, but magnesium is a very important nutrient for children. So are the B vitamins.

"The child's brain or the child's body is like an automobile and if an automobile is putting out blue smoke and getting six miles to the gallon and jumping and jerking, would you not look at the kind of fuel you're putting into the gas tank? We should look at the same thing for our children."

Dr. Mary Ann Block finds that 90 percent of the time, low blood sugar and food allergies or hypersensitivities are the underlying causes of behavior and learning problems. "You find behavior problems commonly in a child who eats too much sugar, doesn't eat enough protein and doesn't eat frequently enough. When they get hungry, they get irritable and agitated and when they eat, they calm down. The number one most likely food allergy—for behavior, eczema or asthma—is cow's milk. From there, it can be many other things—wheat, corn, certainly sugar—usually the food the child likes best and eats the most that is causing the symptoms."

Nutritional supplements are the backbone of her practice. "I recommend magnesium to all my patients because it has a calming effect, it relaxes the body, and if allergies are part of the problem, it can help with that as well. Seventy to eighty percent of the American population is deficient in magnesium, but for the ADHD child, it's imperative. Essential fatty acids are extremely important as is vitamin E—those work together. The mineral chromium is an important nutrient, often referred to as the blood glucose tolerance mineral. It helps the blood sugar stabilize. Almost every single hyperactive child I've seen has had a B vitamin deficiency too.

"I also recommend osteopathic manipulation. This is directly working with the nervous system of the body, very, very gently—it almost doesn't look like they're doing anything—so it's a nice treatment for children. The sympathetic nervous system causes the release of chemicals in our body that make us more hyper and sometimes osteopathic manipulation can help slow that down and get the nervous system more in balance."

Many practitioners, myself included, reserve our severest criticism for the drug industry, using the case of Ritalin as a prime example. In 2005, more than 31 million prescriptions were filled for stimulant ADHD medications in the United States, including about 10 million for Ritalin. Fueled by the magic bullet notion that popping a pill can solve a problem, sales of Ritalin and related drugs have soared more than 500 percent since ADHD became an official diagnostic category in 1980.

Ritalin does provide temporary answers—65 to 70 percent of the children show positive reactions—but the question is, what are the side effects?

As the experts explain below, we've known about the dangers of Ritalin for years. They include cardiovascular complications, strokes, heart attacks, anemia, psychosis, anorexia, and even death. Tragically, it took the FDA until 2006 to urge doctors to monitor for these complications, and until 2007 to order manufacturers of Ritalin and all other ADHD medications to include a "black box" warning label listing the risks. The move came after data revealed that fifty-one deaths in the United States between 1999 and 2003 may have been linked to use of Ritalin or Adderall.

Howard Pleper says, "This is scary. As I lecture around the country, parents come up to me and say 'my child has been on Ritalin and here are some of the side effects.' One of the biggest is anorexia—children absolutely lose their appetites, they stop eating. Anorexia is an extremely dangerous disease that weakens the immune system. It starts to look like chronic fatigue syndrome. Because Ritalin is a class 2 drug, like cocaine, withdrawal is extremely difficult when somebody has been on it long term, whether it is a child or an adult. The drug stunts growth. We have found children who have stopped growing, and I've seen some adults on Ritalin for several years who have stopped growing and are close to dwarfism.

"Ritalin causes serious depression. Children become little robots, they sit in class, and teachers love it because they don't cause problems, but the children become so depressed that they go back to the doctor and get put on another psychotropic drug for depression. A lot of children on Ritalin are not able to sleep at night, either."

Dr. Peter Breggin is even more angry. "We used to beat our kids and we used to think that was okay," he says. "Now that it is no longer generally considered okay to whip the daylights out of a child, more bizarre and potentially more destructively, we think it's fine to give a child toxic substances while the brain is growing.

"We have data on the dangerousness of these drugs. We know they can cause psychosis in children. Animal studies show that when you give amphetamines to animals in the same dose that you give to kids, after only a few times, you get brain cell loss and permanent changes in the brain. That is how these drugs become addictive.

"We have studies showing that if you take Ritalin as a child, you are more likely to abuse cocaine as a young adult. These stimulant drugs are considered so addictive that they are in a more addictive class than Valium and Xanax, which everybody knows are addictive sedative tranquilizers. It's astonishing to think that we are willing to do this to our kids.

"When you see what Ritalin does to an animal, it really demolishes the myth that the drug is correcting a biochemical imbalance in the child because there is the same effect on a monkey or a dog or a cat or a rat. These drugs suppress all spontaneity, all autonomy, all searching and exploring behavior. They suppress socializing behavior, they suppress the desire to escape and they enforce—probably because of their effect on the basal ganglia of the brain—compulsive, narrowly focused behavior. An animal like a monkey that was previously desperate to get out of its cage and play with its neighbor will instead sit quietly behind the bars picking at its own skin compulsively instead of grooming another monkey. That's what we do to our kids. We are making good caged children.

"I don't have language strong enough to describe how outrageous it is that literally multimillions of our children are already being suppressed with psychiatric drugs instead of having their needs met. Their needs for everything from nutrition to inspiring education, consistent discipline in the home and unconditional love. They are having their needs unmet while we drug them into submission instead."

Dr. Peter Tractman sees yet another grievous repercussion. "Among the children I have seen, 90 percent or more of those who have been diagnosed ADHD and are on Ritalin have a vision problem. They have trouble processing information through the vision system and into the brain. Once we give them some remediation and teach them how to process information properly, within about 10 weeks, they are usually reading on grade or very close to grade and the problem is gone.

"The reading problem can actually be caused by the drug. Ritalin's side effects include stunted growth, loss of appetite, baldness, Tourrette's syndrome, nervousness, rapid and irregular heartbeat, and insomnia. It also affects the eye's focusing. So Ritalin inhibits a child's ability to focus on print that is up close, for reading. So a drug with no proven efficacy to improve either cognitive ability or academic ability is given to a child, who suffers these terrible side effects, including his inability to see clearly so he can read."

18

Autism Spectrum Disorders

■■■

Patient Stories: Autism

My son Jamie is now three and a half years old. At about 15 months, he began to lose a lot of the qualities seen in normal children. He stopped talking, he stopped interacting, and he stopped making eye contact. All of this pointed toward autism. Before that, he had been very, very healthy and had developed well ahead of his milestones, except for a very long period of ear infections, which were treated by an equally long course of antibiotics. Over time, we became more and more concerned about him.

At about 18 months, he was diagnosed with severe language delay, meaning that he was not doing anything that the average 18-month-old child does to communicate. Also, he had developed a number of rather bizarre behavioral traits, including spinning and staring at the walls and only playing by himself. We saw a child psychiatrist in Maryland where we live. He thought we had a very serious problem, but he wasn't sure it was autism. He wanted us to look into the possibility of allergies and yeast infection. So we found various people to address those issues and Jamie began to improve.

As the improvement continued, he began to speak again, after about six months. But the improvement was somewhat limited. He still didn't interact with other children, even though a lot of the bizarre behavior had receded and he had perked up quite a bit. Looking for further help with the allergies and the developmental problems, because it still seemed as though there was a missing piece, we went to Princeton to see Dr. Baker. Dr. Baker has very thoroughly investigated Jamie's biochemistry and provided treatment and a lot of suggestions and support. Jamie experienced another big jump forward to the point that now his allergies are of relatively little concern, his development is almost on track (about six to eight months behind), and his behavior and his speech are vastly improved. In the fall, he will go to a normal nursery school, although the children will be six to eight months younger than he is. Aside from this, he will be back on track.

We realize that we are able to turn his symptoms on and off by simply modifying his diet, so we try to be careful with what we feed him. Sugar is the biggest offender. He can take it in very small amounts periodically. But if he gets too much of it, it is like shooting a rubber band across the room. He just flies around the house, becomes totally unreasonable, somewhat destructive and very aggressive. He also becomes overly emotional. He realizes that we are going to try to discipline him for acting out, even though he is aware that his behavior is not really within his control. So I think he feels unjustly persecuted when he is punished.

—Jamie's mother

I saw a four-and-a-half-year-old boy recently. His medical history showed that he had ear infections and multiple exposures to antibiotics, and that regression started around 20 months. Within two weeks after we put him on a milk-free and wheat-free diet, with no sugar and no obvious sources of mold or yeast, he began to talk and play with toys, to make eye contact and to relate to other people. I put him on a mild antifungal agent and he regressed markedly. His mother cut down the dosage to about a quarter of how much I had given him, which was already a small dose, and in about 10 days he brightened up. When he came back five weeks after the first evaluation, he walked in with a little spaghetti machine that he was pushing play dough into and cranking out play dough spaghetti, and he said, 'I'm making spaghetti.' He acted like a typical child, asking numerous questions of his parents about everything in the place. He had become a toy fanatic. They joined a toy-lending service, to meet his insatiable desire for toys.

The child, who is now about six, is reading, drawing and can sound out some words. He is still mildly hyperactive because he's reacting to the mold in the air, especially in the spring, but he is markedly improved. We also use nutritional support and his mother has him in an intensive tutoring program.

—Dr. Leander Ellis

Autism spectrum disorders are a group of developmental disabilities that typically appear during the first three years of life. They range from a severe form, known as classic autism, to a milder form, called Asperger's syndrome. Often, the term autism is used to refer to all of the spectrum disorders, as it will be in this chapter. People with autism vary widely in their abilities and behaviors, but all have some degree of impairment in verbal and nonverbal communication, and social interactions, as well as restricted, repetitive, or stereotyped patterns of behavior or interests. In addition, they often have atypical sensory responses to things they see, hear, touch, and feel.

According to the US Center for Disease Control and Prevention, one in every 150 children has autism. It is three to four times more common in boys than girls. The numbers of children being diagnosed have increased in recent years; some estimates say autism has grown at an annual rate of 10 to 17 percent since the late 1980s. Treatment options include speech, occupational and physical therapies; applied behavior analysis (ABA); highly structured, specialized programs; and dietary interventions. Medications are often used to address severe behavioral problems, anxiety, depression, inattention, or hyperactivity. With the exception of Risperdal—which was approved by the FDA in 2006 specifically to treat aggression, deliberate self-injury, and temper tantrums in children with autism—the medications are prescribed "off label."

Dr. Sidney Baker, a physician and researcher at the Autism Research Institute, offers insight into the nature of autism and the limits of our understanding of it. "All doctors are taught that if you get the right diagnosis, then you'll know the treatment for that person. My patient Jamie illustrates an essential problem with this belief. He was originally diagnosed as being autistic and there was relatively little discussion questioning the accuracy of that diagnosis. He really exhibited the classic symptoms of autism. But to say that because we know the diagnosis, we know the treatment for all the people in that illness group, is not a very useful approach. In Jamie, the pattern of biochemical abnormalities was not especially characteristic of autism. Jamie had a subset of problems that may go with that group, including disturbances of digestion (probably a disturbance of the germs that live in his digestive tract, which may be the mediators of the sugar response) and a bunch of other biochemical markers. My approach to treating him was simply to find everything that was out of balance and, keeping an open mind, to say, 'Let's measure as many things as are reasonable to do, step by step, and fix the imbalances where they occur.'

"I don't think that we entirely understand autism, even using this approach. I think that autism is the single most elusive diagnosis to make, at least in terms of finding the key to it. But when you approach children with what you could call this naive approach of fixing imbalances where you find them, it really works quite well. Part of the corrective action involves helping the child to stay away from things that he or she is bothered by—either foods to which he or she is allergic or sugars—and helping him or her get enough of the nutrients that seem to satisfy a particular biochemical need. Early intervention really helps a lot in the future of such children."

There has been an increase in research in recent years into the diagnosis and treatment of autism. In 2003, the US Interagency Autism Coordinating Committee introduced its congressionally mandated ten-year agenda for autism research. Clinical trials and research studies are now being conducted at various sites across the country.

Dr. Michael Schachter, one of the nation's pioneers in Complementary Medicine, describes what the natural medicine community has been doing: "There is some really good research, especially in France, that shows that magnesium and B6 will help considerably—though not cure—autism, much more than some of the drugs that are commonly used, and with fewer side effects. Some 10 or 12 double-blind, placebo-controlled studies have shown that magnesium and B6 are helpful for autism in children. I'm working with one young man now who's autistic, and we seem to have run up against some interactions with some of the drugs that he was on (including Inderal and Haldol). But the controlled studies indicate that autism can be helped with magnesium and B6. DMG, dimethyl-glycine, also seems to be helpful, not only with autism but also with reducing aggressive behavior."

According to Dr. Jay Lombard, director of the Brain Behavior Center in Pomona, New York, autism is associated with neurotransmitter abnormalities, in particular serotonin, which is derived from the amino acid tryptophan. "Autistic children have too much circulating serotonin, but it is not performing its duties properly, so you get symptoms such as anxiety and sleep disorder. One of the strategies of treating autism is to enhance the beneficial effects of serotonin. This can be done either nutritionally or pharmaceutically. Some of the nutritional compounds that increase brain serotonin levels include L-tryptophan, obviously, because it's a precursor to making serotonin; the herb St. John's wort, which acts as a serotonin enhancer in the brain; and a relatively new compound that has gained wide popularity—the modification of the amino acid SAMe or S-adeno-syl-methionine, which has also been shown to increase brain serotonin levels.

"The other part of treating autism has to do with the immune system, which is over-activated in a lot of children with autism who have chronic ear infection and chronic bowel problems. One of the things that we look at in our practice is excessive yeast involvement. We use probiotics like acidophilus, which helps increase the natural intestinal bacteria in the gut and reduce the amount of yeast.

"There is some evidence that autistic children have problems with the mitochondria in the brain, that they are not making enough brain ATP levels. Two compounds that are particularly effective are cretonne—which should only be given under a doctor's supervision—and a compound called CDP cauline, a form of cauline that helps build up brain cell membrane."

Dr. Alan Cohen is a prominent physician in Environmental Medicine who agrees that many children with autism have immune system abnormalities. "They have an increased sensitivity to infection, hyperactivity to vaccinations and as a result, they need to be on repeated courses of antibiotics," he says. "This leads to a whole cascade of effects which need to be addressed.

"Number one, there could be problems with the gastrointestinal tract as a result of the repeated courses of antibiotics and poor diet. There could be abnormal digestion, pathological alterations in the bowel flora and, as a result of an upset in the normal bowel flora, increased permeability to antigens, peptides and microbial toxins, which are produced by the abnormal bacteria in the intestinal tract. The gastrointestinal tract is directly related to the brain because the circulatory system connects both areas. If these toxins, antagonists and peptides that normally should be secreted are reabsorbed into the bloodstream, they can go to areas in the brain and cause disturbance in normal brain function."

Children should be assessed for certain biochemical abnormalities. "Autistic children may have low levels of certain sulfur amino acids or, very importantly, their livers may not be functioning well either," Dr. Cohen says. "We always build up our own internal toxins from the food that we eat and also external toxins that we take in from the environment. The main organ that handles all these toxins is the liver.

"The system needs amino acids, vitamins and minerals and other such nutrients to function properly. If this is not functioning properly, these toxins will again build up; instead of being excreted into the stool as they should, they will be reabsorbed into the bloodstream. Again, the circulatory system connects our entire body and these potentially harmful molecules and chemicals can end up in the brain, where they cause local inflammation and interfere with normal brain function. You see the effects of this in autistic children, as well as hyper-activity and attention deficit disorder."

Tests also are available for mineral deficiencies, especially zinc and selenium. Dr. Cohen says that children with autism "may have problems with heavy metal toxicity, which at times can be noted on hair analysis, and these include anti-mony, aluminum and arsenic. They also may have a history of subclinical hypothyroidism. The thyroid is extremely important for brain function. I have a number of children who had hypothyroidism detected based on their body temperature and when they were treated with natural thyroid hormone replace-ment, their will to concentrate, their behavior, their focusing and overall abil-ity to function improved as well.

"There are certain treatment modalities that people can do. I would have to say this should be supervised by a medical professional. There is a very impor-tant consensus report called *Defeat Autism Now* that people can get information from. Some basic, simple, inexpensive approaches can be tried that may bring a response from the child within 30 to 60 days."

Dietary interventions are often used in autism. "The diet should be very fresh, varied, totally free of additives and preservatives." Dr. Cohen says. "Avoid gluten, which is in wheat, oats, barley and rye, as well as milk protein. These sometimes cause food allergies, which can also affect the brain. Inflammatory components from allergies can end up in the brain, causing inflammatory reac-tions. I also suggest eliminating yeast and mold.

"I would advise a trial of avoiding certain common food allergens, including milk, corn, soy, eggs, tomatoes, beef, peanuts, and there are several more, but that should be individualized. Sometimes these children have difficulty breaking down protein and they reabsorb these peptides which are amino acids that tend to mimic or exacerbate neurotransmitter difficulties within the brain. Simply utilizing the enzymes that you get from papaya or pineapple can help to a cer-tain extent."

Many researchers have demonstrated the benefits of vitamin B6, as well as mag-nesium, calcium, zinc, selenium, and other nutrients. "At least 18 studies show 30 to 40 percent of children with autism respond to B6 replacement," Dr. Cohen says. "That dose depends on the child's size and age but could be from 100 to 600 milligrams a day. Also magnesium is extremely important, approximately 200 milligrams a day. Calcium, approximately 200 to 300 milligrams a day. Zinc, between 20 and 40 milligrams a day. Selenium, between 100 and 200 micrograms a day. A multivitamin is important, as well as essential fatty acids, including flaxseed oil or fish oil. There is also a vitamin-like compound called dimethylglycin which helps oxygenation to the brain.

For yeast overgrowth caused by repeated courses of antibiotics, Dr. Cohen recommends a trial of antifungal medication or either Nystatin or Diflucan, or natural substances such as garlic and citric seed extract and caprolic acid.

"I have seen a large percentage of children treated with traditional means, not benefiting, then switching to a more complementary or holistic approach and making major improvements," Dr. Cohen concludes. "This is a little bit more difficult to follow because it requires a lot of input on the part of the patients and the children to follow these dietary recommendations and the supplemental regimes. This takes a family effort and children very much have role models in what their brothers and sisters and their parents are doing. Everyone really needs to follow this approach. All I can say is that it is a very healthy approach for anybody to have a diet free of additives and preservatives, organic as much as possible, pesticide-free. A lot of these children have problems with the detoxification process in the liver and toxins build up. You want to minimize the amount of toxins that they are exposed to, by using organic food, with no pesticides and increased nutrients. A number of vitamins and minerals I talked about are increased in organic foods. All these things could be helpful for a lot of people in the family."

Orthodox medical opinion claims autism is caused by genetic defect, but many people have been looking at the possibility that vaccines are at the root of autism. Specifically, the concern centers around thimerosol, a mercury-based preservative that was used in several childhood vaccines until 1999, at which time thimerosol was removed or greatly reduced. An estimated 80 percent of children show significant improvement after detoxification of poisonous heavy metals from their system. Mercury is known to depress zinc, which simultaneously elevates the body's copper levels, the result of a dysfunction in metallothionein. According to Dr. William Walsh, senior scientist at the Pfeiffer Treatment Center in Illinois, 99 percent of children with autism show disorders in metallothionein: "Autism results from a genetic defect in metallothionein functioning followed by an environmental insult." Metallothionein is a protein that binds heavy metals and is responsible for the body's natural detoxification of many metals. Dr. Walsh reports that his center has used metallothionein-promotion therapy on many patients with autism, with good results. He warns that care must be taken to avoid the possibility of zinc depletion.

In 2006, the Autism Genome Project, a collaborative research effort of over fifty research institutes, sequenced DNA samples of over 1,200 families with multiple cases of autism and noted a chromosomal region with a common gene that might contribute to autism. While this study was hailed as a breakthrough by medical researchers, a strict genetic etiology for autism remains controversial.

What the research does not conclude is whether the identified gene is the direct cause of autism or whether one or more external agents—a toxic substance such as a heavy metal—affected the genetic chromosomal region.

Although mainstream medicine, citing the results of several large studies, appears convinced that there is no autism-vaccine connection, there are natural medicine practitioners, parents, and others who strongly disagree. A group of international researchers are finding evidence to support the measles vaccine as a potential cause for autism. Dr. John O'Leary, a highly respected molecular biologist in Ireland, discovered the presence of the measles virus in the intestines of 96 percent of autistic children. Normal children range around 7 percent. The statistical discrepancy cannot be associated with measles as a natural disease and can only be contributed to the vaccine. In one study published in the *Journal of Infectious Diseases*, one-year-old infants inoculated with the measles vaccine showed a dramatic reduction in their alpha-interferon levels, a biochemical produced by the blood lymphocytes. The result is a weakened immune system.

The debate goes on, and people continue to press their points at conferences, in medical journals, and even in courts of law. In June 2007, the US Court of Federal Claims in Washington, DC, heard the first of nearly five thousand pending cases filed by parents who believe their children's autism was caused by vaccination. The court will determine whether the family is eligible for compensation from the National Vaccine Injury Compensation Fund, which has paid out nearly $750 million for other vaccine injuries since 1986.

Defeat Autism Now, better known as DAN, is one of the US's preeminent organizations comprised of private physicians and researchers exploring novel biomedical protocols for the recovery of autistic children. DAN's therapeutic philosophy focuses on the treatment of the underlying causes of autism's symptoms. The method of screening is based on thorough medical testing, scientific research, and clinical experience. For the reason that recent research shows over

50 percent of children with autism having gastrointestinal symptoms, food aller-gies, and malabsorption, an important component of DAN's protocol is a com-prehensive nutritional assessment. The protocol also meticulously questions who the DAN theory believes are best suited for defining the autistic child's symptoms and behavior. Consequently, the protocol is based on the survey find-ings of over 23,000 parents, including parents' evaluations of the treatments prescribed to their children.

Through DAN's research arm, the Autism Research Institute, the following ele-ments are believed to make up the most complete and concise protocol for treat-ing autism.

IMPROVE DIET: A healthy, wholesome diet that avoids sugar and junk food. The DAN protocol recommends parents feed their children organic foods that are free of toxic chemicals such as artificial colors and flavors and preservatives.

FOOD ALLERGIES: Many autistic children have food allergies that hinder proper function of their digestive tract and/or immune systems. A significant study by Dr. R. Cade found that 87 percent of the autistic children tested had the pres-ence of IgG antibodies, which is indicative of an allergy to gluten. The autistic child is also frequently susceptible to dairy allergies. Identifying those foods that adversely affect the child's health are an essential component of a proper treat-ment regimen.

VITAMINS AND MINERAL: DAN research indicates that autistic children have additional metabolic needs. Supplementing the child's diet with vitamin and mineral supplements greatly improves metabolic activity as well as digestive function and sleep patterns.

High Dose Vitamin B6 and Magnesium: Research in over twenty studies shows that high dose supplementation of vitamin B6 and magnesium benefits enzymatic reactions associated with hyperactivity by 45 to 50 percent.

Vitamin B12 and Folic Acid: Vitamin B12 is essential for proper metabolism of fats and carbohydrates and for the synthesis of proteins. B12, along with folic acid, also have important roles in the repair of damaged villi in the gut, which are necessary for proper absorption of nutrients from food.

ESSENTIAL FATTY ACIDS: Infants and toddlers raised on infant formulas rather than mother's breast milk are deprived of the omega-3 and omega-6 essential fatty acids. Low levels of essential fatty acids have been associated with a wide range of psychological disorders and a couple of studies reveal that omega-3 deficiency is nearly always present in autistic children.

DIGESTIVE ENZYMES: Autistic children sometimes have decreased digestive enzyme levels, which contributes to the body's inability to digest food sufficiently. Supplementing the diet with these enzymes, particularly peptidases, has been considered an important element of the DAN protocol.

ANTI-FUNGALS AND PROBIOTICS: A frequent observation in gut analysis of autistic children is a low presence of beneficial bacteria and high levels of harmful organisms such as yeast. Supplementing the child's diet with probiotic formulas strengthens the good bacteria that are essential for proper digestion. According to the experience of DAN physicians, antibiotics should be avoided because they kill off the bacteria an autistic child needs.

MELATONIN: Digestive problems have been associated with poor sleep patterns. Sufficient, sound sleep is an important time for the body to heal itself, including the gut. The hormone melatonin is a commonly known sleep regulator and melatonin supplementation improves the autistic child's sleep.

SULFATION: Insufficient sulfation—the presence of sulfates—diminishes pancreatic enzymes necessary for digestion that in turn can lead to leaky gut syndrome. This disorder can be devastating for the child and can have a direct, adverse affect on neurotransmitter function. Autistic children frequently have low levels of sulfate. In such cases, the DAN protocol encourages sulfate supplements in the form of oral MSM or Epsom salt baths.

GLUTATHIONE: Glutathione, found in red blood cells, is an important biochemical for protecting the body from the toxic affects of metals, especially mercury. A 2006 study published in the *American Journal of Genetic Biology and Neuropsychiatry Genetics* confirmed frequent low levels of glutathione in autistic children.

CHELATION: The DAN philosophy is convinced that toxins, such as the heavy metals mercury, aluminum, and cadium, aggravate autism and in some instances might be the cause of autism's onset. Chelation therapy has been shown to be an effective, safe method for removing toxic heavy metals from the body.

IMMUNE SYSTEM REGULATION: Although seemingly less common, some autistic children have been found to have abnormal immune systems and evidence of autoimmunity disease. While the causes for this remain uncertain, the thoroughness of the DAN protocol takes this into account during its screening process for determining the best customized treatment for each child.

19

Behavioral and Learning Disorders

∎∎∎

Patient Story: Behavioral Disorder

My daughter, Maria, has been helped in a dramatic way by alternative medical approaches. A couple of months ago, Maria became wildly uncontrollable. She's only nine years old, but she was going out at 5:00 and 6:00 in the morning to shop with homeless people. She would go into violent rages and would sleep only about four or five hours a night. Finally, I couldn't keep her home anymore, so I put her into a psychiatric hospital where they determined that she was suffering from manic-depression. They started her on lithium but she wasn't herself; she wasn't conversational the way she usually was, and she was still depressed. She had elevated liver enzymes which, at the hospital, they failed to follow up on. She also had elevated levels of thyroid hormone, which they also failed to follow up on. After three weeks in the hospital, she had calmed down somewhat, and I was able to take her home. She still wasn't well.

I had been consulting with Dr. Slagle while Maria was in the hospital because I have the utmost respect for her and knew that if anyone could figure out what was wrong with my daughter, she could. As soon as Maria came out of the hospital, she had several blood tests done, that showed she had antibodies against her thyroid and that her thyroid levels were fluctuating up and down. Also, she had probably had some sort of liver virus that had precipitated this autoimmune reaction in her thyroid. Dr. Slagle prescribed amino acids, B vitamins and several other vitamins, as well as a homeopathic cortisone and baby aspirin to help shrink the swelling of her thyroid.

On the second day of her taking the aspirin and the homeopathic cortisone, her behavior became completely normal. It was a miracle. For close to a month and a half, my daugh-

ter had been completely out of control, unable to have a conversation, alternating between being hysterical and being completely quiet. I had been so terrified. It was as if I had lost her. And on the second day of the medication, she began to be able to hold conversations; she was completely normal—like herself again. I know that had I not gone to Dr. Slagle, she would have continued on lithium and been somewhat controllable, but not herself.

Dr. Slagle also found that my daughter was highly allergic. She had very allergic reactions to various foods that she was eating on a regular basis. It was clear that her problem had been her immune system and not a psychiatric disorder, which never would have been taken care of had she just stuck with traditional medical doctors, even though she was being seen by some of the best in the country. So thanks to Dr. Slagle and the alternative medical field in general, I have my daughter back.

—Maria's mother

Behavioral and learning disorders in children can be caused by a variety of factors, including problems during pregnancy and delivery, illnesses, injuries, genetics, and environmental conditions such as abuse, neglect, food or environmental allergies, and dietary deficiencies. There are many ways to help these children overcome their problems without padding the pockets of the pharmaceutical industry.

Approximately 5 percent of school-aged children in the US are diagnosed with learning disabilities each year, and the number is rising. A learning disability is defined as lack of academic achievement despite average to above-average intelligence. These children struggle with acquiring, retaining, and processing information needed to succeed in reading, writing, and math, and often have associated problems with self-esteem, depression, aggression, and more.

Behavioral disorders in children are often caused by chemicals. Dr. Harold Buttram explains: "Parents often use the term Jekyll-and-Hyde to describe their children. When they're doing well they may be sweet and lovable little children. Then, if they eat something to which they're allergic, very often a junk food, you get the Jekyll-and-Hyde transformation. They become ugly and belligerent. What actually happens here is the cerebral cortex, the higher center of the brain, literally shuts down and control gets thrown back to the more primitive centers. There is a center at the base of the brain, for instance, that has been shown to be a center for anger. What stimulates this center? Chemicals."

Dr. Buttram says there's a link between an increase in environmental toxins over the years and a corresponding increase in behavioral disorders in children. "What has happened in the past 50 years that has brought about this increase in behavior disorders? According to published reports, before World War II, less than 1 billion pounds a year of organic chemicals were produced in the United States. By 1963, that number had increased to 163 billion pounds per year. Today it is somewhere around 250 billion pounds per year.

"According to an official publication, approximately 70,000 chemical compounds are now in commercial use. Of these, only about 10 percent have had any testing at all for neurotoxicity. Among this 10 percent, only a handful have had thorough testing."

"Volatile organic chemicals are lipid or fat soluble. Therefore, they have an affinity for the fatty or lipid tissues of the body. The brain is a primary target because it consists largely of lipid or fatty tissues. It is also a target because of its rich blood supply. The primary symptoms of volatile organic compounds are therefore cerebral. They include headaches, dizziness, difficulty with concentration, memory lapses, feelings of fogginess or spaciness, drowsiness and fatigue."

It has long been known that behavioral changes are one of the first signs of chemical toxicity. "Therefore," Dr. Buttram says, "I think there are very good reasons for tying in environmental chemicals with the epidemic we're having of behavioral problems such as attention deficit disorder and hyperactivity. The massive increase of environmental chemicals to which these children are exposed is connected to their symptoms."

There are other factors as well. "A combination of subtle brain damage from environmental chemicals, nutritional deficiencies, a crippling of the detoxification systems of the body, food allergies, and an overgrowth of Candida in the system will produce a very sick child," Dr. Buttram explains. "The manifestation of this will be a crippled immune system. This means the child will have more allergies. He or she will be sick a lot of the time and on antibiotics. The brain function cannot possibly be normal; it would be a miracle if it were. The hyperactivity, attention deficit, and behavioral problems, in my opinion, are all actually a continued spectrum of the same thing."

Dr. Buttram identifies several specific groups of environmental chemicals. "Group one consists of toxic heavy metals, of which lead, of course, is the best known. This category would also include mercury, cadmium, aluminum and others. Our concern here is more with the other category, the volatile organic compounds, which are made up of carbon molecules. The commercial uses of volatile compounds break down into three major classes: formaldehyde, organic solvents and pesticides.

"Formaldehyde is present in many, many commercial products. It is present in new homes in the building materials, paneling, floors, and ceilings made of plywood or particle board. It's also present in the carpets, fixtures and furnishings. The bad thing about formaldehyde in a building is that it is very slow to dissipate. Its half-life may be 6, 7 or even 10 years. It takes this long before it is dissipated to the point at which the building is safe to live in. Formaldehyde is also used in fabrics and is found in many of the clothes we wear.

"Organic solvents are present in hundreds, if not thousands, of products. They are found in perfumes made from synthetic musks, for instance, and in caulking, paint, varnishes and cleaning solutions, which are often very toxic.

"Pesticides, our last category, may be the most dangerous of all. They are used, of course, to exterminate in homes or out of doors. If you live in a farm or orchard area, you may be subject to pesticide drifts. There are also often significant residues in foods, especially in foods imported from countries where there is no regulation in the use of pesticides."

Treatment of the wide range of illnesses arising from environmental chemicals must include education, enhanced nutrition, and nutritional supplements. "The pioneers in this field used to be called clinical ecologists, but they've now changed their name to the American Academy of Environmental Medicine," Dr. Buttram says. "These are the people who have really broken ground in this area. They're leagues and leagues ahead of the more conventional medical doctors, and they've set the standard for several of the approaches to treatment we recommend."

The initial step in treatment is parent education. "We educate parents on how to avoid chemicals," Dr. Buttram says. "For virtually all of them this is a first, because nobody has ever talked to them about these things before. Identifying and eliminating poisons in the home is not usually that difficult. We take a history of the home environment in regard to the building of the home and other possible sources of chemical exposure to the child. We teach parents how to reduce exposure to the more toxic chemicals, such as formaldehyde and volatile sprays.

"The problems that arise often occur due to exposure in school. If you have a cooperative school administration, the problems can usually be solved. But from what I have seen, school staff and administration don't usually recognize the potential hazards to children of chemical exposure and their ignorance of the risks sometimes presents additional obstacles."

In nutritional counseling, Dr. Buttram says, "we emphasize just plain simple food without chemicals. I detest the term 'health foods' because it's so misleading. I think 'plain foods' is a better term. I ask parents, who are now in their 30s and 40s, to think back about how their grandparents ate two generations ago. In many instances it wasn't ideal, but it was vastly superior to the way people eat today. They ate mostly plain, unadulterated food.

"So the prime emphasis on diet is the avoidance of chemicals. I attended a meeting in Dallas one time where Dr. William Rea was the speaker. He is certainly one of the most highly respected men today in the field of environmental medicine. Dr. Rea said that it's secondary whether a person is a vegetarian or a meat eater. What is far more important today is the avoidance of chemicals—both chemical additives and residual chemicals.

"For children I think it is imperative to get organic fruits and fruit juices even if you can't do anything more than this. From the figures I've seen, fruit and fruit juice tend to be more highly contaminated with pesticide residues than other classes of foods. Children eat more fruit and drink by far more fruit juice than adults. From this source alone, they could very easily ingest toxic levels of pesticide residues."

The third aspect of treatment is nutritional supplementation. "For practically all children, we recommend a high-quality hypoallergenic multiple vitamin," Dr. Buttram says. "We use one by Klaire Labs, which makes vitamins separate from minerals. We don't recommend giving large doses. We offer other nutritional supplements in special situations. When Candida is present from antibiotic overuse, lactobacillus acidophilus and bifidus are given. When lead and other toxic heavy metals are found, we add a very simple detoxification component to the program, which includes vitamin C and garlic. Garlic is added because it is high in the sulfhydryl amino acids.

"We recommend using a high-quality flaxseed oil. This provides the essential fatty acids for the development of the brain, nervous system and cell membranes. We emphasize nutrient minerals such as calcium and zinc since we know that these minerals can replace the toxic metals in the body. We particularly recommend beans and lentils, which are also high in sulfhydryl amino acids, because of their detoxification potential. The sulfur in these amino acids actually binds with the lead or other toxic heavy metals and helps to carry them out of the body."

Another important component in treatment is food allergy testing. "Most of these children are allergic to certain foods and some of their major symptom complexes can be related to their food allergies," Dr. Buttram says. "We can approach this either through elimination diets or else through skin testing, which we commonly do. We find neutralizing doses and treat with sublingual drops. This can work very well. When it does work you have some very grateful parents."

20

Chronic Depression in Children

■■■

Like behavioral disorders, chronic depression in children is also on the rise. According to the National Institute of Mental Health, it has only been in the past twenty years or so that childhood depression has been viewed as a serious problem. Among the symptoms are pretending to be sick, refusing to go to school, clinging to a parent, getting in trouble at school, being irritable and feeling misunderstood. However, these are also completely normal to every child in America and should not be pathologized. But regrettably, Big Pharma—working with the mental health community, pediatricians, psychologists, and nurses—have pathologized normal behavior as a result of this pernicious effort, and virtually any child can be diagnosed with a mental disorder.

Dr. Lendon Smith attributed the increase in cases to the toxic overload created by environmental chemicals. He was particularly adamant about the magnesium deficiencies that have occurred in many children as a result of environmental poisoning.

"Today there are more children who are chronically depressed than there were in the past," Dr. Smith said. "Our chemistry seems to indicate that chemical deficiencies are involved, e.g., magnesium deficiencies. Mr. Kitkoski, the chemist from Spokane, Washington, whose research I've shared, has spent a lot of time studying the function of electrolytes in the human body. He figured out that we all need the right amount of electrolytes to act as a buffering capacity for the blood. The electrolytes—sodium, potassium, bicarbonate, chloride, a little bit of sulfur, a little bit of magnesium and some calcium—are all the things that become electrically active when they are dissolved. Electrolytes have to do with controlling the pH, the acid/base balance, which controls what the minerals are doing, which brings us back to magnesium levels.

"I think that all the artificial chemicals that are in our environment and food are exerting a toxic overload on children. It's not just lead, but all the things that we are inhaling and eating, that are in our water, and all the things that are in our food that shouldn't be there, as well as the things that are removed from our food that we need. All these things are having an effect on our children.

"For example, I've visited classes of 25 or 30 children sitting there, restless, shuffling their feet, and I ask, 'How many of you have headaches once or twice a week?' and every hand goes up. I look around and see this sea of pale faces with circles under their eyes, as if they had all just been hit in the stomach. I ask them what they had for breakfast, and while they all said that they had eaten breakfast, it turns out to have been a donut or some other cake or pastry because their parents had no time to fix them a decent meal. Or, if the parents did fix them a decent meal, they wouldn't eat it anyway because they chose to get some candy on the way to school instead."

21

Food and Environmental Allergies in Children

■■■

Patient Story: Food Allergy

As Alison's mother, I can honestly say that Alison was born crying. She cried for the first two years of her life. I took her to a clinic at the time and found out she was allergic to corn, wheat and bananas, which caused her to cry every day, all day long. I took her off those foods, and she became a normal, happy two year old. She did well for quite a while until she got a problem with a vitamin deficiency, which caused her to be uncontrollable. I couldn't do anything with her. If I wanted her to get dressed she would scream, rant and rave. It would take me three hours just to get her dressed.

After reading an article on vitamins, I put her on vitamin supplements. That's when we realized that she hadn't smiled in six months. Then she was fine again, until two years ago, when she started to scream at me all the time, day in and day out, no matter what I wanted her to do, over absolutely nothing. She would scream at me that her shoes were wrong, her hair was wrong. It would take me all day long just to get her into the shower. At this point she was ten years old. She should have been bathing on her own. I would go pick her up at school and when she was seventy feet away from me, she would scream, "Mom, you are early!" And she would go on and on about why I was early. The next day she'd look at me and she'd scream, "Mom, you are late!" And she would scream the whole way home, until she went up to her room and I would go off somewhere else to get away from her. She got worse and worse all summer, and in the fall, almost two years ago, I took her to Dr. Buttram.

Dr. Buttram diagnosed my daughter as having food allergies: to corn, potatoes, chicken, egg yolks, rice and chocolate. They put her on these sublingual drops and now I have my normal, happy daughter back again. It was a dramatic change. She had become extremely difficult to live with. She would just scream at me about the most ridiculous things. Nothing was ever right. If she got out of bed—Why didn't I wake her up?—Why didn't I let her sleep?—And she would shriek at the top of her lungs. Some days were worse than others. Now I know that on the days she had a combination of foods or a lot of the foods she was allergic to that she was at her worst. The way that I figured out it was food again was because every once in a while we would have a great day or two and every once in a while her diet just happened to not include these things. Then she would be fine. But the next day she'd be right back again with the behavior—totally out of control for long periods of time.

When my mother found out about Alison's behavior, she told me that I myself had been an absolutely horrendous child. Now that Alison had been diagnosed, she understood that I had had food allergies too. Now I understand that children's behavior problems are not always due to what the parent is doing with the child, as far as discipline is concerned. I've had a lot of children; I've been a foster parent for years. When Alison first started this behavior I tried everything in the book and nothing worked. And the thing that told me that something was controlling her, instead of her doing this, was the fact that we would have good days. And it didn't matter what we were doing on a bad day. If I would sit and play with her all day long, and it was a bad day, we would have a bad day. And discipline meant absolutely nothing, because something was controlling Alison. It was a chemical imbalance in her brain that was controlling her because she had absolutely no control over what she did. It was like the food was controlling her. I related it to the behavior of a manic-depressive or a paranoid schizophrenic who has no control over what they are doing.

Now, when I go to the shopping mall, I see kids who I know have food allergies by the way they are crying. My husband used to say I was crazy, but when Alison was two years old and she would cry, I could tell if it was a food-allergy cry or a two-year-old cry by the sound of her voice. It was a different kind of crying. I have friends who complain about their kids constantly and one child in particular I know has food allergies. And the mother will not take him in to be tested. She'd rather complain about it. The biggest obstacle I see to helping children with behavior problems caused by allergies is making parents understand that there is an alternative. You don't have to live like this. You have to ask yourself, "Do I really want my child to live like this?"

I feel bad that Alison was so miserable for so long. There are so many kids out there that are this miserable. There are kids in learning disability classes and the parents just don't look any farther than their noses. Some parents do make an effort and take their kids to standard allergists who test them, but those doctors may not be able to locate the problem. A friend of mine took her child to a regular allergist who tested him for all the standard things and said he was fine. But he never tested him for half the things to which Alison is allergic and the doctor never questioned the mother about the child's diet.

—*Alison's mother*

When people think of childhood allergies they think of hay fever, asthma, eczema, and hives. But there are many other areas of the body that can be affected by allergies. As Dr. Doris Rapp informs us, "Allergies can cause headaches or stomachaches; they can affect the bladder, causing your child to wet the bed or to have to run to get to the toilet in time. Allergies can cause leg aches, muscle aches, joint aches, sleep problems, behavior problems and learning problems. Some children will become tense, nervous and irritable. Others will become withdrawn and unreachable, hiding in corners and pulling away when you go to touch them. Still others will become very hyperactive and aggressive. Often they will bite, hit, scream and do all kinds of nasty things.

"Most allergists—including myself for my first 18 years in practice—would not recognize this host of physical and emotional symptoms as having been caused by allergies. But I now recognize that dust, molds, pollens, foods and chemicals can affect almost any area of the body and can cause all of the problems mentioned above in some individuals.

"Now it would be going too far to suspect that every time a child has a headache it is an allergic reaction, or that every time he has a bellyache it is due to food sensitivity. But currently, with conventional medical practitioners, this diagnosis is never even considered and is therefore missed too many times. People will have headaches for years and never once consider whether there might some underlying reason for the headache.

"Environmental medicine wants patients to start to take more control of their health. We want you to pay attention to how you feel. If you don't feel well, or you suddenly can't think correctly; if you're confused, or unusually irritable or emotionally volatile; if you cry or become upset or angry for no reason; you have to start to ask, 'Why am I having this reaction now? What did I eat, touch, or smell?' Our whole society is geared to go to the medicine cabinet for a painkiller or an antihistamine when we should be geared to get a pencil and paper to record what could be causing this problem at this time."

Dr. Rapp tells how a little knowledge and awareness can go a long way. "After we have educated the parents," she says, "they often come in to see us knowing exactly what is causing their child's problems. They can tell if it's something inside or outside the house, if it's a food or a chemical. They can pinpoint the cause."

Among the reasons why a child may have allergies or environmental illness is an impaired immune system. "One way to strengthen the immune system so that your child is less prone to environmental illness or allergy is by using various nutrients. A helpful resource is the book, *Super Immunity in Kids*, which says, basically, if you take the correct nutrients in the correct amounts, you can strengthen the immune system so that you are less apt to become ill from natural things such as pollen, dust and mold exposures. You will also be less apt to become ill from exposure to infections.

"Now how can a parent tell if their child's learning problems are related to environmental factors? Think back. Does your child say, 'When I go to school in the morning I feel great!'? Or does the child say, 'I feel great when I leave the house and by the time I get to school I don't feel right'? Or does he say, 'I feel nervous or tired or irritable,' or, 'I have a headache'? If that happens, you have to think, it might be the fumes on the school bus, or what he ate for breakfast, or what he uses to brush his teeth, or the soap that he uses. You've got to think of everything that he came in contact with before he got on the bus, and then what happened when he was on the bus."

Dr. Rapp suggests driving the child to school. "If you find he can eat, bathe, wash and do everything else in the usual manner in the morning and you drive him to school and he's fine, then it's probably the bus that is causing problems. And you can check back and forth a couple of times and try to confirm or negate your suspicions. Now, children who are sensitive to things in the school will frequently notice that their headache starts within an hour. And the headaches frequently become more intense during the day. By Friday afternoon, the headache will be much worse than it was on Monday morning or on Sunday night. At first the headaches may disappear one to four hours after your child leaves school, but later on, if there are too many exposures during the week, you may notice that they don't get better at night and that it might take the whole weekend for the headache to go away."

A heightened sense of smell is also a sign that something is not right.

"Another clue that certain exposures are making your child feel worse is when your child can smell everything before anybody else. She smells natural gas, or smells that perfume across the room, or she can smell food cooking before anybody else. She can smell disinfectants. If these odors bother your child and she can perceive them faster than anybody else, it means that she is probably becoming sensitized to the abundance of chemicals that we have now managed to put in our food, air, water, clothing, homes, schools and workplaces.

"What else do you notice if a child is sensitive to something in school? The child may get an A one day, and an F the next day in the same subject. It isn't that your child lost brain cells within 24 hours, but it does indicate to me that you should investigate that school to try to find out what could be causing the problem. Is the school dusty or moldy? Are the ventilation ducts open and clean? Was the basement of the school ever flooded? Does it smell worse on damp days? There is nothing worse in present-day schools than some of the synthetic carpets. They are made of chemicals that cause problems. In addition, they use adhesives that are full of other chemicals that cause even more problems. Many of these chemicals are neurotoxic, which means they damage the nervous system, or carcinogenic, which means they can cause cancer."

Other symptoms include impaired ability to hear, talk, or speak clearly; difficulty writing, reading or seeing clearly; red earlobes or cheeks; wriggly legs; and dark circles under their eyes.

"If you suspect that your child may have been exposed to neurotoxic substances—those that actually damage the nervous system—ask your doctor to send you to specialists who can tell you whether the nerve conduction time in your child's body is normal or not," Dr. Rapp says. "They can do a variety of blood tests to find out if the chemicals that are in the carpets and the adhesives are in the blood.

"The doctor may even make an allergy extract of the air in a room that smells of chemicals. Sometimes when the child is exposed to just one drop, we can actually reproduce a headache, a stomachache or problems thinking. The doctor makes the allergy extract the same way one would bubble air through a fish tank: Using a pump to bubble the room air through a salt solution in a tiny test tube. The air bubbles for about eight hours and at the end of this period a solution remains that contains some of the chemicals that were in the air. Then an allergy extract is prepared from this solution which can be injected in the skin, or placed under the tongue. If it causes numbness in the arms, tingling in the fingers, a headache, stomachache, problems with remembering, or a change in activity or behavior within 10 minutes, we have probably collected the problem chemical from the air within the solution."

Provocation/neutralization testing also may be used. "The doctor can then make dilutions of that chemical solution and probably eliminate those same symptoms with one drop of the right dilution of that solution," Dr. Rapp explains. "In other words, if the child develops a headache in a certain room, you can put a drop of the air allergy extract under the tongue and provoke the headache in 3 to 8 minutes. Then you can give the child a five-fold weaker dilution of that same solution and often you can eliminate or neutralize the headache in less than 10 minutes.

"After you have done a skin test with the allergy extracts, and shown that there is a cause-and-effect relationship between the child's behavior or physical symptoms and a chemical in the school, the next thing is to determine what the school can do to eliminate the problem. One of the things they can do is not put carpets in schools. If they do have carpets and they're causing problems, they can take the carpets up and put in hard vinyl tile. In such cases, it is important to insist that they use adhesives that are safe when installing the tile."

Poor ventilation can cause problems. Dr. Rapp says, "Due to the energy crunch we had in the '70s, many schools closed down their ventilation systems to save money and to cut down on the cost of heating. Dust, molds and chemicals have accumulated at very high levels in these schools. The windows don't always open, and the result is that there has been a gradual build-up, so that more and more children and teachers seem to be adversely affected when they go to school."

Parents should insist that school administrators check the ventilation system, Dr. Rapp says. "There are fast and easy ways to measure the amount of carbon dioxide in a classroom, which can tell you whether the ventilation is good or not. The level should be 800 ppm or less. Relatively simple tests can also be done to measure for certain chemicals, such as chlorine and formaldehyde. Sometimes, because of poor cleaning of the ventilation systems in schools, the problem is dust and molds, not chemicals. Other times, they put chemicals in the ductwork while cleaning, which really causes trouble because the chemicals then circulate throughout the school, causing illness. Sometimes the intake for the ventilation system is too close to the area where all the school buses line up. The bus drivers let the engines idle for long periods, resulting in all the gasoline fumes and hydrocarbons entering the ductwork intake and circulating throughout the school.

Dr. Rapp describes some of her cases involving environmental allergies. "In one case I encountered, a school had a printing press, and the exhaust pipe from the printing press was at exactly the same level as the ventilation intake on the roof, with the result that all the chemicals from the printing press were going right back in and circulating throughout the school. Some printing press chemicals are toxic to the nervous system and cancer-causing.

"A patient I saw last week has three sons who came home smelling of mop oil, which is used to clean the school. The mother said that the children's clothes smelled so badly that she had to use very hot water to eliminate the smell. One of the boys developed a headache and a burning sensation in his throat. So I asked her to bring some of the mop oil and I just put it underneath his nose and let him take one whiff of the odor. Within seconds, he was complaining of a headache around his forehead on both sides of his temples and he said it was throbbing and that his throat was burning. I gave him oxygen for about 10 minutes and the headache, throbbing and burning in his throat gradually subsided. We videotaped this reaction.

"There was another child who had trouble only on the two afternoons a week when he went to school. He would be weak and tired, hardly able to stand; he couldn't hold a pencil, clung to his mother, but only on those two days. I sent the mother to the school and asked her to try to figure out what's different in the schoolroom that might be causing her son's problems. It turned out that they used a very common disinfectant aerosol in the room, six times a day on the tabletops, to reduce infections. Then they used the same solution on the cot that he napped on. All she had to do was ask the school to stop using that disinfectant and install an air purifier, and the child improved remarkably.

"Then the mother noticed that he had similar problems when he went into the gym, and it turned out that they were using a certain kind of floor wax in the gym. We suggested that they use something that had fewer petrochemicals in it and the result was that he can now be in the gym for 20 minutes. That child had tics and twitches, which is another thing that you see in some children with these allergies. The symptoms disappeared after environmental allergy care."

Food allergy must also be ruled out. "Ideally," Dr. Rapp says, "your child should eat only organically grown food because it is less contaminated with pesticides, food coloring or other chemical additives that may be causing adverse reactions. However, in some places, it remains difficult—and expensive—to buy foods uncontaminated by chemicals. I encourage people to grow their own vegetables so that they will have their own source in the winter and one which they know does not contain any chemicals.

"There is one very important and simple thing you can do to tell which area in a school or in your home, or which food, might be causing your children a problem. Ask your children how they feel before they eat a meal, or before they enter a particular room. Also ask them to write their name and to draw. You should do the same thing. And then, if you have asthma, blow into something called a Peak Pocket Flow Meter, which is a plastic tube with a gauge on it. If you blow 400 before you eat and half an hour later you blow 200, one or more of the foods that you ate is causing asthma or spasm of your lungs. Check out each food separately five days later and find the culprit.

"Another thing to do is to take your child's pulse before eating. If the pulse is 80 and suddenly after eating it is 120, a food has set off a silent alarm in the child's body, which has caused her pulse to increase. So check the writing, the drawing, the pulse rate, the breathing, and how your child feels and looks before a meal and then a half hour or so later. If any of these variables indicates a change for the worse after a meal, one of the foods your child ate may be the cause of the problem. If the change occurs after being in a particular room or area, something in there may be at cause."

Dr. Rapp says to wait before trying to identify the problem food. "It is critical that you wait five days to get all that particular food out of the body. So for five days, if you have noticed your child had a reaction after eating corn, don't feed your child corn (and tell her not to eat any at school either). Then at 8:00 a.m. on a Saturday, give her the first of the foods she may have been reacting to, and at 10:00 a.m. give her the second possibility, and at noon the next one. In this way, you check each food all by itself. Again, check the breathing, the pulse, the writing and drawing, and how your child feels and looks before and a half hour or so after each food.

"You can apply the same principles of food isolation to every room in your house and at school or every room at work. Check your breathing (or your child's breathing) before you enter a room, do all the things that I suggested above, and then do them again several hours later. If you find that a particular room is a problem, then you have got to ask, 'Why? What do I smell in this room, what am I touching in this room, what is in this room that could be bothering me? Is it the heating system, the covering on the furniture, the carpet, the floor wax, the furniture polish? Are there items that have been dry-cleaned in this room? Is there an odor?' You'll be surprised at how much you can figure out on your own."

The car and other things outside your home should also be checked. "Notice how you and your children feel before you get in the car, then check again half an hour later," Dr. Rapp says. "Compare indoors with outdoors and you'll be able to tell whether it's the outdoor pollution, the lawn spray next door, the mold, pollen, or pollution in the air that is causing problems outside versus inside. You can easily figure out many, many answers by checking your child's pulse, his breathing, and how he writes, draws, feels and looks. Check these same parameters on yourself as well. If you have high blood pressure, you can even use a blood pressure cuff and check your pressure before and after each of these exposures and you'll turn up answers. By keeping detailed records, you can often figure out the reasons why your children are ill, and many times you can then get rid of the cause and make them feel much better.

"Keep in mind: The indoor and outdoor factor that causes more problems than any other is molds. If you live in a moldy house and you are always wheezing, on cortisone, always sick and in and out of the hospital, it could be the moldy house that you are living in that is causing the problem. Sometimes if you live in too much mold, it doesn't matter what kind of treatment you're on. You have to move or get away from the thing that is causing the problems.

"There are some new ways of doing brain imaging that can actually show changes in the brains of some of the people that are exposed to neurotoxic substances. For example, if a child sniffs glue or hair spray or aerosols, you can actually show a characteristic pattern of change in the brain imaging-pattern on the particular individual, which will look different from somebody who has epilepsy or someone who has schizophrenia or depression. They actually produce different brain pictures. I'm sure in a few years, many people who say they are always depressed, or tired, or nervous will be able to have a brain-image pattern taken that will show that specific areas of the brain have been affected by certain exposures or foods."

PART FIVE

Organic Conditions Commonly Misdiagnosed as Mental Disease

22

Blood Sugar Instability (Hypoglycemia)

∎∎∎

Patient Story: Hypoglycemia

I had been seeing a psychiatrist for depression and was on medication—and still am. I noticed that while the medicine took care of certain symptoms, it seemed to have no effect on an enormous number of them. I used to be a body-builder back in the early 1980s, so I had some experience with nutrition. I went to see Dr. Spreen because I noticed that my hypoglycemia was acting up; I noticed a direct correlation between what I ate and how I felt. When I went to see him, I was complaining of really severe panic disorders, irritability and difficulty in concentrating. I went from having an excellent memory to no memory at all. Also I had such fatigue it felt like I was walking in Jell-O all the time. I'd sleep 12 hours a day and get up with no energy at all after sleeping. I'd be tired the whole day.

The first thing Dr. Spreen did was to give me injections of B12. Immediately I noticed a difference. As soon as I'd walk into the gym to work out, my energy was there. In the morning I felt really good. But I was still plagued sometimes by panic attacks. So he put me on a high dose of tyrosine, which is one of the free-form amino acids. I took up to 7 grams a day and noticed a real strong response. Tyrosine is also related to the thyroid because one of the products the thyroid needs for normal functioning is tyrosine. He also put me on a low dosage of thyroid, a quarter grain a day. I took that and noticed immediate results. With that and the tyrosine, I felt like a new person.

This experience showed me that even though a doctor may be treating you for depression, he might be missing the things that might have led to the depression or that might go hand in hand with it. Many books that I've read—in particular, Carlton Frederick's

New Low Blood Sugar and You—*say that when there is any mental disorder present, hypoglycemia is going to be right there along with it. But the medical community doesn't accept that hypoglycemia is as predominant as some nutritionists say it is because the doctors are thinking about the organic forms, which are much rarer. But with the diet that we are eating today, which is high in carbohydrates and low in basically everything good for you, hypoglycemia is manifesting itself in great numbers.*

As a child, I ate a diet that was full of simple carbohydrates—all sorts of sweets and sugars—and had a lot of the symptoms that are associated with hypoglycemia: I was hyperactive and had asthma. You see, hypoglycemia can trigger asthma attacks. Since I started working out and watching my diet, the asthma went away.

For the panic attacks, Dr. Spreen suggested vitamin C. I took vitamin C powder, which is ascorbic acid, in the morning. I probably took 15 to 20 grams a day. It was almost like taking a sedative. It calmed me right down. My thought patterns straightened out; I was calm; and I wasn't as irritable and fidgety as I had been. I balanced out the rest of my nutrients with a mineral supplement and a good vitamin supplement high in the B spectrum. I take an additional B complex with pantothenic acid on the side because Dr. Spreen thinks that most people don't have enough B vitamins in the diet. I'm inclined to agree with him, since I've followed his advice and noticed an enormous positive response.

—William

Hypoglycemia occurs when a person's blood sugar concentrations are abnormally low and not sufficient to meet the body's needs. Dr. Hyla Cass elaborates: "Hypoglycemia can result from a combination of stress and poor eating habits, particularly in people genetically predisposed to this condition. The disorder can present itself in a variety of ways: depression, irritability, anxiety, panic attacks, fatigue, 'brain fog,' headaches including migraines, insomnia, muscular weakness and tremors, all of which may be relieved by food. There can be cravings for sweets, coffee, alcohol or drugs.

"In fact," Dr. Cass continues, "many addictions are related to hypoglycemia. Coffee and sugar consumed by recovering alcohol or drug addicts only prolong their problem, though in a less dangerous, more socially acceptable form. (It is interesting to note the large amount of these substances consumed at Alcoholics Anonymous meetings, for example, and on psychiatric wards.)

"Such individuals can often overcome coffee, drug and alcohol addiction through correcting their hypoglycemia, with minimal withdrawal symptoms or later cravings. For recovering alcoholics, for example, I recommend the hypoglycemic regimen described below plus the amino acid glutamine, 500 milligrams, three to six times daily, which is particularly useful to counteract cravings.

According to Dr. Cass, people with hypoglycemia are often diagnosed as though they have simple depression and anxiety, and then treated for a psychological condition. "They are put on antianxiety agents such as Valium or Xanax. If they are extremely depressed as well as anxious, they are put on antidepressants such as Prozac. I've had people come to me on medication who wanted to go off of it. It turned out that they were hypoglycemic.

"You can replace antidepressants with amino acids, minerals and cofactors, vitamins for amino acid metabolism," Dr. Cass says. "When depressed patients come to see me who are also hypoglycemic, I put them on a hypoglycemic diet, which is approximately six small meals a day. Also, I have them take chromium for balancing their blood sugar levels. I also give them magnesium, glutamine and tyrosine. Tyrosine is an excellent natural antidepressant. It's a precursor to the neurotransmitter norepinephrine, which is one of the brain chemicals that helps us feel good."

Dr. Cass recommends the following hypoglycemia program, which is designed to both strengthen the adrenals and maintain adequate blood sugar levels: elimination of refined carbohydrates (sugar, white flour), coffee and alcohol; small, frequent meals of complex carbohydrates, high fiber foods and protein; and daily supplementation with a multivitamin/mineral complex that includes 200 to 600 micrograms of chromium, 200 to 400 milligrams of magnesium, 10 to 20 milligrams of manganese, 500 to1,000 milligrams of potassium, 50 to 75 milligrams of B vitamins, 500 milligrams of pantothenic acid (vitamin B5), 3,000 milligrams of vitamin C. Dr. Cass says that these supplements can be divided into doses taken two to three times daily.

Dr. Leander Ellis suggests that hypoglycemia can be brought on by a variety of causal factors, some circumstantial, others stress-related, still others environmental. "Hypoglycemia," he explains, "is a phenomenon that can be triggered by allergy, infection, exhaustion, or large amounts of sugar that encourage the growth of yeast in the intestinal tract, which then, in turn, gives rise to some allergic effects and a variety of other subtle effects. I see hypoglycemia as a symptom of a larger problem, rather than as a disease.

"Most of the time there are other important causes to account for the rollercoastering of the blood-sugar levels. The most common one is probably Candida, yeast. The next most likely cause is food allergy. Often, a person is not only gorging on sugar, but is allergic to sugar, is not only gorging on chocolate, but is allergic to chocolate. So you get a curious combination of Candida, yeast mold, fungus allergy and allergy to foods. You usually have to control these several elements, as well as get adequate nutritional support, in order to quiet these symptoms down."

Although Candida is a major factor in hypoglycemia, as well as other chronic conditions, the mainstream medical profession has continued to ignore it. "The major reason for this," Dr. Ellis says, "is that medicine is taught by prestige suggestion, meaning a doctor needs someone he or she trusts to tell him what is important. Unfortunately, the people that we doctors have the most contact with after we leave medical school are drug company representatives. Therefore, until a learned professor at an Ivy League medical school tells us that Candida is a problem, it doesn't exist."

Dr. Warren Levin explains the basic physiology of hypoglycemia, as well as some of its special characteristics. "Hypoglycemia is a basic problem that is frequently stress-induced. When people take a large dose of sugar into the body (and one cola drink contains more sugar than the entire bloodstream), the level of sugar in the body goes way up. Now, the body's entire commitment is to maintain balance or equilibrium (the technical word is homeostasis). The body produces a basic hormone called insulin that is supposed to take the sugar from the blood and deliver it into the cells, and when the sugar goes up very rapidly the body reacts excessively, resulting in too much sugar being driven out of the blood, and that produces low blood sugar, or hypoglycemia. The body then has to correct the balance again, and it can be an emergency. If the blood sugar goes too high, it is not an emergency; the body can tolerate it. But the brain requires a certain level of blood sugar to function, so when the blood sugar starts plummeting—and it can sometimes drop at a frightening rate—the body calls forth its emergency hormone, adrenaline.

"Adrenaline was designed to protect us against the saber-toothed tigers back in the primitive world. It mobilizes all sorts of bodily functions. One of the things it does is to dump sugar from the liver into the blood very rapidly. However, adrenaline also causes what we call the fight-or-flight reaction, associated with the state of fear. We get a rapid heartbeat, dry mouth, sweating, fear, and a sense of impending doom."

Dr. Levin concludes with a cautionary tale that contains precisely the kind of great wisdom and knowledge that the medical community needs to hear: "Now, suppose someone has an ice cream sundae and a few hours later he or she sits down to read the funny papers and all of a sudden he or she gets this terrible reaction. The individual goes to the doctor and explains that while just sitting there, reading the paper, all of a sudden the skin got sweaty and the heart started pounding. The doctor says that the problem is all in the head and that the patient must have a Prozac deficiency. 'With this Prozac prescription,' the doctor adds, 'you'll be fine.' We have to stop thinking that way. Headaches are not a Darvon deficiency, depression is not a deficiency of Elavil, and until doctors realize that the body's biochemistry is an exquisite balancing act, and start treating it with great respect, we are in a lot of trouble. Hypoglycemia is not a disease; it is a symptom requiring a search for an underlying cause."

23

Candidiasis

■■■

Patient Stories: Candidiasis

I have suffered from chronic candidiasis since I was about 13. We think it might have been linked to my taking massive doses of sulfa drugs for kidney problems when I was younger. I can't remember a time since I was 13—and I'm 31 now—when I didn't have a yeast infection. There may have been 2- and 3-week periods when I wasn't suffering from symptoms, but I always, to some extent, had a very severe yeast infection. I went to conventional doctors and they gave me the typical vaginal and topical cremes, and basically patted my hand and told me to come back and see them in two weeks. These medications seemed to help during the time that I used them, but invariably the infection returned, and was often twice as bad after I stopped the treatment. So after a while, I simply avoided going to see any physician and just lived with the problem, except on the occasions when my symptoms got so severe that I just had to go see someone.

Eventually, I went for a Pap smear and a nurse practitioner suggested that I read a book called The Yeast Syndrome. *It wasn't until I read the book and got Dr. Stoll's name out of it that I even connected my physical ailments with my mental health. I had always been moody and prone to periods of depression and there was a history of depression in my family. I never needed to be hospitalized, but I felt that some of these bouts, especially during my adolescent and college years, were extremely severe. I suffered mood swings and would have described myself as having a very volatile personality. But after going to Dr. Stoll, who started me on oral Nystatin, changed my diet, and used various supplements to correct my nutritional and physiological deficiencies, within about 60 days I felt like a totally different person. In fact, my husband commented that it was like being married to a different person. In hindsight, I can see that as my candidiasis symptoms were eradicated, my mental symptoms disappeared. So I use mental symptoms now as a red flag. If I start seeing personality changes within myself, I take a look at what I've been eating lately and how I've been feeling, and make some changes there. Then I seem to get back on track.*

I have learned that conventional treatments that just treat the symptoms are not going to help you. You have to look for the root cause of your ailments. There is help out there to be found. You simply have to find someone like Dr. Stoll who knows how to treat your illness, and comply with their recommendations. You will get better.

—Ellen

My youngest child was born with a lot of health problems—nothing life-threatening, he was just sick all the time. He lived on antibiotics from the day he was born until he was about five years old. He cried all the time and never slept. Most people don't think of an infant as being depressed, but when a baby cries all the time, you could say he's depressed, or in an anxious state, or in a state of pain. It was certainly very stressful for the both of us. As it turned out, most of his problems were allergy-related. He had ear infections, bronchitis, very severe eczema, and his digestive tract had become very permeable.

Within a month after I had taken my son to Dr. Stoll, and we had begun regenerating his intestinal lining through treating his candidiasis and watching his diet, I began seeing some improvement. Six months later, he was a totally different child. We were a totally different family.

My child had inherited his allergy problems from my mother-in-law. She had severe asthma and emphysema, and she was extremely depressed because she thought that she was dying. She was so sick that she would crawl out of bed in the morning to a chair, and just wheeze and cough all day long in that same chair. She could do no housework, she no longer had a driver's license, and she didn't go anywhere. She spent more time in the hospital than she did at home.

So I took my mother-in-law to Dr. Stoll and within a month or two, she started showing tremendous improvement. Within about four to five months, she was a totally different person. The care she received literally turned her life around. She took the driver's test and got her driver's license again. She bought herself a car and became very active among senior citizens. The depression was gone. She had been on 13 different drugs, and he probably got her off three-fourths of them.

—Nancy

Dr. Ken Korins explains that Candida is a yeast, which is a normal part of the constitution. "Usually, it lives harmlessly in the GI tract or the skin. However, overgrowth can affect the GI tract, the genital-urinary tract, the endocrine system, and the nervous system. Some of the symptoms that yeast or Candida can cause are fatigue, decreased energy, problems with libido, problems with thrush (a white coating on the tongue or esophagus caused by overgrowth of the yeast), bloating and gas, intestinal cramps, rectal itching, altered bowel function, vaginal yeast, urinary tract infection, menstrual complaints, depression, irritability, and problems with concentration, as well as allergies, chemical sensitivities and decreased immune function in general.

"People with Candida often crave sugars, alcohol and various carbohydrates. The patient is most often but not always a woman between the ages of 15 and 50. There might be a past medical history of vaginal yeast, antibiotics, birth control and steroids. Antibiotics are particularly important in causing problems with yeast. It used to be that antifungals were commonly given with antibiotics because of this reason. Many other drugs such as oral contraceptives, anything that interferes with hydrochloric acid and a lot of simple sugars in the diet can cause problems with yeast.

The diagnosis of candidiasis is often made by a history of the symptoms. Stool cultures and antibody tests also may be used.

The mechanism of candidiasis is explained by Dr. Korins: "Although Candida is usually a normal part of the constitution, stress interferes with the secretions, with the immunity, with the nutrition or drugs or impaired liver function. When this happens, the yeast products are absorbed by the body. On the one hand, toxins are produced, which creates a metabolic stress on the body, interfering with liver function and the elasticity of enzymes. Also, antigens are produced by the yeast which in activity with the toxins, cause activation and depression of the immune system. Antigens cause auto antibodies to develop, which can wreak havoc with the body, causing rheumatoid arthritis symptoms, among other things.

"So we have a condition that causes problems in the immune system, hormonal imbalances, and in general, multi-system involvement, including problems with food and other chemical sensitivities. This leads to a situation where people are more prone to infections. Therefore, they get put on more antibiotics, which gives the Candida more opportunity to proliferate. It develops a vicious cycle."

Dr. Korins has several suggestions for addressing the factors that predispose someone to candidiasis. A diet with a low component of simple sugars, especially refined sugars, is recommended. "It is also important to limit foods containing honey, maple syrup and milk because of the lactose," Dr. Korins say, because "even these simple sugars, the Candida can thrive on. Foods containing yeast or mold such as alcohol, cheese, dried fruits and peanuts and known allergens should be avoided since they also weaken the immune system and leave less reserve to deal with these conditions."

In terms of digestion, supplements are beneficial. "Supplementing with hydrochloric acid, pancreatic enzymes and other herbs, such as bitter herbs, which can help secrete bile, may prevent Candida overgrowth," Dr. Korins says. "Pancreatic enzymes can be particularly important because incomplete digestion of proteins may cause food allergies. Also, the pancreatic enzymes help keep the intestines free of yeast, bacteria, protozoa, worms, and help break down the immune complex.

"The immune system is extremely important to address. Treatment for AIDS, cancer, or diabetes or treatments such as chemotherapy, steroids, or radiation greatly affect the immune system. Nutrition has to be addressed. Technically, a nutrient can cause problems with Candida because there is no known nutrient that doesn't have some effect on the immune system. However, studies have shown that nutrients that are especially low in patients with Candida are vitamin A, B6, zinc, lignum, magnesium, essential fatty acids, folic acid and iron. Of course, a high potency multi-vitamin should be added to the supplements."

If a person is taking medications that compromise the immune system, Dr. Korins says, "Treatments are not going to work because you are going to be continually perpetuating Candida overgrowth. Drugs like Tagament and Ranitidine, that are used for gastric ulcers and gastritis, decrease hydrochloric acid secretion, which is essential to control Candida and also for absorption of nutrients."

A healthy liver is critical in the control of Candida. "If the liver is overwhelmed with toxins, it cannot detoxify the body properly," Dr. Korins explains. "These toxins are released into the system, creating problems like psoriasis and premenstrual syndrome. The liver is also important because of something known as the die-off effect. As the Candida is being killed by the body, more toxins are released, causing an exacerbation of symptoms, even if the person is on the way to healing. So the liver must be in optimal function during the healing process."

Many natural herbal remedies can be very effective in treating candidiasis. Caprilic acid is a fatty acid with a lot of antifungal properties. One gram with meals can be very effective. Lactobacilli are well-known bacteria; they are good bacteria that can decrease Candida growth. Garlic is extremely active against many fungi and in fact some studies have shown that garlic is more active against Candida than Nystatin. Barberry, in tincture form, stimulates blood supply to the spleen and activates macrophagen. It can be very helpful in maintaining the normal floor of the gut. It's active against many pathological bacteria including Candida, as well as E-coli and salmonella. Common spices can even be beneficial—ginger, cinnamon, thyme, and rosemary.

Dr. Aubrey Worrell also approaches the Candida problem holistically: "The body is the source of the Candida allergen. When there is more Candida than there should be in the gastrointestinal tract, the body absorbs more of the Candida antigen. You accelerate the problem by eating sugar and foods with mold, and by breathing mold in.

"Over a period of years, I noticed that patients with Candida manifest multiple symptoms. As an allergist, I would of course see patients with asthma, hay fever and skin rashes. But I began noticing that many of these patients with allergies had other problems such as respiratory and gastrointestinal symptoms. Another complaint I see quite frequently is people just not feeling good. They're tense or headachy. They're tired and weak. They have a tendency towards depression and fatigue. They're forgetful and unable to concentrate.

"In actuality, these problems are often manifestations of a subtle disruption of immune function in which there's an overgrowth of yeast and an increasing allergy to the mold."

Dr. Worrell uses a combination of approaches in treating patients with Candida. "Number one," he says, "you have to have a good, nutritious diet. It can't be loaded with alcohol and sugar. It has to be composed of broad-spectrum healthy foods. Number two, you put them on the mold-free diet. Number three, you have to place them on Nystatin therapy for approximately two to six weeks."

Dr. Richard Tan confirms many of Dr. Worrell's insights. Dr. Tan also emphasizes a systemic and holistic approach: "I have been diagnosing a large number of patients with Candida, and sugar affects them greatly. Quite a few patients that I am seeing have memory lapses, are forgetful and depressed, and they have seen other doctors who diagnose the depression and give them anti-depressants. When I go over all the system reviews, I find that it is more of a systemic problem; along with the Candida, they also have some sinus problems, achy bones and joints, stomach upsets and gas. They often say that they have cravings for sugar or foods that contain sugar, as well as bread.

"I have a survey form that I go through. In my scoring system, after awhile, if the score is high, then I strongly suspect that they have Candida. So then I explain my hypothesis and start to treat them. I put them on a diet program plus some antifungal medication. When they come back after two weeks, they usually say that they haven't felt so well in a number of years.

"This quick recovery is a revelation to me. I keep on seeing this type of patient. And every time I treat one, I am still amazed at how different they become after awhile, at how much they improve."

Dr. Tan has a few more recommendations. "Patients with Candida should avoid all processed foods, and especially those with sugar, such as soft drinks. Get back to the basics. Grow your own garden if you can. If not, maybe go to a health food store, where you can buy organic, unprocessed foods. While most Americans eat too much fat, people with Candida need to be more concerned with sugar than with fat. If you eliminate nutritionally poor foods, you will often be surprised at how your taste for things changes as your diet changes."

Dr. Ray Wunderlich emphasizes the link between depression and candidiasis. "A very high percentage of the people I see who are depressed also have imbalances, such as an overgrowth of Candida. Thyroid disease is another example. If you considered all the women whom I treat in my practice, from 70 to 75 percent of them would have thyroid disease, and an even higher percentage would have some form of Candida."

"A good example is a TV reporter I saw this morning. After coming into my office to film a segment on my approach to medicine, she got personally interested in what I do. She is 40 years old. We did a mineral analysis on her and found that she is deficient in five nutrient minerals. She is a perfectly normal, functioning individual of 40 years of age. But when you examine her carefully, it turns out that she has recurrent vaginal yeast infections, some bloating, some gas and indigestion, and she has taken antibiotics: a classic profile of a Candida patient, which is all too common. In a place like Florida, where the weather is so humid and molds and yeasts grow so readily, problems associated with recurrent yeast infections are almost an epidemic."

Dr. Walt Stoll brings his understanding of the body's immune system to bear on his clinical approach. He describes his clinical experience using examples from candidiasis patients, with references to rheumatoid arthritis patients and others. As he explains: "The immune system sees the world in black and white. Something entering your body that it comes in contact with is either you or it is not you. If it is you, the immune system is not supposed to attack; if it is not you, then it is supposed to attack. One of the things that your digestive tract does is to break down things from the environment into particles small enough for you to absorb without alerting your immune system that they came from somewhere else besides you. But if, for example, your gut is not doing the job perfectly, it leaks a particle of protein (a peptide) that is large enough to alert the immune system, in your joints, muscles, or ligaments, for instance. Then your immune system can't tell the difference between the protein particle from outside and the one in your tissues, so it attacks both. Let's imagine that every time you have corn, for example, you don't break it down perfectly and one of those peptides leaks out of your intestine. Your body attacks the corn peptide, but it's also attacking the peptide—that is identical to the corn peptide—in your muscle, ligament, and joint. You'll feel that immune response as arthritis, tendonitis, or other conditions.

"If you stop the process," Dr. Stoll continues, "the immune system settles down in three and a half days, and you begin showing improvement. The first example I heard of was about 10 years ago. If you took someone with rheumatoid arthritis or took a group of these patients and put them on a fast, 75 percent of them would improve within a week. You can't keep someone on a water fast forever, of course; but here was a dramatic illustration of the fact that there was another cause of rheumatoid arthritis that we could address. We didn't necessarily have to limit our course of treatment to gold shots, cortisone, and a crippling future for the patients.

"There are a number of things that make the gut more permeable to peptides. Stress is one of them. We know not to go swimming right after we eat, because there is not enough blood supply in the body to adequately supply both the intestinal tract and the muscles. When your blood supply is concentrated in your intestinal tract digesting your meal, going for a vigorous swim risks not getting enough blood in the muscles, resulting in cramps and, possibly, drowning. When you are chronically stressed—and most stresses are not psychological but environmental—your body deals with it with a fight-or-flight response, which makes your muscles get a little more chronically tight and active. Your body concentrates more blood supply into the fight-or-flight area and then takes away the blood supply from the intestinal tract. The intestinal lining replaces itself on average about every 14 hours, so it requires a heavy blood supply. If you are chronically stressed for long enough, eventually the intestinal lining functions less normally, which of course produces other imbalances. The normal bacteria that are supposed to grow sometimes get out of balance and allow Candida to move in and flourish. This damages the lining further and so things leak even more."

Dr. Stoll says that this food absorption syndrome is the main cause of brain fatigue. "By the time I see most of my patients," he explains, "they have had everything else tried unsuccessfully on them and a large percentage of them have this syndrome as their basic cause. If the patient is willing to follow directions, within a few weeks they already see enough improvement so that they know they are doing the right thing. Within a few months, they've usually improved enough so that they can handle it from there on their own.

"My procedure is to first collect all the medical records that the person has accumulated up to that time, so I don't have to repeat any tests that have already been done. If some things have obviously been missed, then I try to fill in the gaps. There are labs around the country that do a pretty good job of looking for parasites, candidiasis, low magnesium, and other disorders that are either not done or done poorly by conventional labs. I look at the entire chronological history of the patient for a couple of weeks before their appointment and try to think of any factor that might have influenced their health and that might be indicated as a pattern of change over time. Then we have the regular databases that we use in conventional medicine to look for other kinds of patterns. I'll also ask the patient to keep a record of his or her usual diet and anything special that they ingest for a week or so. Then I put all those pieces together with a general physical exam and see if the pattern suggests some of these other causes."

Patient education is key at this point. "Finally, when I get a picture and it's pretty obvious what is happening, I educate the patient sufficiently so that he or she can make an informed decision about going forward with the therapy," Dr. Stoll says. "I tell patients to make their decision very carefully, so that once having decided to go ahead they then are able to maintain that commitment. That way, we are sure that if the patient doesn't get well it is because we were wrong, and not because the patient was careless about sticking to his or her diet and regimen. Generally, I can predict within a few days how long it is going to take for the person to start feeling better. I have patients keep a record of their symptoms so that they can track their own progress and improvement. As you get better, frequently you forget how badly you were feeling before. Unless someone lives with a patient, it's hard to assess exactly where you are once a patient begins to improve.

"The treatment depends upon the cause, of course. If the person has candidiasis, then the treatment is relatively simple and straightforward. A strict diet is necessary for a while. I will probably have to give them some digestive enzymes to correct the poor protein metabolism, until they can do some relaxation techniques to get the blood supply back to the intestinal tract, which usually takes from three to six months. In the presence of candidiasis, I usually use some Nystatin, a prescription antifungal agent, to try to directly attack the Candida problem. If the person hadn't been absorbing things too well for a while I might use some concentrated nutrients with antioxidants to try to replenish the body with what it needs to repair itself and to improve the immune function."

24

Chronic Fatigue

■■■

Patient Story: Chronic Fatigue

I did an experiment. I wanted to see how far I could push my body before it would collapse. I kept very detailed records. My diet was absolutely the same, the amount of protein, fat and carbohydrate, the amount of vitamins and minerals and enzymes, the amount of juices, nothing changed. Then I raced every single week. I did about 50 races a year. For 81 races, I had a personal record each week, faster than any that I had done up to that point and I had not changed anything. One day, there was a race in Central Park, a short little three mile race. I couldn't run that race as fast as a slow training session. I charted that. I said to myself maybe it was lack of sleep, maybe it was the flight, maybe it was all these things. The next week another race, same thing. I could not do it. I did not have the energy.

I had a full blood chemistry done. I tested for every virus, bacteria, parasite, hepatitis, everything. My blood was clean as clean can be. I had to ask why I had no energy when I stressed myself in competition. I realized that there is something that medicine does not talk about, science does not look at. I had looked in the Western model first, being a scientist, wanting to see if I had a virus or blood sugar imbalance. No, everything was normal. What I found I was deficient in at that point was the essential chi energy.

The chi energy is life force energy. It had been diminished by nearly two and a half years of training and pushing nonstop. It doesn't show up in our blood or in our cells, but something is missing. It took almost six months before that was able to rebalance itself and rejuvenate. Then I was able to start all over again and, this time, compensate for it. The rule of health is compensation. We all cannot move out of a city that is polluted, move away from a job that's got high noise and dust particles or even away from working around sick people, as I do. By rebalancing and rejuvenating and compensating, that's how we are able to be healthy. If you live in a very polluted environment, you put in antipollution devices. You balance yourself, give yourself time and peace and quiet. Training for a marathon is very immune depressive. Understanding the compensation factor, now I take some vitamin C drips. The amount I will have in my system is different than anyone else's because it's unique to my own system. Each person has their own unique needs. It deals with the energies and I'm not talking about viral or bacterial or blood sugar or glandular depletion.

—Gary

Even when you rest and the muscles are recovered and the blood chemistry is normal, liver enzyme is normal, everything is normal, it's possible that that vital energy still isn't completely balanced. That takes time, you cannot rush that. People who are working on things they really enjoy spend an inordinate amount of energy working—not just physical but emotional energy, spiritual energy— and that is not in and of itself depleting. I remember some friends who were building themselves a home and they would have friends up for work weekends. We would all chip in and help them. Everybody else would be exhausted after six hours, and they would be happy working twelve hours later. There are ways that we can tap into inner resources within our body and within our mind that allow us to compensate for fatigue. It's the compensating energy of the chi, the submeridian that engages us in life. When you suddenly think about doing something you have not done that you are excited by, you have all the energy in the world. If we can keep ourselves positively focused and have goals each day to achieve something that is obtainable and within our reach, it gives us more energy. That helps us with other things that could be depleting us.

You can deplete your energy and become exhausted just by consumption or by the thought of consumption. At other times and in other cultures you don't find people as likely to be overstuffing their closets with an obscene amount of clothes. When someone tells me they have fatigue, I don't stop with just bacteria and viral panels, or the blood sugar examination. I look at other things— what they've done in their life, what they're feeling, what they're believing, because that will affect an energy system that we can't measure, but is there. By rebalancing that system, you can frequently help a person improve their overall life energy; then you work on the individual glands and organs and blood chemistry.

I measure fatigue backwards, in increments. You felt tired, but you didn't have the flu and you were not sore in your muscles or joints. You had intermittent fatigue: more energy in the morning, less in the evening or afternoon. You go to exercise or you want to stay up a little later and go dancing, but you just don't have any energy. You wake up and just don't seem to be rested no matter how much sleep you get. You really have to look at levels of fatigue. From that very mild form of fatigue, to the very major, the information in this chapter will help all because someone who has full-blown chronic fatigue syndrome may have multiple factors at work in their system, whereas someone else may only have two or three.

It is difficult, but possible, to distinguish between feeling overtired and constantly worn out, and having chronic fatigue syndrome. All of these states affect our mental and emotional life. Sometimes, fatigue is caused by other diseases of either mind or body.

Most fatigue-centered conditions begin slowly. A person gradually feels less energized than in prior months or years. They just can't do the things they did before.

Dr. Jacob Teitelbaum actually lost a year in medical school due to his contracting chronic fatigue syndrome. For over a decade he's worked with chronic fatigue and fibromyalgia patients. He identifies chronic fatigue syndrome as a group of symptoms associated with severe, almost unrelenting fatigue. "Disordered sleep is classic—trouble falling or staying asleep. Severe achiness is usual in a lot of different parts of the body. For some people the most disabling and scary part of the disease is the brain fog—confusion, poor memory, trouble finding words, even names. Increased thirst is very common because of the hormonal problems, bowel disorders, recurrent infections. So if you have several of these together, I think you have the disease. The new fibromyalgia and chronic fatigue criteria show that there are about 6 million in the country with this disease." Other practitioners include, on the list of symptoms, recurring sore throat, lymph node swelling, headache, intestinal discomfort, depression, and decreased concentration.

The first thing people do is usually the worst thing. "When people feel horribly tired and can barely function, they try to take coffee or caffeine to boost their energy," Dr. Teitelbaum says. "It feels better for a little while, but caffeine is a loan shark for energy. You'll feel better for a couple hours, and then crash four or five hours later. When people crash, they drink more coffee and then more, up to 8 to 12 cups a day. They're wiped out. It's really important for people to come off the coffee so their energy levels can start to come back up.

"Also, caffeine aggravates hypoglycemia, which is very common in this disease because of the underactive adrenal gland. This can put people on an emotional roller coaster. The average American gets 150 pounds of sugar added to their food each year, which is 18 percent of their calories. This plus white flour, having lost most of its vitamins and minerals, results in a diet that truly is destroyed before people ever get started, and then this sets them up for chronic fatigue syndrome."

The B complex vitamins are critical. "Get one that has at least 25 milligrams of B complex, selenium, zinc, chromium, copper," Dr. Teitelbaum says. "If your iron is low, treat that. The lousy diet decreases the immune function with this disease, so bugs that most people wouldn't get, like Candida overgrowth, parasites, abnormal bacteria growing in the bowel, are common. These things get to the B12 before you can absorb it. Because digestion is poor, people are not absorbing the B12 they need. The body overutilizes the B12 to try to heal the damage, and both of these things drive the B12 level down to very low levels. This causes fatigue and a lot of other problems. The B12 deficiency can also aggravate allergies, such as sulfite sensitivities. So getting B12 shots, even if your doctor says the levels are technically normal, would be a very important part of the treatment. B12 shots—1000 to 2000 micrograms once a day to once a week—a total of 12 shots can make a big difference, regardless of your level."

The hypothalamus is often implicated in chronic fatigue. "Current evidence suggests that a major portion of these symptoms are manifestations of a poorly functioning hypothalamus," Dr. Teitelbaum explains. "This is a very exciting area of research. If you had to look for the missing link that ties this whole disease together, the hypothalamus is a good one. It is a very small area, called the master gland, in the brain that controls four major functions: different glands; temperature regulation (if you have this disease, your temperature is almost never up to 98.6, it's usually 97); sleep; and blood pressure, pulse and blood flow. You usually find low blood pressure with this disease, which is why your spouse jumps to the other end of the bed when you put your cold feet on them. These all stem from the hypothalamus.

"The glands are critical. You see low DHEA because of the underactive hypothalamus in about 70 to 80 percent of people with the disease. The thyroid will often be low—even if the blood tests are normal, because blood tests look different if the thyroid is low from the hypothalamus not working than most doctors would expect them to be. So you have to go by the symptoms: fatigue, cold intolerance, dry skin, confusion, achiness, and a low body temperature. These call for a triatal thyroid hormone. Low adrenal function causes, a loss of stamina and low estrogen in women (people often get this disease a year or two after a hysterectomy or tubal ligation) and low testosterone in men."

Often there is a history of respiratory infection. "Major respiratory infections are frequently unrelenting because the immune system is overactive and poorly functioning," says Dr. Teitelbaum. "Because of the change of blood flow to the nose, chronic nasal congestion is very common and so is sinusitis. People get antibiotics for these from their doctors and then they get yeast or Candida overgrowth. I say avoid antibiotics if you have chronic fatigue. Zinc lozenges are effective—at least 10 milligrams of zinc five to eight times a day during the infection. Vitamin C should be boosted to high levels—anywhere from 5,000 to 10,000 mgs a day. Use nasal rinses—half a teaspoon of salt and a cup of lukewarm water, sniffed maybe an inch up each nostril. Blow your nose so you wash out the infection. Echinacea—about 325 micrograms—is more effective than antibiotics. Don't use it for more than three to four weeks at a time because then it stops working.

"Because nutritional deficiencies are rampant with chronic fatigue, magnesium is a key player, but the form of magnesium is important. I would take about 300 micrograms a day of magnesium or succinate, aspartate. Malic acid 300 micrograms four times a day is important for the muscles. Also coenzyme Q10, 100 micrograms a day; NADA, 5 micrograms twice a day; and potassium magnesium aspartate, 1000 micrograms, maybe one to two times a day. These help the energy factories a lot.

"These things are simple, cheap, nontoxic, and if you do them and cut out the sugar and coffee, for a lot of people suffering from fatigue, sometimes that's all it takes."

As Dr. Allan Spreen tells us, "Physical and emotional fatigue go hand-in-hand. Fatigue tends to affect mental functioning, so that a person suffering from fatigue feels that his or her memory is not as good as it once was. I consider that type of fatigue biochemically based. I'm sure it's in the genes that some people wear out faster than others.

"Because food sensitivities often manifest themselves as cravings, we try to get people off the foods they crave. Chances are they may be sensitive to these foods, such that their sensitivity can manifest itself as fatigue and mental states tied to fatigue, such as irritability or frustration."

Depression is often a reaction to fatigue. "People think they're getting old or sick, or that they're dying, because they don't have the energy they once had," Dr. Spreen says. "And depression causes a domino effect. Once people are depressed, they don't care to do anything. If they don't do anything, their self-worth decreases. They feel worse and worse.

"We try to take a complete approach. We find that as digestion improves, with proper foods and supplemental digestive enzymes, fatigue tends to diminish. Subsequently, energy levels and clarity of mind improve. People can concentrate better. The patient can remember things better because his or her mind isn't experiencing brain fog from all of the toxic junk floating around in the body."

Dr. Spreen's approach should show results in a relatively short time, he says. "We ask people to give us two weeks. We want them to stop eating the foods they crave the most. If there is anything they feel the day just isn't complete without, we tell them that that's what they need to give up first. Once they give that up, if their fatigue worsens for the next two or three days—if they become more irritable, pick fights with family members, their self-worth diminishes, feel like they're not getting anywhere, have more intestinal problems—I can almost guarantee that that food is a major part of their problem.

"Once they get past that hump, which I call withdrawal, they tend to feel much better and everything seems to improve. Their peace of mind improves; they are less fatigued; their depression tends to decrease, if it's not true clinical depression from some other cause; their energy level increases; sleep improves; and the quality of their relationships improves. Their state of mind seems to dominate the other way where everything becomes better. It's not a panacea but it's a place to start."

Dr. Spreen outlines a nutritional approach to regaining energy: "Our efforts here are to optimize a person's biochemical intake nutritionally so that he or she can make the best use of whatever genetic disposition and overcome fatigue. Of course, there's always the possibility that fatigue represents the onset of something serious like cancer or something else. Our approach to treatment is to consult on a nutritional basis, complementing whatever diagnosis a patient might have from their primary physician. We don't seek to replace a primary physician.

"Normally I start by taking the known stressors out of the diet. The first three are sugar, sugar and sugar. When people eat a lot of refined sugar, the body tries to bring the sugar level down. Their sugar levels bounce up and down, up and down. They're getting highs and lows, which make their mind fog up and prevent clear thinking and memory."

Dr. Spreen follows up with other recommendations. "We ask people to eat foods in their natural state, not processed foods. If a person stays on junk all the time—eats 12 candy bars a day, three soft drinks or more (with seven teaspoons of sugar in each soft drink), and smokes and drinks and gets stimulants in other bad foods—taking a multivitamin just isn't going to do the trick. I try to get people off caffeine. I give them vitamins and supplements which, hopefully, their bodies will absorb. If their absorption is not good, they may require digestive enzymes, additional acidophilus, or hydrochloric acid supplements."

Finally, Dr. Spreen uses two naturally occurring substances: B12 and B complex. He starts with a B12 shot, "the old 'quack' remedy that most doctors consider a placebo and don't even like to talk about. I'm batting about three out of four that just with a B12 shot, you'll feel more energy within a day. And B complex, is needed today more than ever before because of the American diet. The B vitamins work together, predominantly to help with the assimilation of carbohydrates. When complex carbohydrates are removed from the diet, people use up the B complex stores in the body, which are somewhat limited, being water-soluble. If people consumed more unrefined foods, they would have what is required in food for the assimilation of that food. So I give both B complex in a supplement and extra B12 if fatigue is a problem. Plus I try to get people off refined sugar, refined white flour, refined pasta, and anything else that might stress the body."

Herbs also are beneficial in chronic fatigue. "To boost mental function, I use ginkgo biloba, probably the number-two herb after ginseng," Dr. Spreen says. "We'll give a trial of that to people who say they don't remember things the way they used to, and to children with learning disorders. We'll try the herb for about 6 weeks. If the person doesn't feel a noticeable difference in that time, it probably doesn't work for them. The nice thing about this type of remedy is that it's harmless. If it doesn't work, you've only lost a few dollars; it hasn't done any harm. I think that herbs with a 2,000-year history have done people some good, that herbalists, dating back to the Indian medicine men and ancient Chinese herbalists, knew what they were doing.

"If we can help a person sleep, we can help him or her to think and feel better when awake. Valerian is an herb that has been used for years to help with sleep. Sometimes we mix that with taurine, which is not an herb but an amino acid. These two agents together tend to help people relax, although this does not work all the time.

"Some botanicals that worry us are at the opposite end of the spectrum. We want to get these substances out of the body. Nonherbal teas and coffee are artificial stimulants. They make people feel good momentarily, but harm them in the long run. We compare it to the difference between feeding a horse right and whipping a horse. You can make a horse work harder for awhile with the whip, but you'd better feed him or he won't continue to work. We try to get the whips out of there and enhance nutrition instead."

Dr. Ken Korins explains how homeopathy works in the case of chronic fatigue. "Homeopathy," he said, "is a type of energy or vibrational medicine. It works by stimulating the person's innate healing forces. In some traditions, for instance Chinese medicine, that's called the chi. In homeopathy, we call it the vital force. It relates to chronic fatigue because chronic fatigue, as well as many other conditions, represents a disbalance in the person's system, particularly on their energy level. When that is corrected, many things fall into place.

"I treat chronic fatigue and Candida together, since many of their symptoms overlap. Although the cause of chronic fatigue is not known, the Epstein Barr virus, a member of the herpes virus group, is often involved. The symptoms may persist for months or years. All these viruses have one thing in common—they establish a lifelong latent infection in the host. In fact, by the end of adulthood most adults do demonstrate antibodies against the Epstein Barr virus, indicating a past infection. Those with the most serious symptoms generally have the highest antibody levels to Epstein Barr. This may actually indicate that the chronic fatigue syndrome is a problem of decreased immune function and not just a disorder caused by a specific virus.

"Susceptibility is a very important issue because the presence of the virus is not enough to cause the syndrome. The terrain must be fertile to enable the virus to propagate and cause disruption to the organism. Any condition that compromises immune function such as AIDS, cancer, chronic kidney failure, rheumatoid arthritis or other primary, or secondary immunodeficient states."

Detoxification is important in chronic fatigue. Dr. Korins says we must look at "external toxins such as chemicals and drugs as well as internal toxins such as Candida and free radicals. Stimulation of the elimination organs, such as the bowel, liver, kidney, lymph nodes and skin are extremely important. The immune system must also be addressed. There are many nutrients that can help address this but at least people should be on a good multi-vitamin, with carotenes, vitamin C, and zinc; this is extremely important for the immune system and also for the glandular system. Glandular extract such as thymus, spleen, and liver can be very beneficial, as well as certain botanical support such as goldenseal, echinacea, licorice, astragalus and aloe vera, to name a few."

Homeopathy works by stimulating the body's innate healing potential and the goal is to be curative, not just to suppress the symptoms, Dr. Korins says. "The trick is to find the right remedy. I suggest you pick two or three symptoms that are most disturbing, even though you might have a list of 20 or 30, and then find the remedy. If the indicated remedy does not seem to be working, try using what we call a nosode, the homeopathic remedy for Epstein Barr virus or Candida. This can be very effective in and of itself.

"Gelsemium is a major remedy for chronic fatigue syndrome. It is good for patients who get extremely tired with the least exertion. They may always want to be in bed. Their limbs tremble with exhaustion; there is a lot of muscular soreness; the eyelids may feel heavy to the point where they droop. Blurring of vision and double vision is not uncommon when gelsemium is indicated. Gelsemium is also a remedy for acute flu. It is a good remedy for people that have never been well since the flu. It reduces the thirst that often accompanies fever."

Phosphoric acid is good for weakness and debility, which usually moves from mental to physical. "The phosphoric acid condition seems to result from loss of bodily fluids, particularly sexual bodily fluids," Dr. Korins says. "If you've had a very promiscuous period, feel drained sexually and are chronically tired and fatigued, phosphoric acid can be particularly helpful. People who respond to this remedy are usually mentally apathetic and indifferent, and have tearing pains in their joints, as if the bones were scraped. They are better with short naps. There is a craving for sodas and carbonated drinks. Phosphoric acid is also a major remedy in diabetes.

"Arsenicum album is good for people who have anxiety and restlessness with their exhaustion, who fear death and disease and despair of recovery. The sensations often revolve around burning pains in the stomach, hay fever symptoms with excretions that are thin, watery and burning. They have other gastronomical, intestinal symptoms, such as weight loss, and chronic conditions with a lot of diarrhea, especially after eating watery fruits. Shortness of breath with exertion is very common. The skin tends to be dry, rough and scaly. Arsenicum is also indicated during acute Epstein Barr virus or flu-like symptoms especially when there is great thirst."

Kali phosphorica also helps with anxiety and fear. Compared with arsenicum, it is more effective against brain fog. "People who need this cannot recall names or words," Dr. Korins says. "They have problems with memory.

"Baryt carbonica brings focus and helps with slow mental grasp, a lot of confusion, difficulty learning. People in this state often have an enlarged tonsil. The glands are enlarged almost to the point of touching each other and they get colds very easily."

Another remedy for brain fog is anacardium. It is helpful for people "who are very forgetful and have developed a tendency to use foul language after the development of chronic fatigue. They also tend to have a lot of fixed ideas. There is an obsessive component to the anacardium syndrome.

"Lycopodium is a very important remedy for brain fog with weak memory, confused thoughts, dyslexia, loss of words. There are abdominal symptoms with noisy flatulence, especially after eating and a lot of bloating. They desire sweets, are excessively hungry, have sensitivities of the liver and sore throats that begin on the right side and spread to the left.

"Nux vomica is another remedy that has a lot to do with impaired liver function It is good for problems after eating, like the sensation that the food is stuck in the stomach like a rock and just sits there for hours. Also irritable bowel-like symptoms like constipation alternating with diarrhea.

"The idea is that homeopathy is very specific. It is important to remove the obstacles to the cure. Diet, stress and toxins must be addressed in order for the homeopathic remedies to work most effectively. When we look at health from this mind set, we can help the body to heal and rebalance. With this approach, it is less important to address a particular virus, bacteria or fungi because the immune system is strong and can heal most of these things, including ones yet to be identified."

Dr. Alan Pressman believes that glutathione may be the key to chronic fatigue. First, he explains how the liver works to detoxify the body: "When our body has to combat environmental pollution and free radical damage, the major organ responsible is your liver, the largest organ of the body. One of the liver's major jobs is to keep you clean, to remove and destroy tremendous amounts of some of the 5 trillion pounds of chemicals that we are exposed to every year."

The liver completes its job in two phases. "The toxin will come into your system and into your liver and will then be oxidized. We call that activation. That is the phase in which the toxin is being made ready to be taken out of your body in your feces and in your urine and perhaps in your saliva and your perspiration. Mostly in your feces and urine. The second phase—this is a crucial phase—is the removal of this toxin out of your body. If you do not remove it, it builds up and creates problems. When a toxin is made ready to be eliminated from the body, it is actually bio-activated, meaning that it becomes more toxic that it was before. But now it can be packaged in nice little bundles and taken out of the body. That is the responsibility of phase two of liver detox, to take this toxic garbage out of your body.

"Phase 1 and Phase 2 must be coordinated. The toxins—mercury, lead, and all the chemicals that accumulate in your system—are taken out of your body through Phase 2, which is totally under the control of your levels of glutathione and glutathione enzymes. In order for your body to be clean, to be pure, to be detoxified, you have to have a high level of glutathione in your liver at all times. Glutathione gets used up, so you have to keep replacing it with supplementation. If you do not, you can wind up with symptoms ranging from Parkinson's disease to Alzheimer's disease to neurotoxicity of a number of different brain pathways, all the way down to chronic fatigue syndrome and fibromyalgia. There is new proof in the research on nitric oxide, that in all cases of fibromyalgia and chronic fatigue syndrome, there is a marked deficiency and depletion of glutathione, lypoic acid, and n-acetyl cysteine.

"If you are suffering from brain fog, if you are mentally confused, if you are disoriented, if you have body pain, if you have frequent illnesses, if your energy is gone, if your zip is gone, if you are having trouble learning, trouble concentrating, having constipation or diarrhea or gastrointestinal discomfort, even cardiac arrhythmia—all this could be related to abnormal detoxification in Phase 2 by the liver."

Dr. Pressman says that this condition is relatively simple to detect. "A functional liver detoxification profile measures glutathione activity in the liver through urine and saliva. We basically challenge you by having you take a prescribed amount of caffeine, of aspirin and acetaminophen and we watch the urine and saliva to see how successful you are at detoxifying those three substances. From that, we can tell you exactly how your glutathione is functioning. The foods high in glutathione are avocado, asparagus, watermelon, squash, potato, and vegetables like spinach and parsley."

Dr. Andrew Gentile explains that people suffering from chronic fatigue often have cognitive impairment. "Intellectual functioning wanes," he explains. "People say, 'I go from one room to another and I just don't remember why I went into the first room,' or 'I see a colleague I have worked with for a number of years and I'm quite embarrassed because I can't remember their first name.' There is also simply an inability to respond to physical and emotional stress. So many patients say, 'I seem to be feeling better and then as soon as I take a brisk walk or go swimming, within 72 hours, I begin to experience what seems like a flu—chills, sore throats, fevers. I get exhausted and go into a relapse and I don't feel well for anywhere from a week or two to months on end.'

"Fatigue is usually a symptom of depression. Because there is no known cause of chronic fatigue, you might see your general practitioner and complain of a list of symptoms and he would diagnose depression. But we now know that chronic fatigue simply is not depression."

Chronic fatigue strikes people of all ages. "It was a misnomer when it was called yuppie flu," Dr. Gentile says. "Age clusters, however, do tend to be around the mid 30s, with women getting it twice as much as men do. It is worldwide—in Japan, they call it 'low natural killer syndrome.' Some believe that the number of affected people could be as high as 5 million. The prevalence rates vary depending on the study—at first it was 2 to 7 out of 100,000, but we now know it is much higher, more like 1 out of 100.

"There appears to be a higher percentage of physicians, nurses and teachers who get it. I myself contracted this disorder in the late '70s, early '80s. I was a clinical psychologist working in a group home with many disadvantaged, multiply handicapped children. Most of the other workers experienced a nondescript, flu-like illness and then would pick up and seem to feel well. I also experienced that and then I took a vacation down south and did a lot of running. I was an avid runner and swimmer and I got a flu. This is what most people say, they got a flu and they just simply never recovered. It took me several years to recover."

Dr. Gentile has a distinct way of looking at chronic fatigue. "I think of it as an endpoint on a continuum," he says. "There are a lot of points along the continuum where people feel tired, they know something is not right, they're not sleeping right, yet we couldn't technically diagnose them as having chronic fatigue. Nonetheless, it's very important to look at what's going on for them so they can get to rebalancing.

"Traditional medicine searches for a single cause—in this case they were looking for single viral agents or several viral agents that cause the whole body to lose it's functional capabilities. In the early '80s, researchers were in a flurry looking for a connection to the Epstein Barr virus. This turned out to be a wild goose chase, as all such simplistic single agent studies will be, because Epstein Barr is widely distributed in the normal population by about age eight. Eighty-five to 90 percent of the population has caught Epstein Barr and recovered and therefore it could not be the causative agent or else why wouldn't everybody being coming down with the syndrome? Human Herpes Virus 6 fell upon a similar fate. It is widely distributed in the normal population and therefore could not be the distinguishing virus. Nobody is now thinking that a single viral agent or a combination of viruses really explain all the data. We are beginning to think that viruses are just a small part of this. I would like us to think about multi-causal arrangements such as allergy, environmental toxicity, Candida, stress, attitudes, some behavior such as rushing and too great involvement and being non-self rejuvenating."

A holistic approach is much more revealing. "A naturopath would look at everything in a person's life—their stress levels, behaviors that cause stress, a slightly compromised immune system, foods causing allergies, a higher toxic load," Dr. Gentile says. "They work with a computer—one wonders why they get a headache three or four hours later? They keep complaining about stale air and everybody in that office is complaining about the same stale air. We look at the long standing nature of these factors. The body tries to meet all these demands, tries to manage the total toxic load on the immune system as if it were a rain barrel. Water was filling up in the rain barrel and it got to the brim and then the slightest drop overflowed the barrel. That's the point at which a person begins to show some real signs of illness.

"The point where one drop in the rain barrel let it overflow is the proverbial straw that broke the camel's back. Traditional medicine will spend millions of dollars investigating the straw. They will not look at the fact that the camel walked for 100 miles with a 100 pounds on its back, which is where the answers are. If we were to carefully investigate an individual who has come down with chronic fatigue, we would find the unique things about that individual's life—they were drinking alcohol and had a lot of marital stress and at the same time, they were doing a lot of running. There were a lot of things suppressing their immune system. They had lost the connection with the general harmony.

"Many of my patients frequently tell me, 'I go to Arizona and I feel different, I come back and I get sick again. I go to Colorado and I can bicycle, I come back here and I can barely walk from my chronic fatigue.' It's not just that they took vacations. We need to look at illness in its total ecological environmental sense— that illness could be seen as a disharmony or disconnection with one's environment."

At issue here is a patient's connectedness, or lack of it. "We are talking about this on a level of disconnection," says Dr. Gentile. "The person's own response to their illness, once contracted, that's disconnected if they cannot develop higher ways of understanding how their life has lead them to this point of illness. If they view their illness as the outside superimposed in—"I caught a germ"— that's typical disconnected, linear, analytic thinking, very much the way our medical sciences approach problems. They're on to traditional medicine, doing lots of tests and finding nothing. If they switch thinking and begin to say 'my organism became imbalanced in some way, it could no longer meet the total toxic load and that has to do with the way I live my life,' they could take a different path. They could tie themselves back into the loop of life and make more lifestyle changes, which lead to healthier patterns in living and shorter remediation of their illness and shorter relapses.

"What I believe has been missed with this particular illness is predisposing factors. People say, 'For years before I became diagnosed, I had a problem with sleep' or 'I have always been pushing it.' There are a lot of personality variables here that need to be researched."

Many of these patients have high cytokine levels. "When you begin to look at the body's inability to meet the total toxic load, you notice that the cytokines— a messenger cell in the immune system which carries instructions to other cells—seem quite high for this group," Dr. Gentile says. "The cytokines themselves may be responsible for causing a lot of the neurologic symptoms, the inability to think clearly. We know that the bowel has certain receptors for these cytokines and high numbers of people with chronic fatigue have bowel symptoms. It's as though the immune system designed to take care of this total lifestyle/viral/bacteriologic load has turned on itself. There were so many demands made on it from the way the person lived, just from sheer external toxicity, that the system could not keep up those levels. The immune system is designed to say, 'this is an alien, let's attack it and get rid of it' and 'this is part of a normal cell in my body, so let's not attack it.' You get into disturbances when this detection is not accurate any longer. You have a perfect metaphor for the body maiming the self."

"Some things are energy depleting and some things are energy rejuvenating. What we know in terms of the mind-body connection from Hans Sele, a landmark physician and researcher in stress, is that the body tries to support energy expenditures by reorganizing itself. It gets much more economical about distributing cholesterol, distributing blood to vital parts of the body and so forth. It continues to do this in a step wise fashion as long as you continue to make the demands. In those early studies, the more demands that were placed on animals, the more they thrived. Researchers scratched their heads and said, 'What's the limit? These animals are being placed in challenging if not untoward levels of demand and they are doing better and better.' As soon as they stopped the experiment, the animals started to die. Autopsies showed swollen spleens, shrunken thymus, and enlarged adrenal glands."

"There is a way of being with our experience and not losing our own functional integrity, the boundaries where we end and something else begins. It's like singing in a chorus. The product is the sum total of all the voices. The unique contribution you are making needs to be maintained, but you are also in larger harmony with others. It is much what a cell has to learn in order to stay healthy in its environment. It needs to learn how much to take in and only what it truly needs. If it becomes too permeable, it takes in too much toxicity that it can't break down and it will die. If it closes off too much, it will not get what it needs and it will die. That's a metaphor for a way of being with something without losing your own functional integrity. There are situations in which the emotional discharge into what you are doing is depleting and it's not going to be replenished. Your body will actually forget how to self rejuvenate. In chronic fatigue, I see this all the time."

25

Hormone Imbalance

■■■

Patient Story: Hormone Imbalance

A 40-year-old woman was having marital difficulties and had been seeing a counselor for a couple of years. While she did need to straighten out her relationship, that wasn't causing her physical and emotional problems. She was deficient in adrenal hormone. She was tired and irritable, and couldn't get through the day. She couldn't manage the children. They would get on her nerves and she'd lash out at her husband. I tested her blood level of DHEA and found that it was more than two standard deviations below the mean. I put her on a very minimal dose of DHEA, and within two or three months she had discharged all of her counselors and her husband called me to tell me what saviors we were. These are some of the miracles we see.

—Dr. Ray Wunderlich

Disturbance of the hormonal cycle can play a major role in the development of various medical conditions. Hormone imbalances are often misdiagnosed as mental disease.

"Mental functioning is impaired in people who are low in the adrenal hormones, especially in DHEA," says Dr. Ray Wunderlich. "When these hormones are down, people become chronically fatigued. They have difficulty getting into mental gear, making decisions, seeing options, and fighting off the chemical assaults found in their environment. We can measure adrenal function in the saliva and the blood, and we can show that it increases with DHEA supplementation."

Dr. Wunderlich says the hormone DHEA can work wonders. "It's probably the closest thing to a panacea in medicine that we have found as of yet," he claims. "It is the so-called 'mother hormone' of the adrenal gland, an antidepressant that seems to be able to counter a lot of the allergic reactions that we see in people who are accumulating toxic insults as they age, decade after decade. This adrenal hormone declines from the age of 20 to death, due to illness and aging. By intervening with appropriate doses of the adrenal hormone DHEA, we can reverse many of the allergies and immune susceptibilities that we see in people over 25 years of age.

"Some cases of chronic depression, irritability and premenstrual syndrome are related to adrenal dysfunction, with low levels of the mother hormone of the adrenal gland. This is particularly so in people with low-blood-sugar symptoms We believe that this DHEA is kind of a baseline hormone. It feeds all the other systems, including the ones that regulate the sugar balance in the body. It can also serve as a precursor to the sex hormones—both female and male—as well as to the electrolytes, the salt and water hormones of the adrenals. It is highly individual in its response, but it is a major reactor that we didn't know about some years ago. The effects of DHEA have been well-researched; it has an anti-cancer, antiviral and antidepressive effect in animals. People have improved through the use of herbs, vitamins and minerals, which have probably been supporting the functioning of this hormone in the body, among other effects." Among the vitamins and herbs that help support adrenal function and the precursors of adrenal function are vitamin C, pantothenic acid, B complex, licorice, and Siberian ginseng.

Dr. Joseph Debe has also helped patients with hormonal imbalance. He provides a brief overview: "If we take a look at the stress hormones, these are epinephrine, which is commonly known as adrenalin, cortisol and DHEA. Epinephrine is a short-acting hormone that is released in the fight or flight reaction. For example, if we are almost involved in a car accident our heart starts pounding, racing, and we feel shaky. This is from the release of a lot of adrenaline. Cortisol and DHEA are long-acting stress hormones, which are released over a longer period of time. They all have slightly different effects on the body."

There are several ways that diet can cause imbalance in these hormones. "One very common way for Americans," Dr. Debe says, "is eating too much refined carbohydrate. We are getting a big burst of sugar in the bloodstream. When you eat pasta, cookies, cakes, there is an unnatural spike in blood sugar that results from this. The body is not meant to be exposed to such a sugar load all at once. What happens is the blood sugar spikes, the body tries to control it by releasing insulin and often the body releases too much insulin, the blood sugar dips too low and this has all kinds of consequences.

"A drop in blood sugar causes confusion, mood swings, irritability, anxiety, lightheadedness, headaches, blurred vision. Glucose is a primary fuel source of the brain. It's critical that the brain has a steady supply of glucose so when we are eating excessive convenience foods or refined carbohydrates we have a seesaw of blood sugar. That has a direct impact on the brain but then it further imbalances the stress hormone that I was mentioning. With regard to adrenaline, the blood sugar drops, the adrenaline goes up, and it's interesting that adrenaline when oversecreted over a period of time reduces the brain's production of dopamine. Dopamine is one of the neurotransmitters that has been found to be low in children with ADHD."

Low blood sugar also causes oversecretion of cortisol. "Cortisol damages the brain in a number of ways," Dr. Debe says. "It literally causes brain damage when it is oversecreted for long periods of time. Studies done with rats have found that injecting the animal with cortisol causes them to be unable to find their way through a familiar maze. Upon autopsy, they were found to have physical signs of brain damage.

"Cortisol, specifically, damages part of the brain called the hippocampus, which is involved in Alzheimer's disease. One of the causes of high cortisol and low DHEA is eating refined carbohydrates on a regular basis. And indeed people with Alzheimer's disease have been found to have high cortisol and low DHEA levels."

Mixing protein with carbohydrates may be helpful, Dr. Debe says. "People addicted to eating carbohydrates who don't want to make any drastic change right off can start by not eating the carbohydrate by itself. If you eat several cookies, that is pretty much pure carbohydrates and will cause a big swing in blood sugar. If you have some protein with the cookies—let's say instead of having the cookies between meals, you have them immediately after consuming a balanced meal that has protein (fish, legumes, lentils)—the negative effects on the body are much less. The protein causes the body to release another hormone called glucogen, which helps to balance out the blood sugar. We don't have that big seesaw in blood sugar that is detrimental in itself and also causes imbalance in the stress hormones."

According to Dr. Debe, estrogen levels fluctuate tremendously in response to dietary intake. "There are so many things that influence our estrogen levels, which men also produce. One very important factor is meat intake. If a woman is eating a lot of meat, her body produces more estrogen levels. One way this works is seen in the connection between our diet and the bacteria that live within the intestinal tract. Each of us has about 100 trillion organisms within the intestinal tract. Most medical doctors don't consider the intestinal flora, but they have metabolic activity on par with the liver. The metabolic byproducts are absorbed into the bloodstream partially and influence all aspects of our physiology, including the brain. There are bacteria in the intestinal tract that cause estrogen to be recirculated into the bloodstream instead of eliminated. These bacteria feed on meat. So if we are eating a lot of meat, we have more of these bacteria and we have more estrogen returning to circulation.

"Another thing that raises estrogen levels is constipation. If food is in the intestinal tract longer, there is more time for these bacteria to work on the estrogen and recirculate it into the bloodstream. Not only does low fiber cause constipation, but fiber finds the estrogen and drags it out of the body."

There are nutritional ways to reduce estrogen levels. "A woman can effectively lower the active estrogen in her body by consuming ground flaxseeds," Dr. Debe says. "Flaxseeds contain compounds called lignins, which increase binding proteins that take active estrogen out of circulation. Estrogen exists in the circulation in protein-bound form, which is inactive, and in free form, which is the active hormone. One way to effectively lower the biological estrogen is to increase protein that binds it and that is done by consuming ground flaxseeds."

Soy is also beneficial. Dr. Debe explains, "Soy contains estrogen-like compounds that compete with the body's own estrogen for binding to receptor sites. If we have a lot of these isoflavones, as they are called, in circulation, they compete with the body's estrogen and reduce the estrogen stimulation of the brain. Because these isoflavones are weaker, they can normalize estrogen activity."

Women who are not producing enough estrogen can increase their estrogen activity without taking hormones, which carry risk. "If they are vegetarian, they can consider adding some animal products to their diet," Dr. Debe says. "If that goes against their beliefs, there are other options. Licorice contains compounds that allow the body to retain more estrogen in circulation longer. So do soy isoflavones—the soy substitutes for the woman's inadequate estrogen. Soy has been found to have the same impact on neurotransmitters within the brain as the body's own estrogen does."

Dr. Debe recommends that women consider being tested with the female hormonal panel, "a test that uses 11 salivary samples over the course of a month to measure fluctuations in estrogen and progesterone. When you go to your doctor and he takes a single blood sample for estrogen or progesterone, that tells you nothing about what is going on with your cycle over the course of a month. With 11 salvia samples on different days, we can determine if your estrogen is too low at a particular time in the cycle, progestogen is too high at another part of the cycle and have therapy that is much more specific and we can take steps to rebalance the hormones with that detailed information."

26

Nutrient Imbalances in the Body and Brain

■■■

Dr. Priscilla Slagle has made a unique and important contribution in her medical practice. For nearly thirty years, she has treated patients with mood disorders, depression, anxiety, memory loss, and other health problems using amino acids to correct nutrient imbalances in the body and brain. "I continue to be amazed at their efficacy," she says. "I usually use them in combination with proper diagnosis and treatment of other conditions.

"Usually, by the time people get to me, they have already been many places and tried many drugs, and I am the end of the road for them. So these patients don't have simple, straightforward kinds of problems. They usually have multiple-symptom problems, for instance, chemical sensitivities, viruses, food sensitivities, autoimmune problems, parasite problems, fungus problems, and so on.

"So first I find out what is going on. When a patient comes to me, I often do an amino acid panel so that I can measure 42 different aspects of amino acids in their body. There are 22 amino acids, but I am also measuring metabolic breakdown products. Their patterns suggest connective tissue or autoimmune disease, chronic viruses, chemical or food sensitivities, or Candida. While it is an extensive diagnostic process, it does seem to find the root cause of some very puzzling complex physical and mental problems which patients are experiencing."

After making the diagnosis, Dr. Slagle focuses on removing the offending agents. These may include chemicals, yeast-inducing foods, drugs, or other substances. Then she embarks on the rebuilding process.

"For depression," she says, "I use tyrosine, which is an amino acid that raises norepinephrine, a major brain chemical that maintains good mood, drive, motivation, and concentration. Glutamine makes glutamic acid, one of the two major brain fuels, and is important for memory, focus and concentration. I use these two amino acids to treat depression. They must be combined with the active form of B6, which controls the absorption, metabolism and conversion of amino acids into all their various end products, such as neurotransmitters, antibodies, digestive enzymes, muscles and tissues in the body.

"I also give my depressed patients a basic multivitamin with minerals. Many depressed people are magnesium-deficient, so I've been using a relatively large amount of magnesium in my practice. I've also incorporated a fair amount of potassium for chronic fatigue syndrome patients. Many of them have potassium problems that are not necessarily picked up by a standard blood test. I check cellular potassium levels rather than the regular blood tests. I use some home-opathic cortisone with certain people with autoimmune disease."

Taurine and cysteine also may be used. "Taurine is a neuroinhibitory neuro-transmitter which has a calming effect," Dr. Slagle says. "It also controls heart rate and helps with fat metabolism. Many of the people who have chemical sensitivities and yeast problems (probably 90 percent of the ones I see) have a reduced taurine as well as a reduced cysteine level. Cysteine, like taurine, is an amino acid that helps the body to detoxify."

Dr. Slagle describes what happens in many people with chemical sensitivities. "The detoxification processes in their bodies has broken down due to overload, or deficiencies of various nutrients, or a liver dysfunction. So they aren't able to handle the same kind of toxic load that other people might handle who aren't dealing with the same variables. I use large doses of vitamin C and multi-amino acids, as well as certain other products which support detoxification pathways.

"At the risk of sounding fanatical, I believe we are poisoning this earth," Dr. Slagle concludes. "Many people with chemical sensitivities, autoimmune disorders and immune deficiency problems are early victims of what is happening to the planet, harbingers of what may later grow into a more serious and more obviously recognized problem. I have begun to see in my practice a vast number of autoimmune problems that I feel are environmentally or chemically induced. This problem is significant and deserves to receive national and international attention. I really appreciate the work that Dr. Rodgers has done and I recommend that people, particularly those with chemical sensitivities, read her books."

When treating nutrient imbalances that manifest as mental disease, Dr. Sidney Baker emphasizes magnesium deficiency and yeast problems. He provides some historical background, starting with his presentation of a paper on magnesium at a conference years ago. "At this colloquium, there were magnesium experts from all over, mostly academic people, and mostly people who had jobs like running an intensive care unit or a cardiac care unit, or a department of immunology or obstetrics and gynecology. Everyone there from every medical specialty was saying, 'Isn't it amazing that our colleagues are not aware of the very lengthy published information on the prevalence of magnesium deficiency in America, and its very widespread picture in clinical practice?' Any ordinary person would have come away from the conference saying, 'Well, how come this problem is being overlooked?' The cynical answer may be the truth: Magnesium deficiency research has no corporate sponsor.

"I've become convinced that magnesium deficiency is a major epidemic, one that we are experiencing right now in North America. Magnesium deficiency is widespread in its pattern of symptoms. It affects cardiovascular disease, allergies, tension, panic attacks, premenstrual syndrome and hyperactivity in children, to name just some of the conditions. The underlying theme behind many of the symptoms is what you might call being 'uptight.'

"Both magnesium and yeast problems probably began around 1950. The magnesium problem probably has its roots in the widespread use in agriculture of fertilizers containing potassium. The yeast problem probably arose because of the widespread use of antibiotics in the population.

"Many people come to see me specifically because they think that I am a yeast specialist, and so perhaps I see these patients in disproportionate numbers. But I think that this epidemic, which is being disregarded by many people in mainstream medicine, is simply overwhelming in its prevalence in the United States. Many people's medical histories show a quite obvious yeast problem. They started getting sick soon after they started taking antibiotics; they have bloating and difficulty concentrating; they have intolerances to foods, gastrointestinal disturbances and recurring vaginitis. Unfortunately, when they seek help from most doctors, they are told, 'Gee, we're very skeptical about this whole yeast idea; it isn't proven and so therefore we won't put you on simple remedies to see if you might have it.' The dogma has overcome the simple observation of nature."

Dr. Lendon Smith also confirms the importance of the magnesium factor, both in his clinical practice and in research studies in both animals and humans. "I've been working with a chemist out of Spokane, Washington, whose name is John Kitkoski. He started doing experiments with horses by taking blood samples and then testing for mineral and other nutrient deficiencies. He discovered that some of these horses were low in calcium or magnesium, for example. So he would put standard feed out in the corral, and then he would put standard feed plus calcium, or magnesium, or zinc, and let the animals go out and freely eat. They would smell everything and eat only what they needed. If they were low in calcium, they would eat just the calcium-supplemented feed, and then when they had had enough he noticed that they would come back to the standard feed. He would take a blood test and find out that their body chemistry had returned to normal. He figured out that the reason why the nose is placed in front of the mouth is to tell us 'don't eat that' or 'do eat this.' The sense of smell, along with taste, is a monitoring system."

Dr. Smith determined that people who are low in magnesium are more likely to have emotional distress. They more often experience anxiety, tension and irritability, which can lead to additional problems. "If the body chemistry is balanced," he says, "then the body can handle almost any kind of stress or stressors that come along. If it is not, then stress can exacerbate the problem."

Blood tests are used to determine the levels of chemicals in the body. Dr. Smith says, "If the GGT [Gamma glutamyl transferase] level is low, a person is low in magnesium because it's a magnesium-run enzyme. If a person has high levels of GGT, they often have too much magnesium. Mr. Kitkoski uses the standard 0 to 40 to 50 on the testing, going by the deviation from the mean. If somebody has around 20 on their GGT, then they are probably all right. But if they are low, and they have signs of anxiety and tension, if they can't relax, get spooked by people, and can't seem to handle the stresses of the world, then magnesium will help."

27

Premenstrual Syndrome (PMS)

...

Patient Story: PMS

A 30-year-old woman came to see me recently, two months after she had broken up with her boyfriend. She was depressed. She'd gained weight. She was exhausted. She had trouble keeping up with her work as a secretary. Psychotherapy wasn't helping. I asked her what she was eating and it turned out that there were a number of dietary patterns that were contributing to her emotional state.

I took a careful history which revealed that, while she wasn't overeating, she had developed the habit of drinking coffee and eating sweets to counter fatigue. Not only did this cause her to gain weight, but the coffee and sweets induced a hypoglycemic cycle. Her blood sugar levels were irregular, and this caused her to feel anxious. It was as though at a certain time of the day she was going into a withdrawal phase and the caffeine and sugar would help bring her back up.

So the first part of her problem was this hypoglycemic cycle. Her other problem was PMS, which had grown worse over the past few months. Her symptoms included mood swings, irritability, water retention, craving sweets and weight gain. She had always thought that PMS was normal, that this was what women (and their hapless partners) had to live with—a misconception held by too many women.

Her lab work revealed that she did have a fairly low fasting blood sugar level. To handle the hypoglycemia, I prescribed a specific diet and supplement program. For the PMS, I recommended the following regimen: For the first two weeks of her cycle, a dong quai herbal combination; for the second two weeks, a specific PMS combination containing extra vitamin B6, magnesium and ingredients that detoxify the liver, an important compo-

nent in treating PMS. (The specific ZAND herbal formulas are particularly effective.)
I also recommended regular exercise.

After a month on this regimen, she was feeling much, much better. She started to feel
like she had some control over the break-up with her boyfriend and over her work prob-
lems. She was able to take control of her problems rather than allowing these factors in
her life to control her.

—*Dr. Hyla Cass*

In the twenty-first century, premenstrual syndrome (PMS) has finally been recognized by most orthodox physicians as a legitimate disease, not "just something in a woman's mind" for which she needs a tranquilizer. We now know that
women with PMS are often allergic to their own progesterone hormone. We also
know that overgrowth of yeast is a big contributor.

Women with PMS need to build themselves up nutritionally. They can do this
with magnesium (800 to 1200 milligrams), vitamin B6 (from 25 to 50 milligrams), and vitamin E (400 to 800 units). It is best to take these nutrients in the
higher quantity during the second half of the menstrual cycle.

In addition, women can help to alleviate PMS by participating in aerobic
exercises. Whether it is power walking, jogging, bicycling, or swimming, a lot
of people feel the symptoms of their PMS subside when they engage in exercise.
They are improving their immune systems. Also, their central nervous system
functions are changing.

Dr. Hyla Cass emphasizes how often biochemical imbalances and psychological problems coexist. In her practice, she combines her work as a holistic
psychiatrist with use of naturally occurring substances to restore biochemical
balance. She begins with nutrition, as described in the patient story above. "In
cases where this nutritional regimen is not sufficient, I prescribe natural progesterone cream from day 14 until day 28 of the menstrual cycle. The kind of
progesterone I recommend is a natural progesterone, not the progesterone that's
in the regular pharmaceutical birth control pills or the hormones that are administered by prescription. It's a derivative from the wild Mexican yam and is available in health food stores. It's also useful for menopausal symptoms. It is applied
topically to the skin on fatty areas of the body, where it can be easily absorbed."

Dr. Cass uses the example of another woman to further illustrate how hormonal imbalance can be corrected naturally.

"Not long ago, a 48-year-old woman came in to see me complaining that her life 'just wasn't working.' She was a very successful professional. She had a great marriage. Her children were grown and in college and they were doing well. Her husband was successful. She really had a very good life, and yet she was unhappy. Now you could simply call this a midlife crisis, and do psychotherapy.

"However, when I took a psychological history—aware that this was a time of life for her to start looking inward, to evaluate her life—at the same time I asked her about her menstrual cycles. She said she was still menstruating. Her periods were changing in frequency and amount, but with no other symptoms. I sent her to the lab and it turned out she was very low in progesterone, low in estrogen, but particularly low in progesterone.

"I prescribed the natural progesterone cream, which helped to alleviate most of her psychological symptoms. Her irritability went way down. She realized that her uneasiness was metabolically based. It wasn't simply a personal psychological issue. She was peri-menopausal." In addition to the progesterone cream, Dr. Cass also prescribed herbal formulas.

"Even though people do have psychological issues—and it is important to deal with them—it's equally important to look at and treat the underlying chemistry," Dr. Cass says. "Often the psychological problems will lessen in severity or even disappear with treatment of biochemical imbalances."

Dr. Doris Rapp emphasizes the role that food cravings can play in the development of premenstrual syndrome. "The foods that you crave premenstrually are the foods that could be causing you to feel sick. I know one mother whose premenstrual chocolate cravings were so powerful that she would put the chocolate bars in the freezer to at least slow down the pace at which she would eat them when she was premenstrual. If you are a chocoholic and you can't manage without eating chocolate, it's a good bet that chocolate is a food that is causing you a problem."

28

Thyroid Disorders

■■■

Patient Stories: Thyroiditis

I first followed the conventional route in medical treatment. I was in my fifth year of infertility treatments, had taken multiple infertility drugs, and wound up severely depressed. I'd lost 35 pounds in two months. I couldn't sleep, I had panic attacks. Doctors put me on the conventional Xanax treatment for three years. I had hair loss, skin problems, nail-biting problems and aches all over my body, especially in my legs.

Dr. Spreen got me on a vitamin regimen, which made me feel somewhat better. Then, last summer, he put me on very low doses of thyroid and immediately—within two to three weeks—all the problems were gone. I'd had thyroid checks three times while I was being treated for infertility, and the blood tests had always come up negative. But I knew that my family had thyroid problems. At least six members that I can think of have thyroid disorders, but mine just never showed up on tests.

After taking very low doses of thyroid, my skin problem cleared up, I stopped biting my nails and my legs stopped aching. The mild depression I was still suffering from vanished. I felt great. I slept like a normal person again. I had energy. People started commenting on how I seemed to be like my old self.

I feel rather fed up with the original doctors. They treated me like I was a hysterical woman who needed to get a grip on things. I have never told them about my recovery using alternative methods because I don't think they'd be receptive to it. I did tell my therapist who has been very receptive to these new treatments and is most interested in the thyroid treatments. But I'd say that the medical community is not open-minded about alternative treatments at all.

—Jenny

I had hives, some kind of an allergic response, about five years ago and it progressed to the point where I had hives on my vocal cords. It was a pretty serious allergic reaction, for which I was treated with antihistamines. Later, I was treated with prednisone. When small doses of prednisone given every other day didn't help, my doctor began increasing the dosage until I was taking 70 milligrams every day. After about six weeks, I started declining physically from taking this tremendous dose. I gained about fifty pounds. I had conjunctivitis in both eyes. I had open sores. I was so weak that I was almost bedridden.

I found another doctor, who slowly weaned me off of the prednisone. But, my immune system had been damaged. I had a lot of viral illnesses that are usually associated with chronic fatigue syndrome. I could scarcely get out of bed, and I couldn't lose all the weight I had gained. I went from doctor to doctor. Many of them said, "Your metabolic system has been altered by prednisone. Too bad, but you will never lose that weight. Too bad, but your immune system has been damaged." No one could offer me any help at all.

Dr. Atkins finally was a lot of help to me. I learned about dental amalgams, because when your immune system is depleted, you are much more susceptible to any kind of toxins, including mercury leaching from mercury amalgam fillings. It was causing me a great deal of trouble and I did have those removed.

Then I moved to California. I had heard about Dr. Slagle and her work with depression and had referred friends to her. They'd had miraculous cures after two weeks of taking B complex and amino acids. But I didn't think of going to her myself because I thought of her as someone who only treated depression. In fact, like many alternative physicians, she treats the whole person.

She had worked with fatigue a lot, and she first tested me thoroughly and found that my thyroid and my whole endocrine system were not functioning properly—most likely a result of prednisone. She picked up subtleties in the test that other doctors had ignored. She believes that a body should be healthy and whole. She doesn't need unusual test results to say something is wrong here. So she discovered a rather unusual problem in my thyroid and was able to treat it.

When I began seeing her I still had very limited energy and I still didn't feel normal. In one day, I could either go to the grocery store or go to a doctor's appointment. That was all. The remainder of the day I had to rest. After Dr. Slagle began treating my thyroid, I had a leap of improvement. I regained my energy. She gave me amino acids, which heightened my mood. Even though I hadn't thought I was depressed—and still don't think I was—the amino acids made me feel healthier. And while I don't have the energy of a lot of people around me, I can pretty much function normally, which is a miracle. It has been a five-year struggle and I'm finally living practically a normal life.

I have learned from my experience that you simply cannot go to a traditional physician and allow that doctor to treat your symptoms with drugs. I learned to use tremendous caution when entrusting my body to someone. If you're going to trust your body to someone, you should know whether that physician treats the whole person and sees you as more than an allergy or a gallbladder.

—Helen

Thyroid disease is fifteen to thirty times more prevalent in women that in men. About 15 million women are being treated for it in the United States. The thyroid gland, located at the base of the neck, is an important component of the immune system. As Dr. Stephen Langer explains, "The thyroid gland puts out a teaspoon of hormone a year which affects the metabolism and acts as a cellular carburetor for every cell in the body—from our hair follicles down to our toenails. As such, the thyroid can be implicated in just about any kind of condition you can think of. As for its relationship to psychological disorders, since it plays a role in the metabolism of the nervous system, people who have thyroid disorders have conditions like depression, anxiety, panic attacks, and bipolar disorders."

Dr. Hyla Cass explains what happens when the thyroid does not function as it should. "When the thyroid isn't working properly, the immune system is impaired, and this sets up a vicious cycle. You have a person whose immune system is depleted and who is anxious; they're told by regular doctors that the problem is all in their head, that there's nothing physically wrong with them. So then they feel worse. I recently saw a young woman who came in depressed, tired, unable to get up on the morning, and feeling overwhelmed by her work responsibilities. Her history revealed that she was often cold, especially in her hands and feet (she even wore socks to bed), had thinning hair, dry skin, constipation, and was losing the outer part of her eyebrows. I suspected an imbalance in her thyroid. When I asked about thyroid disease, she said that it had been suspected before, but her tests had been normal. I checked her thyroid hormones, including thyroid antibody levels.

"Often despite 'normal' blood tests, there is an underactive thyroid. Dr. Broda Barnes's technique of monitoring thyroid function through body temperature is used by many alternative practitioners. Although this patient's thyroid hormone blood levels were normal, she did, in fact, have antithyroid antibodies, confirming a diagnosis of Hashimoto's thyroiditis. This is an autoimmune disease, treatable with thyroid hormone, antioxidants and adrenal support. Her signs were those of hypothyroidism, indicating that the circulating hormone was being rendered ineffective. With Hashimoto's thyroiditis, there are often also intermittent signs of hyperthyroidism, or overactive thyroid, such as irritability or heart palpitations.

"I prescribed thyroid hormone from natural (animal) sources, and asked her to monitor her body temperature, so I could adjust the dosage. She asked whether this supplementation would suppress her own thyroid function, and whether she would be taking it for the rest of her life. The answer was 'no' on both counts. The treatment actually supported her own gland, allowing it to heal. Within 10 days of starting the program she was feeling alive again."

Dr. Cass says that a large number of her patients have thyroiditis in combination with other maladies. "I really can't emphasize the importance of this problem enough because thyroiditis often accompanies the mixed infection syndrome, which can consist of any combination of the following: parasites, Candida, and the viral syndromes—including the Epstein-Barr virus and the cytomegalovirus. Psychological components include depression, anxiety and even panic attacks. To treat thyroiditis, I've done nutritional consults on people that were under the care of other physicians. When I suggested that they had thyroiditis and that it was to be treated with low doses of thyroid hormones, I was met with skepticism from the other doctors."   Dr. Langer says that most of his patients have symptoms that are both psychological and organic in nature. "Many people come into my office with an organic kind of illness that has been misdiagnosed as being either psychosomatic or primarily psychological," he says. "Very rarely do I see a patient who comes in with complaints that are primarily psychological in cause. Very often, their complaints have some organic basis which, if taken care of, allows them to resolve much more easily whatever psychological problems they do have.

"If a person's metabolism is hypofunctioning, everything is going to be slow. In a book I wrote called *Solve the Riddle of Illness*, I explain why upwards of 40 percent of the population may have subclinical hypothyroidism and not detect it by the traditional blood chemistry work that's done at their general practitioner's office. The symptoms of low thyroid include weakness, dry coarse skin, slow speech, coarse hair, hair loss, weight gain, difficulty breathing, problems with menstruation, nervousness, heart palpitations, brittle nails, and severe chronic fatigue and depression.

"Now if you get somebody with a constellation of symptoms like that, they're going to be sick and tired of feeling sick and tired. Plus they're going to feel depressed all the time because they're going from one doctor to another, sometimes with two or three or four pages worth of complaints, and the doctors tell them it's all in their head, or that they should go home and learn to live with it. Obviously you're going to see depression. Now not everything that I see is hypothyroidism by any means. But hypothyroidism is so easy to identify and so ubiquitous in the population, and it can be treated so well and so rapidly for so little money, that it's become a primary interest of mine."

Dr. Langer describes his treatment approach using case examples. "Recently I treated a patient who was the wife of a doctor and the mother of two young children. She basically came in and told me that she didn't want to go on living. She was so tired all the time and so depressed that she couldn't keep her head off the pillow after 2:00 in the afternoon. If she didn't go to bed, she would just fall apart. I did a history and physical on her and we made some dietary changes, but basically this woman was profoundly hypothyroid. We put her on a quarter of a grain of thyroid, which is what I start my patients with before building them up very gradually. A quarter of a grain is the smallest dose available. It's such a small quantity that most pharmacies don't even carry it, because when doctors order thyroid they don't even think to order so small a dose. But a quarter of a grain of thyroid was enough. Within a three-week period, this woman not only regained her mental health, but she was out taking tennis lessons, which was shocking even to me because although the treatment usually works it usually takes a longer period of time. So, just that amount of metabolic support was enough to turn this person's life around.

"Another person I treated was a 62-year-old woman who was a member of the Catholic clergy. She had been a nun for at least 30 years when I met her and I will never forget this woman. She came in bloated, profoundly depressed and fatigued. The only thing that kept her going was basically overworking her adrenal glands. She came in and told me that when she was 12 years old, she went under a dark cloud. When I saw her it was 50 years later, and by that time she had been through 30 or 40 different doctors, including internists, endocrinologists, psychiatrists and psychologists of various sorts.

"One of the first things that showed up in her—which I thought was a very positive sign—was that she was freezing all the time. When we did a basal body temperature, it never went above 95 degrees. Basal body temperature is a person's resting temperature when she wakes up in the morning. However, when I did a blood work-up on her, all her thyroid hormone levels were within normal limits. I empirically placed her on a dose of thyroid that we gradually built up to about four grains a day, which is quite a high dosage. She's one of the few people I've treated who has needed that high an amount. Within three months her depression of 50 years duration was totally gone. Now, obviously she was bitter and angry that she had been suffering for all that time. But the organic feeling that she had of overwhelming fatigue totally disappeared within a three-month period of time, and I've seen that response in thousands of patients over the years. A small dose of thyroid, combined with things like nutritional support and eliminating food allergies, can really turn a person's life around."

Among the psychological symptoms of thyroiditis are depression, anxiety, and panic attacks. Dr. Langer explains, "They could be sitting and reading a book. All of a sudden they will develop a cascade of heart palpitations and fearfulness. I've had a number of patients who have been rushed, almost on a monthly basis, to the emergency room to be worked up by cardiologists because their heart was pounding over 200 beats a minute. Cardiologists would do EKGs and echocardiograms and tell them to go see a psychiatrist who would work them up, not find anything, and then put them on an antidepressant or a tranquilizer, and actually make the condition worse. When you have an undiscovered organic basis for a psychological problem, being put on psychotropic medication is like sitting on a thumbtack and being put on pain pills for the rest of your life. It has about the same effect. It wears the system down, and as a result the patient's condition not only does not improve but will in fact deteriorate, because the underlying cause is not being treated."

Even though middle-aged women are most often affected, thyroid disorders can occur in younger women and in men. "I have seen as many men as women who are suffering from autoimmune thyroiditis and, I might add, from hypothyroidism," Dr. Langer says. "Men are really given short shrift and aren't even given the requisite diagnostic tests in many instances to rule out thyroid disease because the medical profession thinks that this is strictly a woman's disorder.

"Moreover, I have seen teenagers and children who are acting out, who are written off as hyperactive, when they may be suffering from a thyroid disorder. Because thyroid dysfunction often leads to frequent infections, these kids are placed on antibiotics. Then they wind up with an overgrowth of yeast in their gut that in turn causes a low-grade inflammation in their gastrointestinal system. As a result, they don't adequately digest their food, so the body starts regarding the food as a foreign invader and puts out antibodies to the food. The child starts exhibiting the classic symptoms of food allergies, which are psychiatric complaints: anxiety attacks, depression, forgetfulness, inability to concentrate, even full-blown panic attacks. In a lot of these cases, you can actually isolate and eliminate the foods that cause an anxiety attack, but merely removing the food is not enough to get to the underlying cause of the disorder. Frequently patients have food allergies because of a pre-existing condition in their digestive systems which has to be addressed. The presence of such a pre-existing condition can cause immune system alterations which result in autoimmune dysfunction. So this is a vicious circle. One of the chief target organs of autoimmune dysfunction is the thyroid gland. You get autoimmune thyroiditis."

"In my clinical experience, I have found that with the thyroid and nutritional support, very often a person will get better. The thyroid is not a lifetime treatment and can be removed after the person's condition has been stabilized. Thyroid treatment is inexpensive, works rapidly, and when done properly it is absolutely nontoxic."

Dr. Langer mentions one other connection to be drawn between depression and the thyroid dysfunction: poor libido. "One of the classic symptoms of depression is a loss of interest in sex," he says. "Those people who in the past were sexually active, but who all of a sudden or gradually started to lose interest in sex, will be diagnosed as being depressed right away. Men come into my office by the score—many of them young—who have potency problems, and they can't figure it out because they have no apparent organic illness. As a result, they get performance anxiety, and if that continues long enough, they wind up getting severely depressed. But I have found that if you go to the root cause of their depression, very often it's the thyroid that's malfunctioning."

Dr. Allan Spreen reminds us that while thyroid supplementation is an important modality, it is not fail-safe. "I'd love to say that correcting thyroid function is a panacea. While it doesn't work 100 percent of the time, if a patient comes in complaining of fatigue and depression that is linked with the physical findings of foods not digesting well, and cold extremities, then an underactive thyroid may be the root cause. People come and say, 'Oh, my husband says, Don't touch me with your feet at night because they're just ice cold.' These are the same people who are comfortable in a room when everybody else is boiling and they're freezing in a room when everybody else is comfortable. Their thinking seems to have slowed down, they just don't seem to be able to concentrate like they used to, and they don't remember lists the way they used to.

"In this kind of a situation, once I find that their blood levels of thyroid are normal, I go back to the old school of Broda Barnes, who did axillary temperature testing. I ask my patients to keep a record of their early morning basal body temperature. If their basal metabolic rate based on early-morning body temperatures is really low, then I consider them to be candidates for thyroid supplementation. In axillary testing, Broda Barnes talked about temperature ranges between 97.8 and 98.2 degrees Fahrenheit, which is lower than the 98.6 people think of as normal. But the axillary temperature is taken in the armpit first thing in the morning, using a mercury thermometer that stays there for 10 minutes before they get up. If their temperature is, much of the time, down in the 96.8, 96.7, 96.5 range, I at least consider the possibility that the person needs low doses of natural thyroid.

"Thyroid is a prescription drug, but it can be broken down into very low doses. Some doctors who use this type of testing use synthetic thyroid. I prefer to prescribe natural thyroid in very low doses. If a person responds—either their temperature rises or their symptoms lift—then I retest them to see if their blood levels of thyroid have changed. Many times a person with this profile of symptoms who takes thyroid will feel better, and their blood tests will have remained unchanged, including their thyroid stimulating hormone and their actual thyroid hormone levels. So the blood testing has missed the diagnosis, and yet the person feels well with the increased, but undetectable dose of thyroid hormone."

29

Migraines

■■■

If you're one of approximately 30 million Americans who suffer from migraines, you know how debilitating this condition can be. Lasting several hours to as long as a few days, migraines are headaches marked by throbbing pain on one side of the head and associated symptoms such as nausea, vomiting, and sensitivity to light and sound. Shortly before the headache begins, some people also experience auras—flashes of light, blind spots, and tingling in the arm or leg.

Sleep disturbances and depression also may be present. Dr. John Allocca, a medical research scientist and author of *The Migraine-Depression Solution*, emphasizes the connection between migraines and mental health conditions. In an article published in the *International Guide to the World of Alternative Mental Health* (www.alternativementalhealth.com), he explains, "During the headache, one may experience mood changes with feelings of being rejected and often seriously depressed. At times one may be unsociable, rejecting companionship or the presence of others, becoming irritable and rejecting any demand to make a decision." He goes on to say that migraine and depression, as well as insomnia, "have similar mechanisms and pathways, all resulting from a loss of serotonin and norepinephrine."

Migraines typically begin prior to young adulthood, and are three times more common in women than men. They are believed to be caused by abnormalities in certain nerve pathways and chemicals in the brain. Specifically, a decrease in serotonin causes the trigeminal nerve to release neuropeptides. These substances travel to the outer covering of the brain, where they cause blood vessels to dilate. Among the many triggers of migraine attacks are stress, environmental changes, hormones, sleep changes, medications, and sensory stimuli. Foods also may play a role. Foods containing tyramine, such as red wine, aged cheese, and smoked fish; nitrates, including hot dogs and bacon; and monosodium glutamate (MSG);

and caffeine are commonly implicated, as are chocolate, nuts, aspartame, and fermented or pickled items.

Conventional treatment usually consists of pain-relieving medications, preventive medications, and avoiding triggers. Complementary medicine offers a host of other remedies, including dietary and environmental changes; herbal, vitamin, and mineral supplements; homeopathy; acupuncture; and biofeedback.

Dr. Mary Olsen, a chiropractor, suggests general guidelines for treating migraines brought on by different factors. Diet is a good place to start. "Since migraines don't necessarily follow immediately after ingesting a food, it may be difficult to make a connection between a particular food and the resultant headache. We often have patients keep a food diary to record what is eaten and their physical reactions. If we suspect that a particular food is troublesome, the patient is asked to place a sample of that food under the tongue. If there is a sensitivity, a muscle that tested strong previously will weaken. The pulse is also evaluated for such changes as increases in intensity or frequency. Treatment can be as simple as removing the offending food."

If environmental exposure is suspected, houseplants may be helpful. "Different plants have the ability to absorb different toxins," Dr. Olsen explains. "For example, spider plants absorb the formaldehyde released from particleboard, plywood, synthetic carpeting and new upholstery, while chrysanthemum protects against the toxic effects of lacquers, varnishes and glues."

Dr. Olsen also advocates the use of the herb feverfew. "Feverfew has sedative qualities," she says, "and can be taken as a tea. One cup per day is usually effective."

According to Dr. Jennifer Brett, "When feverfew is taken with magnesium in does of 250 to 500 milligrams daily, as well as with ginkgo biloba, most people notice a significant reduction in the number of migraines, even to the point of disappearance. This includes people who suffer daily migraines. Many people come to me who have had no success with more conventional treatments. After I start them on the feverfew and magnesium, they get a significant reduction in the number of headaches and the severity of pain. Even when they have headaches, they tend to be less frequent and less painful." Feverfew should not be used by pregnant women.

Dr. Emily Kane, in an article published by the American Association of Naturopathic Physicians in *HealthWorld Online*, adds her recommendations, with the reminder to first consult with a nutritionist or naturopath: vitamin B-complex injected into the muscle every two to ten days; omega-3 fatty acids (such as raw flax or linseed oil, one teaspoon daily); omega-6 fatty acids, found in fish, and olive oil; vitamin B3, 500 milligrams at the start of the migraine; magnesium in doses of 400 to 800 milligrams daily; and Quercetin, 500 milligrams per day.

Dr. Kane also suggests the following herbal tea, which can cleanse the system and thereby prevent or decrease migraines:

> 1 part hops
> 1 part chamomile
> 1/2 part oatstraw
> 1/2 part catnip
> 1/2 part skuillcap
> 1/4 part peppermint leaf
> You can make this formula yourself by adding a heaping table-
> spoon to a cup of water that has just boiled and steeping it for
> three to five minutes. You can add honey to sweeten. Drink
> this tea two to three times a day.

Among the homeopathic remedies that have been useful in relieving migraines are arnica montana, lachesis, natrum muriaticum, nux vomica, phosphorus, pulsatilla, rhus toxicodendron, sepia, silica, and thuja occidentalis. These substances are matched to the particular symptoms a person exhibits.

Dr. Kane says there are many inventive forms of hydrotherapy that involve applying cold to the head and heat to the feet. For example, cold wet packs on the forehead, back of the neck and head will constrict the blood vessels so that less blood flows into the head. Soaking the feet in a hot footbath that contains peppermint and apple cider vinegar as well as water will bring the blood away from the head and into the feet, and also cool and cleanse the blood. When the headache is severe, try alternating hot and cold, using towels that are soaked and then wrung out and applied to the face and head. The last application should be cold.

Accupressure is based on the principle that a vital energy, called qi (chi), flows through the body. The primary cause of pain is an imbalance in this energy. The goal of the healer is to balance the client's energy so that pain and discomfort do not manifest, or if they do appear, will be relieved. The practitioner concentrates on certain pressure points to modulate the flow of energy. A point known as Wind Gate is effective for migraines related to the change of seasons. It is actually two points located at the highest point of the neck just below the hairline on either side of the muscles that run up the spine. Other points useful in people with migraines are the fleshy area between the thumb and forefinger and the area below the bottom of the big toe.

Biofeedback is a technique that teaches a person to consciously keep regular bodily processes that are normally involuntary, such as heartbeat, brain waves, blood pressure, and muscle tension. The processes may be monitored by electronic equipment or by natural observation, such as holding a finger over an artery. With practice, the person learns to makes changes on his own. Using thermal control, a biofeedback technique, people may be able to control migraines by raising their finger temperatures with a digital-temperature device. This appears to work by increasing blood flow, which is decreased by nervous tension. Another biofeedback technique places sensors on the temples, over the temporal arteries. People learn to diminish their migraines by changing their pulse rates.

PART SIX

What You Can Do: Protocols for Heart and Brain Health

First, a word of caution. When it comes to protocols, or specific programs, it is important to remember that they are designed to be done in an incremental fashion, under medical supervision. It is stated here in the strongest possible way that you must, you simply *must* follow this protocol under a holistic physician's supervision, ideally a board-certified cardiologist.

Remember, please . . . The following caution has been given several times before, and will be repeated later, but it is extremely important. It will be given in the form of an example: If you have high cholesterol, heart disease, and hypertension, and each has a protocol calling for garlic at 1,000 mg, this does not mean that you are to take 3,000 mg. You take only the amount called for in one protocol. In other words, these protocols are not additive.

Generally, you would follow the protocol for the primary condition. Let us say you have five illnesses. Take the illness that seems to be the most threatening, and follow that protocol. Once you have followed this protocol for a year, and you see the condition improving, chances are great that the other conditions are improving as well.

Your whole body, at this point, should be stronger and healthier, and your immune system should be working better. The energy-enhancing vitality of one protocol will, no doubt, help you with your other conditions. However, if you still find you need help, go to the second protocol (the one for the next troublesome condition). Try that one for a year as well. Never take three protocols for three conditions at once. That would overwhelm the system.

I also want to stress again that in suggesting alternative treatments, I am not claiming that these treatments are absolute cures, only that they can have a major, beneficial effect on the conditions. I am not asking you to give up whatever your doctor is suggesting, if you decide to go with any of these protocols. These are complementary, augmentative treatments. That is why they should be followed under medical supervision.

30

A Wellness Protocol

■■■

Before we begin exploring specialized treatments for individual ailments, I want to offer a baseline wellness protocol. This one-size-fits-all program of supplementation is based on the work I did in the health support groups and represents one of the pillars of my Wellness Model. You should work with your doctor to make sure that the supplements listed below are right for you. This is particularly important if you are taking any medications. Moreover, you should not be taking all these supplements at once.

Baseline Wellness Program

Vitamin A	15,000 IU
Vitamin C	10,000 mg
Vitamin D	300 IU
Vitamin E	500 IU
Vitamin B1	75 mg
Vitamin B2	50 mg
Vitamin B3	150 mg
Vitamin B6	102 mg
Folic Acid	800 mcg
Vitamin B12	250 mcg
Biotin	400 mcg
Pantothenic Acid	500 mg
Calcium	282 mg
Iodine	10 mcg
Magnesium	800 mg
Zinc	20 mg

Manganese	25 mg
Chromium	200 mcg
Selenium	100 mcg
Molybdenum	125 mcg
Potassium	50 mg
Copper	2 mg
Astaxanthin	25 mg
L-Carnosine	100 mg
Rosemary Leaf Powder	25 mg
Tocotrienols	25 mg
Raspberry Leaf Powder	5 mg
Citrus Bioflavonoid	300 mg
Rutin	25 mg
Red Wine Concentrate	25 mg
Grape Skin Extract	150 mg
China Green Tea Leaf Powder	200 mg
Licorice Root	25 mg
Cabbage Leaf	25 mg
Carrot Root	25 mg
Para Amino Benzoic Acid	200 mcg
Mushroom Complex	50 mg
Milk Thistle Leaf Extract	25 mg
Bilberry Fruit Powder	25 mg
Lycopene	20 mg
Grape Seed Extract	50 mg
Coenzyme Q10	50 mg
Quercetin	50 mg
Ginkgo Biloba Leaf Powder	60 mg
Broccoli	75 mg
Acerola	100 mg
Hesperedin	100 mg
Glutathione	100 mg
Linolenic Acid	100 mg
Ginger Rhizome Extract	100 mg
Superoxide Dismutase	25 mg
Alpha-Lipoic Acid	150 mg

Trimethylglycine	200 mg
Phosphatidylserine	200 mg
Isoflavone Genistein	200 mg
Inositol	250 mg
Lutein	25 mg
Citrus Bioflavonoids	300 mg
Methylsulfenyl Methane	400 mg
L-Taurine	500 mg
N-Acetyl Cysteine	500 mg
L-Lysine HCl	500 mg
Orthinine Alpha Ketoglutarate	500 mg
Choline Bitartrate	500 mg
Phosphatidyl Choline	500 mg
Acetyl-L-Carnitine	500 mg
Bromelain	15 mg

31

A Cardiovascular Protocol

■■■

Supplements

The following nutrients are needed for the cardiovascular system. It is not suggested that all of these be taken at once. That would be too much for the body, so take only a few at a time over the course of the day.

Coenzyme Q10 is a superstar in protecting the heart. It feeds the cell. It allows the transport of fatty acids to the cell so that the cell's mitochondria have the energy needed to function properly. This is especially important for the heart muscle, for obvious reasons!

I believe that if every American took between 100 to 300 mg of coenzyme Q10 a day, and if people with cardiovascular disease took between 300 to 500 mg of this wonder-nutrient daily, we could be saving hundreds of thousands of lives a year. If you're taking a large amount of coenzyme Q10, do so in divided doses. For example, if you are taking a total of 500 mg of coenzyme Q10, you should take 100 mg five times a day.

Calcium and magnesium from citrate (always taken together) in the amount of about 1,500 mg a day are a crucial pair of nutrients for the heart. There will be more information about magnesium, the most important but sadly neglected heart nutrient, below.

Other important substances include garlic (1,000 to 5,000 mg), onion (a raw onion a day helps keep strokes and heart attacks away), and L-carnitine (500 to 1,000 mg). L-carnitine increases energy by burning fat within the cell's mitochondria. This helps the body to recover quickly from fatigue. And L-carnitine is especially good when combined with vitamin E, another superstar heart disease fighter, phosphatidylcholine (500 mg twice a day), DMG (dimethylglycine)

(100 mg once a day), TMG (trimethylglycine) (200 mg twice a day), Maxepa (fish oils) (1,500 mg), potassium (500 mg), selenium (200 mcg), melatonin (1 to 3 mg), B complex (50 mg), vitamin C (2,000 to 10,000 mg), DHEA (25 mg; do not use DHEA if you have cancer), chromium picolinate (200 mcg), chondroitin sulfate (500 mg two times a day), evening primrose oil (generally at 1,500 mg in divided doses), polycosinol (10 mg), and N-acetyl cysteine (1,500 mg). Alpha-lipoic acid (300 mg) is very important as a free-radical scavenger.

Also very important for heart disease is natural (not synthetic) vitamin E (with tocotrienols and the gamma fraction) generally at 400 IU with tocotrienols at 100 mg. Bioflavonoids are also quite helpful. Make sure you have what are called methylating agents, namely vitamin B_{12}, folic acid (800 units), and TMG. The essential fatty acids are just that—essential! The two types are called omega-3 and omega-6. Fish oils are a source of omega-3 and evening primrose oil is a source of omega-6. Generally, 3,000 mg of omega-3 and 2,000 mg of omega-6 should be divided into three doses, daily.

L-arginine facilitates the body's production of nitric oxide, which has an antiangina and antistress effect upon the arteries, enabling the muscles in the arterial walls to relax. This amino acid is generally taken at 2,000 to 3,000 mg per day.

Lecithin can reduce arterial plaque, lower blood pressure, and lessen angina pectoris. Take lecithin granules in one teaspoon in the morning (they can be sprinkled over cereal). Taurine, an amino acid that acts as an antioxidant, can help fortify cardiac contractions and consequently enhance the outflow of blood from the heart. Take it generally at 500 mg. Niacin (vitamin B_3) has been shown to help prevent heart attacks. It also helps prevent people from dying from them.

Mineral for the Heart

Magnesium is the single most important mineral for the heart. Generally, people don't realize that a magnesium-deficient heart is almost always more susceptible to heart attack. This brings up the ever-important concept of the preventive approaches. Logic suggests that if filling a specific nutrient deficiency in a sick person ameliorates the condition, then giving a healthy person that nutrient in more than adequate amounts should prevent the condition from developing in the first place. In the case of heart disease, we see certain nutrients, such as magnesium, that are deficient in all patients. Common sense would then dictate that giving more than adequate amounts of these nutrients to people will help prevent or reverse heart disease.

Herbs for Heart Health

There are some herbs that are excellent for promoting cardiovascular health. Cayenne is a superstar because it contains the active ingredient capsaicin. Capsaicin lowers blood pressure and cholesterol and prevents heart attacks and strokes. It is a natural blood thinner. However, it is not safe for everyone to take this herb, because for those taking certain medications, such as Coumadin (warfarin), there could be contraindications. So you have to ask your physician if any prescription drug you are taking may prohibit the use of cayenne. This is very important.

Otherwise, cayenne, best known as the spice cayenne pepper, should definitely be used, but carefully, because it is very hot! If you use this as a spice, do not cook the pepper with the food but sprinkle it on only after cooking the food, to avoid irritation.

Hawthorn berry improves arrhythmias, angina, blood pressure, and arterial hardening. It can enhance circulation. It treats valve insufficiencies, irregular pulse, and abnormal acid levels in the blood. In short, it is a really terrific herb! Hawthorn is generally taken at 100 mg twice a day. Bugleweed helps alleviate heart palpitations and lowers blood pressure. Ginkgo biloba, the well-known multipurpose herb, gets more blood flowing into the small blood vessels. It's suggested at 300 mg in divided doses. Motherwort helps secure cardiac electrical rhythm. Tansy is another herb used for heart palpitations, and it can be ingested as a tea. Wild yam enhances the body's production of DHEA, and DHEA is crucial in helping to prevent heart attacks. Arjuna is an Ayurvedic herb that enhances circulation and lowers blood pressure. Indian snakeroot also has anti-hypertensive qualities. Black cohosh, an American herb, helps lower blood pressure.

We've said this before, but let's restate the warnings: It is not at all advisable to take all these substances at the same time. Instead, take one or two of these for a month, as professionally directed. Record the results. Then, under continued guidance, repeat or increase the dosage, or move on to different substances. Do not self-medicate. These supplements are not meant as medicines. These are not meant to treat diseases, but only to augment the body's internal biochemistry, to help strengthen it, so that whatever else you are doing can be better applied.

Intravenous Treatments for Cardiovascular Health

There are several intravenous treatments that have proven very effective in the cardiovascular arena. EDTA chelation therapy is crucial, I believe, for treating coronary artery disease and arterial sclerosis. I have seen many people who were about to receive coronary bypass operations, or some other drastic treatment, improve tremendously, even dramatically, using chelation therapy. If you already have a heart condition, you have to be patient and courageous, because it may take some time, probably upwards of two years, to do this properly, but your life is worth it. We have seen from the literature that this therapy definitely works and that you can reclaim your life!

Vitamin C, taken intravenously, is another extremely important therapy given at a practitioner's office. This lifesaving treatment has been able to help people with cancer and heart disease, among many other conditions.

32

A Protocol to Lower Cholesterol

■■■

Stressed-out baby boomers worry about (among other things!) their cholesterol level. And well they might, since stress tends to elevate cholesterol. Having elevated blood sugar can also contribute to high cholesterol. Generally, most people don't have their cholesterol levels checked. They should. This is done as part of a blood lipid profile.

You cannot eliminate cholesterol from the diet, and, indeed, you should not do so, because, as mentioned previously, cholesterol is important. But it must be kept in check.

We know that high-fiber foods, and the pectin found in apples, will lower cholesterol. Blueberries are very good at this, too. Hot grain cereals, such as oats, barley, and buckwheat are also good. Therefore, having some apples and blueberries in your cereal is exceptionally helpful. Other anticholesterol foods are polyunsaturated oils (in small amounts only!) and linoleic oils from cold fish (but do not eat shellfish), walnuts, almonds, sunflower seeds, and nut butters.

Supplements that Lower Cholesterol

L-carnosine can help rejuvenate the cell and protect it from prematurely aging, going into apoptosis (programmed cell death), and dying, because it protects the chromosomes. (Note: Do not confuse this substance with L-carnitine, another helpful supplement taken at 1,000 mg a day.) Additional recommendations are L-glutamine (2,000 mg a day), vitamin E (400 IU), bromelain as directed, maitake and shiitake mushrooms (generally at 100 mg each), as well as ganoderma (reishi) mushrooms, and bioflavonoids.

Herbs that Lower Cholesterol

The most helpful herbs for lowering cholesterol and triglycerides are ginger, cayenne, raw garlic, and onions; also take ginkgo biloba, gotu kola as directed, and red clover as directed.

Mineral that Lowers Cholesterol

Potassium is the superstar mineral for lowering hypertension and cholesterol. Generally taken at 500 mg a day, it will help significantly.

Phytochemicals that Lower Cholesterol

The healing phytochemicals in fruits and fruit juices are also very important. For people with high blood sugar, there are now concentrates on the market without the fruit sugar in them, so everyone can get the benefits of drinking a lot of fruit juice. Remember that red fruits and their concentrates repair damage to your DNA. This is crucial because once you repair the damage to the DNA, the cell can regain much, if not all, of its previous functioning.

Exercise to Lower Cholesterol

When you exercise aerobically for up to an hour a day, you are increasing the good HDL cholesterol and reducing the bad LDL cholesterol. It may take three, four, or five months, but you will see a noticeable change.

33

A Protocol to Lower High Blood Pressure (Hypertension)

■■■

Hypertension is one of the top killers. It is estimated that 60 million Americans suffer from it. Stress is a major cause. Being under pressure on the job, or trying to do too much, or any of the hundreds of tension-filled situations in life may cause elevated blood sugar and stress hormones. And the unfortunate fact is that elevated blood sugar plus elevated blood pressure is a deadly combination, if ever there was one. One is bad enough. Two together can be catastrophic. If you have these two conditions, you are probably in for some serious consequences. In addition, inflammatory responses are the frequent accompaniment. A heart attack or stroke is just waiting to happen.

Supplements to Reduce High Blood Pressure

When your goal is reducing hypertension, the following will help: the superstar mineral potassium (500 mg to 800 mg); 1,500 mg of calcium magnesium citrate; vitamin C (5,000 mg to 10,000 mg); vitamin B_6 (100 mg); coenzyme Q10 (generally 300 to 500 mg); the omega-3 fatty acids from fish (1,500 mg); L-carnitine (1,500 mg); L-glutamine (1,000 mg); vitamin E with tocotrienols and gamma tocopherol (400 to 800 units); red clover; and again, our tried and true friend garlic.

Phytochemicals to Reduce High Blood Pressure

What can be done about this situation? The advice here is short, but good: first, we have to thin our blood. Green vegetable juices naturally do this.

Stress Management for Lowering Blood Pressure

Keeping all the foregoing in mind, we can end the chapter on a positive and constructive note. Stress management techniques are very important for bringing down your blood pressure. Meditation can play a role here, as can destressing exercises and techniques, prayer, listening to calm music, going for walks, playing with your companion pets, spending quality time in your relationships without arguing, and pursuing hobbies or anything that can bring you joy during the day—or night, for that matter!

Bring your energy to a calm place. Get rid of all excess stimulation around you. Have a candlelit meal with nice soft music. Take a bubble bath, if that is what appeals to you. Do things that are just fun, and watch your blood pressure come down.

34

Supplements for Best Brain Health

■■■

Supplemental vitamins and minerals, as well as smart nutrients and drugs, can be extremely beneficial to our brain health when used in combination with a healthful diet. But I know keeping track of the proper dosages can be difficult. To help you in that goal, I have provided the following chart that summarizes the supplement program I recommend.

The plan that follows is intended to promote brain health and protect your brain. When recommending protocols for specific conditions, as I do later in this chapter, I am assuming that you are already following the supplement program in the chart that follows.

Do not combine this protocol with more than one additional protocol from this book. If you are taking medications, or have any food restrictions, you should consult with your doctor before beginning this or any supplement program. Supplement overdoses are rare, but possible, and certain combinations may affect individuals adversely.

VITAMINS AND NUTRIENTS	DAILY DOSE	COMMENTS
acetyl-L-carnitine (ACL)	2,000 mg in two divided doses	
alpha-lipoic acid	300 mg in two divided doses	
B-complex vitamins	• 100 mg thiamin (B_1) • 50 mg riboflavin (B_2) • 200 mg niacin (B_3) • 1,000 mg pantothenic acid (B_5) • 75 mg pyridoxine (B_6)	A B-complex vitamin should contain the dosages I recommend.

VITAMINS AND NUTRIENTS	DAILY DOSE	COMMENTS
B-complex vitamins (cont.)	• 250 mg inositol (B_8) • 800 mcg folic acid (B_9) • 100 mcg vitamin B_{12} • 60 mcg biotin • 200–300 mg trimethylglycine (TMG) • 45 mg choline • 100 mg para-aminobenzoic acid	
carnosine	1,000 mg	
coenzyme Q10 (coQ10)	100–300 mg with meals	
dehydroepiandrosterone (DHEA)	25–50 mg	Must be prescribed by health practitioner. Individuals with hormone-related cancers should not take DHEA.
dimethylaminoethanol (DMAE)	150 mg	May be overstimulating for some people. Headaches, muscle tension, and irritability may occur. Do not take if you have epilepsy, a history of convulsions, or bipolar disorder. If you have kidney or liver disease, consult your doctor before taking this supplement.
essential fatty acids (EFAs)	• 4,000 mg borage oil (equals 920 mg GLA) • 2,000 mg fish oil extract (equals 1,000 mg DHA) • 400 mg EFP	
glycerylphosphorylcholine (GPC)	600 mg	
hydergine	5–10 mg	
lecithin	1 gram	About 1 heaping tablespoon of granules.
phosphatidylcholine	500–1,000 mg	
phosphatidylserine (PS)	300 mg	Do not use if you have a bipolar disorder. Do not use if you suffer from depression.
pregnenolone	50 mg	Individuals with hormone-related cancers should not take pregnenolone.
proanthocyanidins	80 mg	Naturally occurring in grape seed extract and pine bark extract.
selenium	200 mcg	
vinpocetine	10 mg two times daily with meals	

VITAMINS AND NUTRIENTS	DAILY DOSE	COMMENTS
vitamin C	1–3 grams	
vitamin E	• 400 IU • 200 mg (gamma-tocopherol) • 65 mg (palm oil–derived tocotrienols)	Mixed tocopherols with an emphasis on gamma.

Additional Supplements for Impacting Depression

The following chart summarizes additional supplements I recommend for individuals who suffer from, or are specifically concerned about, depression. If you are concerned about additional brain conditions discussed in other chapters, consult with a health professional about how you can safely impact multiple conditions. As always, if you are taking medication—whether prescription or over-the-counter—or have any food restrictions, consult with your doctor before beginning the supplement program. Your health care provider should always be up-to-date on all vitamins, supplements, and herbal or homeopathic remedies you are taking. Supplement overdoses are rare, but possible, and certain combinations may affect individuals adversely.

SUPPLEMENT	DOSAGE	CAUTIONS
5-HTP (5-hydroxytryptophan)	50–100 mg three times daily	Several months of treatment may be needed for maximum benefit. Nausea is the main side effect, but if it occurs, it usually dissipates within several days. Do not combine with prescription antidepressants. If you are taking prescription medication for depression, you should consult your doctor before taking 5-HTP. Excess levels of serotonin in the blood can be dangerous in case of coronary artery disease.
Adapton (Garum Armoricum)	4 capsules as directed daily for fifteen days; stop for one week, then continue with maintenance dose of 2 capsules daily.	
DHEA hormone	Follow doctor's directions for dosage.	Must be prescribed by your health practitioner. Individuals with hormone-related cancers should not take DHEA.

SUPPLEMENT	DOSAGE	CAUTIONS
DLPA (DL-phenylalanine)	1,000–1,500 mg	Do not combine DLPA with prescription antidepressants or stimulants unless specifically directed to do so by your doctor. Do not take DLPA if you have high blood pressure, or are prone to panic attacks, are taking levodopa for treatment of Parkinson's disease, are pregnant, have melanoma, or have PKU (a rare, inherited metabolism disorder).
DMAE (dimethylaminoethanol)	Increase daily dosage from 150 mg to 650–1,650 mg. Do not exceed a daily supplement of 1,650 mg.	May be overstimulating for some people. Headaches, muscle tension, and irritability may occur. Do not take if you have epilepsy, a history of convulsions, or bipolar disease. If you have kidney or liver disease, consult your doctor before taking this supplement.
Inositol	Increase daily dosage from 250 mg to 2,250 mg. Do not exceed a daily supplement of 2,250 mg. Take in two divided doses.	
magnesium	320 mg (for women) 420 mg (for men)	May take six weeks or more for effect to be felt.
potassium you

out | 500 mg | Do not take potassium supplements if

are taking medication for high blood pressure or heart disease, or if you have a kidney disorder. Consuming foods rich in potassium is okay. Do not exceed a supplementary dose of 3.5 grams daily with-

consulting with your doctor. |
| pregnenolone | Increase daily dosage from 50 mg to 100–250 mg. Do not exceed a daily supplement of 250 mg. | Individuals with hormone-related cancers should not take pregnenolone. |
| SAMe two (S-adenosylmethionine) | Dosage range of

400–1,600 mg | Raise the dose gradually from 200 mg

times a day to 400 mg two times a day, to 400 mg three times a day, to 400 mg four times a day, over a period of twenty days. |
| vitamin D | 400–600 IU daily | Do not exceed 800 IU daily. |

Additional Supplements for Impacting Anxiety

The following chart summarizes additional supplements I recommend for individuals who suffer from, or are specifically concerned about, anxiety. If you are concerned about additional brain conditions discussed in other chapters, consult with a health professional about how you can safely impact multiple conditions. As always, if you are taking medication—whether prescription or over-the-counter—or have any food restrictions, consult with your doctor before beginning the supplement program. Your health care provider should always be up-to-date on all vitamins, supplements, and herbal or homeopathic remedies you are taking. Supplement overdoses are rare, but possible, and certain combinations may affect individuals adversely.

SUPPLEMENT	DOSAGE	CAUTIONS
Adapton (*Garum Armoricum*)	4 capsules as directed daily for fifteen days; stop for one week, then continue with maintenance dose of 2 capsules daily.	
inositol (vitamin B_8)	Increase daily dosage from 250 mg to 2,250 mg. Do not exceed a daily supplement of 2,250 mg. Take in two divided doses.	
magnesium	320 mg (for women) 420 mg (for men)	May take six weeks or more for effects to be felt.
melatonin	300 mcg–1 mg at night a half hour before bed.	
theanine	200 mg	

Additional Supplements for Impacting Memory Loss

The following chart summarizes additional supplements I recommend for individuals who suffer from, or are specifically concerned about, memory loss. If you are concerned about additional brain conditions discussed in other chapters, consult with a health professional about how you can safely impact multiple conditions.

If you are taking medications—whether prescription or over-the-counter—or have any food restrictions, consult with your doctor before beginning any supplement program. Your health care provider should always be up-to-date on all vitamins, supplements, and herbal or homeopathic remedies you are taking. Supplement overdoses are rare, but possible, and certain combinations may affect individuals adversely.

SUPPLEMENT	DOSAGE	CAUTIONS
lecithin	For men: increase daily dosage from 1 gram to 2.5 grams. Do not exceed a daily supplement of 2.5 grams. For women: increase daily dosage from 1 gram to 2 grams. Do not exceed a daily supplement of 2 grams.	Side effects may include nausea, bloating, vomiting, sweating, and diarrhea; extremely large doses can cause a heart-rhythm abnormality; do not use if you have bipolar disorder.
DMAE (dimethylaminoethanol)	Increase daily dosage from 150 mg to 650–1,650 mg. Do not exceed a daily supplement of 1,650 mg.	May be overstimulating for some people. Headaches, muscle tension, and irritability may occur. Do not take if you have epilepsy, a history of convulsions, or bipolar disorder. If you have kidney or liver disease, consult your doctor before taking this supplement.
iron	Consult your doctor.	Have a blood test to determine true iron deficiency, as iron overload can cause health problems. Iron can interfere with a number of drugs, including thyroid hormone drugs, antibiotics, and drugs used to treat Parkinson's disease. Tannins found in coffee and tea can inhibit iron absorption.
NAC (N-acetylcysteine)	500 mg three times daily	Regular supplementation of NAC increases urinary output of copper. If supplementing with NAC for an extended period, add 2 mg of copper and 30 mg of zinc to your daily supplement regimen.
NADH (nicotinamide adenine dinucleotide, also called coenzyme Q1)	2.5 mg twice daily, two or three times per week	High doses (10 mg per day or more) may cause nervousness, anxiety, and insomnia.
PS (phosphatidylserine)	Increase daily dose from 300 mg to 400 mg. Do not exceed a daily supplement of 400 mg.	

Additional Supplements for Impacting Mental Fatigue

The following chart summarizes the supplements I recommend adding to the protocol for overall brain health. This protocol is designed for individuals who suffer from, or are specifically concerned about, mental fatigue. If you are concerned about additional brain conditions discussed in other chapters, consult with a health professional about how you can safely impact multiple conditions.

If you are taking medications—whether prescription or over-the-counter—or have any food restrictions, consult with your doctor before beginning any supplement program. Your health care provider should always be up-to-date on all vitamins, supplements, and herbal or homeopathic remedies you are taking. Supplement overdoses are rare, but possible, and certain combinations may affect individuals adversely.

SUPPLEMENT	DOSAGE	CAUTIONS
calcium	500 mg twice a day	Take with food to increase absorption.
creatine	8 grams per day for five days. Repeat as needed.	
L-glutamine	500 mg three times daily	Take while symptoms persist, but not for more than one month.
magnesium	320 mg daily (for women) 420 mg. (for men)	May take six weeks or more for effects to be felt.
potassium you	500 mg daily	Do not take potassium supplements if are taking medication for high blood pressure or heart disease, or if you have a kidney disorder. Consuming foods rich in potassium is okay. Do not exceed 3.5 g daily without consulting your doctor.

Additional Supplements for Impacting Parkinson's Disease

The following chart summarizes additional supplements I recommend for individuals who suffer from, or are specifically concerned about, Parkinson's disease. If you are concerned about additional brain conditions discussed in other chapters, consult with a health professional about how you can safely impact multiple conditions. As always, if you are taking medication—whether prescription or over-the-counter—or have any food restrictions, consult with your doctor before beginning the supplement program. Your health care provider should always be up-to-date on all vitamins, supplements, and herbal or homeopathic remedies you are taking. Supplement overdoses are rare, but possible, and certain combinations may affect individuals adversely.

SUPPLEMENT	DOSAGE	CAUTIONS
coenzyme Q10 with	Increase daily dosage	Dosage should be gradually increased,
(coQ10) with	from 100–300 mg to 1,200 mg. Do not exceed a daily supplement of	300 mg daily being added over a six-week period until the daily dose reaches 1,200 mg. Individuals supplementing
	1,200 mg. Take with fattiest meal of the day.	coQ10 at high doses should be monitored closely by their doctor.
DLPA (DL-phenylalanine) and	200–500 mg daily	Contraindicated for use with levodopa
		MAOs. Consult with your doctor before taking. Individuals with certain mental health problems should not take this supplement.
glutathione	200 mg two times daily	Glutathione levels may also be elevated through supplementation with cysteine, N-acetylcysteine, or L-cysteine.
melatonin	300 mcg–1 mg two to three nights per week a half hour bed.	Tolerance may develop with regular use. Long-term effects of nightly use are unknown.
N-acetylcysteine	1,500 mg in three divided doses	Regular supplementation of NAC increases urinary output of copper. If supplementing with NAC for an extended period, add 2 mg of copper and 30 mg of zinc to your daily supplement regimen.
NADH (nicotinamide adenine dinucleotide)	2.5 mg twice daily	High doses (10 mg per day or more) may cause nervousness, anxiety, and insomnia.
proanthocyanidins	Increase daily dosage from 80 mg to 380 mg, taken in three divided doses. Do not exceed a daily supplement of 380 mg.	

SUPPLEMENT	DOSAGE	CAUTIONS
vitamin B$_6$	Increase daily dosage from 75 mg to 150 mg. Do not exceed a daily supplement of 150 mg. Take with zinc (30 mg).	Contraindicated for use with levodopa. Discuss supplementation with your health care provider.
vitamin C	Increase daily dosage from 500–1,000 mg to 3,000 mg, taken in three divided doses. Do not exceed a daily supplement of 3,000 mg.	
vitamin E	Increase daily dosage from 400 IU to 800 IU. Do not exceed a daily supplement of 800 IU.	If you have high blood pressure, limit your supplemental vitamin E to 400 IU daily. If you are taking blood thinners, consult with your doctor before taking vitamin E.
zinc	Up to 30 mg daily	Large doses (50 mg or more) can interfere with the body's absorption of essential minerals, impair blood cell function, and depress immune system.

Additional Supplements for Impacting Alzheimer's Disease

The following chart summarizes additional supplements I recommend for individuals who suffer from, or are specifically concerned about, Alzheimer's disease. If you are concerned about additional brain conditions discussed in other chapters, consult with a health professional about how you can safely impact multiple conditions. As always, if you are taking medication—whether prescription or over-the-counter—or have any food restrictions, consult with your doctor before beginning the supplement program. Your health care provider should always be up-to-date on all vitamins, supplements, and herbal or homeopathic remedies you are taking. Supplement overdoses are rare, but possible, and certain combinations may affect individuals adversely.

SUPPLEMENT	DOSAGE	CAUTIONS
acetyl-L-carnitine (ACL)	I recommend increasing your daily supplement from 2,000 mg to 3,000 mg, taken in three equal doses. Do not exceed a daily supplement of 3,000 mg.	

SUPPLEMENT	DOSAGE	CAUTIONS
DMAE (dimethylaminoethanol)	Increase daily dosage from 150 mg to 300 mg, taken in two equal doses with meals. Do not exceed a daily supplement of 300 mg.	Do not take DMAE if you have epilepsy, a history of convulsions, or bipolar disorder. If you have kidney or liver disease, consult with your doctor before taking DMAE. Some side effects associated with DMAE in Alzheimer's patients include drowsiness, high blood pressure, and increased confusion. If you experience these symptoms, stop taking the supplement for a few days, then return to your lower daily dose.
intravenous vitamin B complex	Discuss with your health care provider whether you might benefit from injected vitamin B.	
L-glutamine	500 mg taken three times daily	
magnesium	500–1,000 mg in two equal doses	Take on an empty stomach. If loose stools occur, decrease dosage. May take six weeks or more for effects to be felt.
melatonin	300 mcg–1mg at night a half hour before bed	Tolerance may develop with regular use. Long-term effects of nightly use are unknown.
NAC (N-acetylcysteine)	500 mg three times daily	Regular supplementation of NAC increases urinary output of copper. If supplementing with NAC for an extended period, add 2 mg of copper and 30 mg of zinc to our daily supplement regimen.
NADH (nicotinamide adenine dinucleotide, or coenzyme Q1)	2.5 mg twice daily, two or three times per week	High doses (10 mg per day or more) may cause nervousness, anxiety, and insomnia.
PS (phosphatidylserine)	Increase daily dosage from 300 mg to 400 mg. Do not exceed a daily supplement of 400 mg.	
potassium	500 mg daily	Do not take potassium supplements if you are taking medication for high blood pressure or heart disease, or if you have a kidney disorder. Consuming foods rich in potassium is okay. Do not exceed 3.5 g daily without consulting your doctor.

SUPPLEMENT	DOSAGE	CAUTIONS
SAMe (S-adenosylmethionine)	Dosage range of 400–1,600 mg	Raise the dose gradually from 200 mg twice a day to 400 mg twice a day, to 400 mg three times a day, to 400 mg four times a day, over a period of twenty days.
vitamin C	Increase daily dosage from 500–1,000 mg to 3,000 mg, taken in three divided doses. Do not exceed a daily supplement of 3,000 mg.	
vitamin E	Increase daily dosage from 400 IU to 800 IU, taken in two divided doses. Do not exceed a daily supplement of 800 IU.	Vitamin E may cause increased risk of bleeding, and may have adverse interactions with anticoagulants or other medications. Consult with your doctor before beginning high-dose supplementation with vitamin E.
zinc	Up to 30 mg daily	Large doses (50 mg or more) can interfere with the body's absorption of essential minerals, impair blood cell function, and depress the immune system.

Additional Supplements for Impacting Headache

The following chart summarizes the supplements I recommend adding to the protocol for overall brain health. This protocol is designed for individuals who suffer from, or are specifically concerned about, headache. If you are concerned about additional brain conditions discussed in other chapters, consult with a health professional about how you can safely impact multiple conditions.

If you are taking medications—whether prescription or over-the-counter—or have any food restrictions, consult with your doctor before beginning any supplement program. Your health care provider should always be up-to-date on all vitamins, supplements, and herbal or homeopathic remedies you are taking. Supplement overdoses are rare, but possible, and certain combinations may affect individuals adversely.

SUPPLEMENT	DOSAGE	CAUTIONS
5-HTP (5-hydroxytryptophan)	50–100 mg three times daily	Several months of treatment may be needed for maximum benefit. Nausea is the main side effect, but if it occurs, it usually dissipates within several days. Do not combine with prescription antidepressants. If you are taking prescription medication for depression, you should consult your doctor before taking 5-HTP. Excess levels of serotonin in the blood can be dangerous in case of coronary artery disease.
magnesium	Up to 1,000 mg	May take six weeks or more for effects to be felt.
melatonin	300 mcg–1mg two to three nights per week	Tolerance may develop with regular use. Long-term effects of nightly use are unknown.
vitamin B$_2$ (riboflavin)	Increase daily dosage from 50 mg to 150 mg. Do not exceed a daily supplement of 150 mg.	Must build up to a therapeutic level. May not show results for several months.
vitamin B$_3$ (niacin)	At the onset of migraine aura, take 100–150 mg.	High doses of niacin may cause a "hot flash" sensation. Some varieties are advertised as "flash free" and prevent this effect.

Additional Supplements for Impacting Brain Trauma

The following chart summarizes the supplements I recommend adding to the protocol for overall brain health. This protocol is designed for individuals who suffer from, or are specifically concerned about, brain trauma. If you are concerned about additional brain conditions discussed in other chapters, consult with a health professional about how you can safely impact multiple conditions.

If you are taking medications—whether prescription or over-the-counter—or have any food restrictions, consult with your doctor before beginning any supplement program. Your health care provider should always be up-to-date on all vitamins, supplements, and herbal or homeopathic remedies you are taking. Supplement overdoses are rare, but possible, and certain combinations may affect individuals adversely.

SUPPLEMENT	DOSAGE	CAUTIONS
lecithin/choline	For men: increase daily dosage from 1 gram to 2.5 grams. Taken in two divided doses. Do not exceed a daily supplement of 2.5 grams. For women: increase daily dosage from 1 gram to 2 grams. Take in two divided doses. Do not exceed a daily supplement of 2 grams.	Side effects may include nausea, bloating, vomiting, sweating, and diarrhea; extremely large doses can cause a heart-rhythm abnormality; do not use if you have bipolar disorder.
curcumin	500 mg up to three times daily	
DMAE (dimethylaminoethanol)	Increase daily dosage from 150 mg to 650–1,650 mg. Do not exceed a daily supplement of 1,650 mg.	May be overstimulating for some people. Headaches, muscle tension, and irritability may occur. Do not take if you have epilepsy, a history of convulsions, or bipolar disorder. If you have kidney or liver disease, consult your doctor before taking this supplement.
NAC (N-acetylcysteine)	500 mg up to three times daily	Regular supplementation of NAC increases urinary output of copper. If supplementing with NAC for an extended period, add 2 mg of copper and 30 mg of zinc to your daily supplement regimen.
nimodipine	100 mg taken in four equal doses	
picamilon	100 mg taken three times daily	If taking prescription drugs or MAO inhibitors, consult with your doctor before using
PS (phosphatidylserine)	Increase daily dose from 300 mg to 400 mg. Do not exceed a daily supplement of 400 mg.	
vitamin C	Increase daily dose from 1 to 3 grams. Do not exceed a daily supplement of 3 grams.	

Additional Supplements for Impacting Brain Allergies

The following chart summarizes the supplements I recommend adding to the protocol for overall brain health. This protocol is designed for individuals who suffer from, or are specifically concerned about, brain allergies. If you are concerned about additional brain conditions discussed in other chapters, consult with a health professional about how you can safely impact multiple conditions.

If you are taking medications—whether prescription or over-the-counter—or have any food restrictions, consult with your doctor before beginning any supplement program. Your health care provider should always be up-to-date on all vitamins, supplements, and herbal or homeopathic remedies you are taking. Supplement overdoses are rare, but possible, and certain combinations may affect individuals adversely.

SUPPLEMENT	DOSAGE	CAUTIONS
bromelain	1,000 mg daily while symptoms are present	
calcium	400–600 mg elemental calcium daily	
L-glutamine	1,500 mg daily in three divided doses while symptoms are present.	Take while symptoms persist, but not for more than one month.
glutathione	400 mg daily in two equal doses	
magnesium	500 mg daily	May take six weeks or more for effects to be felt.
manganese	20 mg daily in two equal doses	
methionine	1,000 mg daily in two equal doses	
MSM (methylsulfonylmethane)	1,000 mg taken up to three times daily	
vitamin A	10,000 IU daily	
vitamin C	Increase daily dosage from 500–1,000 mg to 3,000 mg, taken in three equal doses. Do not exceed a daily supplement of 3,000 mg.	

SUPPLEMENT	DOSAGE	CAUTIONS
zinc	30 mg daily	Large doses (50 mg or more) can interfere with the body's absorption of essential minerals, impair blood cell function, and depress the immune system.

Additional Supplements for Impacting Insomnia

The following chart summarizes the supplements I recommend adding to the protocol for overall brain health. This protocol is designed for individuals who suffer from, or are specifically concerned about, insomnia. If you are concerned about additional brain conditions discussed in other chapters, consult with a health professional about how you can safely impact multiple conditions.

If you are taking medications—whether prescription or over-the-counter—or have any food restrictions, consult with your doctor before beginning any supplement program. Your health care provider should always be up-to-date on all vitamins, supplements, and herbal or homeopathic remedies you are taking. Supplement overdoses are rare, but possible, and certain combinations may affect individuals adversely.

SUPPLEMENT	DOSAGE	CAUTIONS
calcium (from citrate)	2,000 mg from citrate taken in four equal doses.	
iron	15 mg daily for menstruating women; 10 mg daily for men and nonmenstruating women.	
L-tryptophan	1,000 mg taken a half hour before bed. May take an additional 500 mg if awakened during the night.	
magnesium	1,000 mg taken in four equal doses along with calcium.	May take up to six weeks or more for effects to be felt.
melatonin	300 mcg–1 mg taken a half hour before bed.	Tolerance may develop with regular use. Long-term effects of nightly use are unknown.

Additional Supplements for Impacting Senile Dementia

The following chart summarizes the supplements I recommend adding to the protocol for overall brain health. This protocol is designed for individuals who suffer from, or are specifically concerned about, senile dementia. If you are concerned about additional brain conditions discussed in other chapters, consult with a health professional about how you can safely impact multiple conditions.

If you are taking medications—whether prescription or over-the-counter—or have any food restrictions, consult with your doctor before beginning any supplement program. Your health care provider should always be up-to-date on all vitamins, supplements, and herbal or homeopathic remedies you are taking. Supplement overdoses are rare, but possible, and certain combinations may affect individuals adversely.

SUPPLEMENT	DOSAGE	CAUTIONS
acetyl-L-carnitine (ACL)	Increase daily dosage from 2,000 mg to 3,000 mg, taken in three equal doses. Do not exceed a daily supplement of 3,000 mg.	
calcium	1,000 mg daily in four equal doses after meals and at bedtime.	
intravenous vitamin B complex	Discuss with your health care provider whether you might benefit from injected vitamin B.	
L-glutamine	500 mg taken three times daily	
magnesium	500 to 1,000 mg in two equal doses	May take up to six weeks for effects to be felt. Take on an empty stomach. If loose stools occur, decrease dosage.
NAC (N-acetylcysteine)	500 mg three times daily	Regular supplementation of NAC increases urinary output of copper. If supplementing with NAC for an extended period, add 2 mg of copper and 30 mg of zinc to your daily supplement regimen.

SUPPLEMENT	DOSAGE	CAUTIONS
PS (phosphatidylserine)	Increase daily dose from 300 mg to 400 mg. Do not exceed a daily supplement of 400 mg.	
potassium	500 mg daily	Do not take potassium supplements if you are taking medication for high blood pressure or heart disease, or if you have a kidney disorder. Consuming foods rich in potassium is okay. Do not exceed a supplementary dose of 500 mg daily without consulting your doctor.
SAMe (S-adenosylmethionine)	Dosage range of 400–1,600 mg	Raise the dose gradually from 200 mg twice a day to 400 mg twice a day, to 400 mg three times a day, to 400 mg four times a day, over a period of twenty days.
vitamin C	Increase daily dosage from 500–1,000 mg to 3,000 mg, taken in three equal doses. Do not exceed a daily supplement of 3,000 mg.	
vitamin E	Increase daily dosage from 400 IU to 800 IU, taken in two equal doses. Do not exceed a daily supplement of 800 IU.	Vitamin E may cause increased risk of bleeding, and may have adverse interactions with anticoagulants or other medications. Consult with your doctor before beginning high-dose supplementation with vitamin E.
zinc fere	Up to 30 mg daily	Large doses (50 mg or more) can inter- with the body's absorption of essential minerals, impair blood cell function, and depress the immune system.

PART SEVEN

Recipes for Natural Healing

35

Breakfast Foods

∎∎∎

Tropical Paradise Rice Cereal

2 cups coconut milk
1 banana, sliced
1 cup pitted fresh or frozen cherries
1/2 cup chopped pineapple
1/4 cup shredded unsweetened coconut
2 cups cooked sweet rice
1/2 cup chopped macadamia nuts, toasted (see note below)
2 tablespoons almond extract
1 tablespoon vanilla extract

In a medium-sized saucepan, combine the coconut milk, banana, cherries, and pineapple. Cook over medium-low heat for 2 to 3 minutes. Add the remaining ingredients, mix well, and cook an additional 2 to 3 minutes. Serve hot.
Serves 2
Note: To toast nuts, preheat oven to 375 degrees and place nuts on an ungreased cookie sheet for 10 to 15 minutes or until light brown.

Banana-Coconut Pecan Rice Cereal

1/3 cup uncooked cream of rice
2 3/4 cups water
1 cup mashed banana
1/4 cup coconut flakes

5 tablespoons monnukia raisins

2 to 3 tablespoons pure maple syrup

3 tablespoons pecans

Combine the rice and water in a medium-size saucepan and bring to a boil over medium heat. Cook 3 to 7 minutes, then add the remaining ingredients and cook another 1 to 2 minutes. Serve with rice milk on top.

Serves 2

Almond Cinnamon Millet

6 ounces millet

1 1/2 ounces almonds, blanched and chopped

1 1/2 ounces brewer's yeast

pinch of cinnamon

Cook millet in a saucepan in 13 ounces water. When water comes to boil, lower heat and cook until water is absorbed. Stir occasionally. Add remaining ingredients. Mix well.

Serves 1

Tropical Sunrise

6 ounces basmati rice, cooked (room temperature)

3 ounces pineapple, cut into bite-size pieces

1 tablespoon honey

pinch of cinnamon

Combine all ingredients. Mix well.

Serves 1

Strawberry Sunshine

6 ounces brown rice, cooked (room temperature)

3 ounces strawberries, halved

1 1/2 ounces sunflower seeds

1 1/2 ounces figs, chopped
sprinkle of coconut, shredded and unsweetened

Combine all ingredients. Mix well.
Serves 1

Nutty Oatmeal

6 ounces oatmeal, cooked (room temperature)
3 ounces pears, cut into bite-size pieces
1 1/2 ounce pecans, chopped
1 tablespoon honey

Combine all ingredients. Mix well.
Serves 1

Sweet Cinnamon Oatmeal

6 ounces oatmeal, cooked (room temperature)
1 1/2 ounces dried apricots, chopped
pinch of cinnamon

Combine all ingredients. Mix well.
Serves 1

Nutty Banana Breakfast

6 ounces barley, cooked
3 ounces banana, mashed
1 1/2 ounces walnuts, chopped
2 tablespoons barley malt

Combine all ingredients and mix well.
Serves 1

Vermont Maple Squash

6 ounces spaghetti squash
1 tablespoon maple syrup
1 1/2 ounces brewer's yeast
pinch of cinnamon

Preheat oven to 400 degrees. Cut squash in half, remove the seeds and discard. Place in baking dish cut side down, with 1/3 inch water. Bake for 40 minutes. When cooled, spoon out squash and place in a bowl. Add remaining ingredients and mix well.
Serves 1

Sweet Spice Amaranth

6 ounces amaranth, cooked (room temperature)
3 ounces peaches, cut into bite-size pieces
1 tablespoon honey
pinch of nutmeg
pinch of allspice

Combine all ingredients. Mix well.
Serves 1

Coconut Nut Rice

6 ounces brown rice, cooked (room temperature)
1 1/2 ounces coconut, shredded (unsweetened)
1 1/2 ounces cashews, chopped
1 1/2 ounces dried apricots, chopped
1 1/2 ounces sunflower seeds

Combine brown rice with coconut, cashews and apricots. Purée half the mixture in blender with 2 ounces water until coarsely ground. Add to the rest of the rice. Sprinkle with sunflower seeds.
Serves 1

Fluffy Raisin Couscous

6 ounces couscous, cooked (room temperature)

3 ounces raisins

1 tablespoon honey

pinch of cinnamon

Combine all ingredients. Mix well.

Serves 1

Amaranth Peach Delight

6 ounces amaranth, cooked (room temperature)

3 ounces dried peaches, chopped

1 1/2 ounces pecans, chopped

pinch of clove

pinch of allspice

Combine all ingredients. Mix well.

Serves 1

36

Nutritious Drinks

■■■

Frozen Cherry Supreme

3 cups orange or apple juice
1/2 cup ice cubes
1 cup frozen cherries
1 tablespoon vanilla extract
1/2 teaspoon ground cinnamon

Combine all ingredients in a blender and blend until smooth.
Serves 2

Carob-Pecan-Banana Shake

2 cups rice or soy milk
2 bananas
1 cup ice cubes
3 tablespoons toasted carob powder
4 tablespoons toasted or fresh pecans
1 tablespoon vanilla extract
1/4 teaspoon ground nutmeg
3 tablespoons rice syrup (optional)

Combine all ingredients in a blender and blend until smooth.
Serves 2

Cider Smoothie

8 ounces coconut milk
5 1/2 ounces apple cider
2 tablespoons granulated dates
1 1/2 ounces sunflower seeds
1/4 teaspoon vanilla
pinch of cinnamon

Place all ingredients in a blender. Blend until smooth and frothy.
Serves 1

Rio Refresher

4 ounces soy milk (unsweetened)
1 1/2 ounces apple cider
1 1/2 ounces Brazil nuts, chopped
1 1/2 tablespoons almond syrup
1/2 tablespoon soy oil
pinch of cinnamon

Combine all ingredients in a blender and blend for 2 to 3 minutes or until
smooth.
Serves 1

Easy Nutritious Soy Milk

8 ounces soy milk (unsweetened)
2 tablespoons barley malt
pinch of cinnamon

Blend all ingredients together in a blender until mixture is frothy.
Serves 1

Tropical Banana Soy Milk

8 ounces soy milk (unsweetened)

3 ounces banana, mashed

1/4 teaspoon vanilla

pinch of nutmeg

Blend all ingredients together in a blender until mixture is frothy.
Serves 1

37

Salads

■■■

Spicy Bulgur Marinade

3 ounces bulgur, cooked (chilled)

3 ounces alfalfa sprouts

3 ounces spinach, coarsely chopped

3 ounces marinated artichoke hearts, chopped to bite-size pieces

2 tablespoons sunflower oil

2 teaspoons cider vinegar

1/2 teaspoon salt

1/2 teaspoon basil

1/4 teaspoon curry powder

pinch of cayenne

Combine all ingredients and mix well. Allow to set in refrigerator overnight for best taste. Serve chilled.

Serves 1

Arugula-Orange-Pepper Salad

1 cup sliced red, yellow, and orange bell peppers

1 cup sunflower sprouts

1 cup torn arugula

3/4 cup chopped fresh Italian parsley

1 cup shredded beets, steamed 15 minutes

2/3 cup shredded carrots

2 seedless oranges sliced
1 cup chopped fresh yellow tomatoes

Combine all ingredients in a large salad bowl, adding tomatoes last as a garnish. Serve with a vinaigrette or light lemon dressing.
Serves 1

Pecan, Walnut, and Pine Nut Salad

1 cup sliced fennel root
3 cups mixed mesclun greens
1/2 cup diced fresh peaches
1 diced pear
2 peeled sliced fresh seedless oranges
1/4 cup chopped pecans
1/4 cup walnuts
1/4 cup pine nuts

Combine fennel, mesclun greens, oranges, pear, and peaches in a large salad bowl. Toss with a light, sweet salad dressing, such as orange vinaigrette, and top with walnuts, pecans and pine nuts. Serve chilled.
Serves 3

Indonesian Sprout Salad

2 cups sunflower sprouts
2 cups bean sprouts
2 cups whole walnuts
1/2 honey
3 cups sliced red cabbage
1 cup diced raw carrots
1 cup sliced nori
1/2 cup toasted sesame seeds

Coat walnuts with honey and place on a lightly greased cookie sheet. Bake in a preheated 375 degree oven for 20 minutes. In a large bowl, toss sprouts, red cabbage, carrots, nori and sesame seeds. Toss with dressing and top with walnuts before serving.

Serves 2

Crunchy Couscous Salad

3 ounces yellow squash, cubed

3 ounces celery, chopped

3 ounces scallions, chopped

3 ounces safflower oil

1 1/2 ounces miso

1/2 teaspoon cumin

pinch of cayenne

3 ounces black-eyed peas, cooked (chilled)

3 ounces couscous, cooked

Combine squash, celery and scallions in a bowl. Set aside. In a blender, combine oil, miso and 2 ounces water. Blend until smooth. Add vegetables to miso mixture and blend until coarsely ground. Add cumin and cayenne. Combine with black-eyed peas and couscous. Mix thoroughly.

Serves 2

Raisin Basmati Salad

3 ounces basmati rice, cooked (chilled)

3 ounces celery, chopped

3 ounces raisins

3 ounces pineapple, cut into bite-size pieces

1 tablespoon safflower oil

1/4 teaspoon cinnamon

Combine all ingredients and mix thoroughly. Serve when rice is cooled.

Serves 2

Nice Rice Salad

3 ounces basmati rice, cooked (chilled)

3 ounces amaranth, cooked (chilled)

1 1/2 ounces watercress, chopped

1 1/2 ounces red pepper, diced

2 tablespoons safflower oil

1 teaspoon minced onion

juice of 1 lemon

1/2 teaspoon salt

Combine all ingredients. Toss and serve.

Serves 2

Chopped Veggie Bean Salad

3 ounces black-eyed peas, cooked (chilled)

3 ounces couscous, cooked (chilled)

3 ounces celery, chopped

3 ounces carrot, chopped

1 1/2 ounces pecans, chopped

1 1/2 teaspoons safflower oil

1 teaspoon chopped fresh parsley

1/2 teaspoon marjoram

Combine all ingredients. Mix well. Place approximately 1/4 of mixture in blender with 2 ounces water. Blend until completely pureed. Return to the rest of mixture and mix well.

Serves 2

Oriental Seaweed Salad

3 ounces hijiki (1 ounce dry)

3 ounces carrots, cut in long thin strips

3 ounces daikon, cut in long thin strips

3 ounces scallions, chopped

2 tablespoons safflower oil

1 teaspoon minced garlic

1/2 teaspoon caraway seeds

1/2 teaspoon salt

3 ounces amaranth, cooked (chilled)

Soak and rinse hijiki three times and place in bowl. Lightly sauté carrots, diako, and scallions in skillet with safflower oil for about 5 minutes, then add to the hijiki. Add garlic, caraway seeds and salt. Combine with amaranth. Mix well.
Serves 2

California Marinade

3 ounces cauliflower flowerets, in bite-size pieces

3 ounces bulgur, cooked (chilled)

3 ounces avocado, cut into 1/2-inch cubes

1 1/2 ounces sunflower seeds

2 ounces shallots, chopped

1 ounce coconut, shredded (unsweetened)

2 tablespoons sunflower oil

1 teaspoon tarragon

1/2 teaspoon basil

1 teaspoon soy sauce

1/4 teaspoon salt

2 teaspoons cider vinegar

Steam cauliflower for 8 minutes. Combine with the remaining ingredients and mix well. Serve chilled.
Serves 2

Mellow Rice Salad

3 ounces basmati rice, cooked (chilled)

1/2 ounce pecans, chopped

3 ounces fresh dill, chopped

3 ounces yellow pepper, chopped

1 1/2 tablespoons safflower oil

2 tablespoons cider vinegar

1/2 teaspoon salt

Combine all ingredients.

Serves 1

Superior Spinach Salad

3 ounces spinach, coarsely chopped

3 ounces cauliflower flowerets, in bite-size pieces

3 ounces avocado, cut into bite-size pieces

3 ounces marinated artichoke hearts, cut into bite-size pieces

1 1/2 ounces peanuts, chopped

1 1/2 ounces shallots, chopped

1 1/2 tablespoons sunflower oil

1/4 teaspoon oregano

1/4 teaspoon sage

1/2 teaspoon salt

Combine all ingredients and mix well.

Serves 1

Cool Garden Noodles

3 ounces brown rice, cooked (chilled)

3 ounces buckwheat noodles, cooked (chilled)

3 ounces avocado, chopped into bite-size pieces

3 ounces marinated artichoke hearts, chopped into bite-size pieces

2 tablespoons sunflower oil

1 teaspoon chopped fresh parsley

1/2 teaspoon minced garlic

1/2 teaspoon basil

1/2 teaspoon salt

pinch of ginger

Combine all ingredients and mix well.

Serves 2

Aduki Vegetable Salad

3 ounces aduki beans, cooked (chilled)

3 ounces onion, chopped

3 ounces tomato, chopped

3 ounces green pepper, chopped

1 1/2 ounces almond, blanched and slivered

2 tablespoons sesame oil

1/2 teaspoon minced garlic

1/2 teaspoon tarragon

1/4 teaspoon basil

1 teaspoon salt

Combine all ingredients. Serve at room temperature.

Serves 2

Mykonos Bean Salad

3 ounces okra, cut into 1/2-inch pieces

3 ounces aduki beans, cooked (chilled)

3 ounces scallions, chopped

3 ounces green pepper, chopped

2 tablespoons olive oil

1/4 teaspoon thyme

1/4 teaspoon sage

1/4 teaspoon chopped fresh dill

1/2 teaspoon salt

Steam the okra for 7 minutes. Combine with remaining ingredients and toss gently. Serve at room temperature.

Serves 1

Italian Mushroom and Potato Salad

3 ounces potato

3 ounces mushrooms, chopped medium fine

3 ounces okra, cut into 1/2-inch pieces

3 ounces onion, chopped

3 ounces tomato, chopped

1 1/2 ounces scallions, chopped

1/4 teaspoon basil

1/4 teaspoon oregano

1/2 teaspoon salt

1 1/2 tablespoons olive oil

Preheat oven to 400 degrees. Bake potato for 45 minutes. When cooled, cut into 1/2-inch cubes. Sauté vegetables, basil, oregano and salt in olive oil over low heat for about 5 minutes. Combine all ingredients and mix well. Serve hot. Serves 2

Tahini Potato Salad

3 ounces potato

1 1/2 ounces sesame seeds

3 ounces scallions, chopped

3 ounces mushrooms, sliced

1 1/2 ounces triticale flour

1/2 teaspoon cumin

1/2 teaspoon basil

1/2 teaspoon salt

1 1/2 ounces tahini

2 tablespoons sesame oil

Preheat oven to 400 degrees. Bake potato for 40 minutes. When cooled, cut into 1/2-inch cubes. Toast sesame seeds in a skillet, without oil, for 3 minutes over low heat. Set aside. In a separate bowl, combine vegetables with remaining ingredients, except oil, and 2 ounces water. Sauté all ingredients, including potato cubes, with sesame oil for 4 minutes over medium heat. Place in a bowl, and add sesame seeds and salt. Mix well. Serve hot.

Serves 2

Malayan Millet Salad

3 ounces aduki beans, cooked (chilled)

3 ounces millet, cooked (chilled)

3 ounces green pepper, chopped

3 ounces onion, chopped

1/2 teaspoon tarragon

1/4 teaspoon thyme

1/2 teaspoon salt

pinch of celery seed

2 tablespoons sesame oil

Combine all ingredients and mix well. Serve hot or cold.

Serves 1

Walnut and Black Bean Salad

3 ounces black beans, cooked (chilled)

3 ounces soybean sprouts

1 1/2 ounces walnuts, chopped

1 teaspoon tarragon

1/2 teaspoon thyme

1/2 teaspoon salt

1 1/2 tablespoons soy oil

Combine all ingredients together and mix well. Sauté for about 5 minutes in soy oil. Serve at room temperature.

Serves 1

Millet and Greens Salad

3 ounces green pepper, chopped

3 ounces onion, chopped

3 ounces collard greens, coarsely chopped

3 ounces millet, cooked (chilled)

1 1/2 ounces pumpkin seeds

2 tablespoons sesame oil

1/2 teaspoon thyme

1 teaspoon tarragon

1/2 teaspoon salt

Steam all vegetables for 3 minutes. Combine all ingredients. Mix well. Serve hot or cold.

Serves 2

Chick Pea and Lima Bean Seaweed Salad

1 ounce dulse, dry

3 ounces snap beans, cut into 1-inch pieces

3 ounces chick-peas, cooked (chilled)

3 ounces lima beans, cooked (chilled)

2 tablespoons corn oil

1 teaspoon dill

1 teaspoon tarragon

1/2 teaspoon salt

juice of 1/2 lemon

Soak and rinse dulse 2 or 3 times in cold water. Steam snap beans for 10 minutes. Mix all ingredients together. Serve chilled.

Serves 2

Sprout and Veggie Salad

3 ounces brussels sprouts

3 ounces lima beans, cooked (chilled)

3 ounces barley, cooked (chilled)

3 ounces soybean sprouts

1 1/2 ounces Brazil nuts, chopped

2 tablespoons soy oil

1 teaspoon soy sauce

1/2 teaspoon chopped parsley

1/2 teaspoon rosemary

1/2 teaspoon salt

Steam brussels sprouts for 10 minutes. Combine all ingredients and mix well. Serve cool.

Serves 2

38

Soups

■■■

Hot Bean Soup

3 ounces kidney beans
6 ounces cauliflower flowerets, in bite-size pieces
6 ounces spinach, coarsely chopped
1 teaspoon minced onion
3 tablespoons sunflower oil
1/2 teaspoon basil
1/2 teaspoon salt
pinch of cayenne

Soak beans overnight in water. In the morning, rinse well and add 32 ounces of fresh water. Bring beans to a boil and lower to medium heat. Place the cover on the pot. The beans should cook for about 2 hours. After 1 1/2 hours, add remaining ingredients and continue cooking for an additional 30 minutes. Puree half the amount in blender for about 15 seconds and return to the rest of the soup. Mix well. Cook for an additional 10 minutes.
Yields 4 to 5 cups

Tomato Potato Soup

9 ounces potatoes, sliced
3 tablespoons sesame oil
1/4 teaspoon cumin
1/4 teaspoon basil

1 teaspoon salt
3 ounces tomato, chopped
6 ounces pepper, chopped
3 ounces scallions, chopped

Boil potatoes for approximately 15 minutes in 4 cups water. Transfer potatoes and cooking water to blender and add seasonings. Puree until smooth. Return mixture to saucepan and set on stove again over low heat. Add in the chopped vegetables. Cook for an additional 10 to 15 minutes.
Yields 4 to 5 cups

Italian-style Pinto Bean Soup

3 ounces pinto beans
3 ounces carrots, sliced
2 ounces mushrooms, sliced
1 ounce arugula, chopped
3 tablespoons safflower oil
1/2 teaspoon cumin
1/2 teaspoon salt

Soak beans overnight in water. In the morning, rinse the beans, pour into medium saucepan and add 32 ounces fresh water. Bring beans to a boil; then lower heat to medium. Cook with lid on. When the beans have cooked for about 1 hour, add the remaining ingredients. Puree half the mixture in blender and blend for 15 seconds or until coarsely ground. Return mixture to the rest of the soup. Cook for an additional 15 minutes over low heat.
Yields 4 to 5 cups

Favorite Vegetable Soup

3 ounces mung beans
3 ounces onions, sliced
2 ounces celery, chopped
2 ounces red cabbage, sliced
1 teaspoon chopped fresh parsley

3 tablespoons safflower oil
1/2 teaspoon salt
1/2 teaspoon oregano
1/2 teaspoon basil
6 ounces basmati rice, cooked

Soak beans overnight in water. In the morning, rinse the beans, pour into saucepan and add 32 ounces water. Bring beans to a boil and lower to medium heat. Place the cover on the pot. After 1 hour, add the vegetables, oil and seasonings. Puree half the mixture in blender for 15 seconds or until coarsely ground. Return to the soup along with the basmati rice. Mix well and allow to cook for an additional 10 minutes.

Yields 4 to 5 cups

Cashewy Bean Soup

3 ounces kidney beans
6 ounces brown rice, cooked
1 1/2 ounces cashews, chopped
3 tablespoons sunflower oil
1/2 teaspoon minced garlic
1/4 teaspoon chili powder
1/2 teaspoon salt

Soak beans overnight in water. In the morning, rinse the beans and add 32 ounces of fresh water. Bring to a boil and lower to medium heat. Cook with lid on. The beans should cook for about 2 hours. After 1 1/2 hours, add the remaining ingredients. Continue to cook for an additional 30 minutes. Puree half of this mixture in a blender for 15 seconds and add back to the rest of the soup. Cook for an additional 10 minutes.

Yields 4 to 5 cups

Jamaican Squash Soup

6-ounce butternut squash
1 1/2 ounces sunflower seeds, raw
2 teaspoons maple syrup
1/2 teaspoon curry
pinch of cinnamon
3 ounces celery, chopped

Preheat oven to 400 degrees. Cut squash in half. Remove seeds and discard. Place in a baking pan, cut side down, with 1/3 inch water. Bake for 40 minutes. When cooled, remove skin and place squash in a blender along with remaining ingredients, except for celery, and 2 cups water. Blend until smooth; add the celery. Mix well. Transfer to medium saucepan. Cook over low heat for about 20 minutes or until thoroughly heated.
Yields 3 cups

Gary's Noodle Soup

6 ounces celery, chopped
6 ounces spinach, coarsely chopped
6 ounces asparagus, cut into 1-inch pieces
3 tablespoons sunflower oil
1/2 teaspoon cumin
1/2 teaspoon basil
1/2 teaspoon salt
6 ounces rice noodles, cooked

Put vegetables in medium saucepan with 4 cups water. Bring to a boil and add remaining ingredients, except for noodles. Lower to medium heat and continue cooking an additional 10 minutes. Puree half of this mixture in blender for about 15 seconds and then return to saucepan. Add noodles and cook for an additional 10 minutes.
Yields 4 to 5 cups

Turnip Black Bean Soup

4 1/2 ounces black beans

3 ounces turnips, chopped into 1/2-inch cubes

3 ounces corn (fresh or off the cob)

3 ounces tofu, cut into 1/2-inch cubes

3 ounces fresh chives, minced

3 tablespoons soy oil

1/2 teaspoon cumin

1 teaspoon salt

Soak beans overnight in 32 ounces water. In the morning, rinse well and add 40 ounces fresh water. Bring beans to a boil and lower to medium heat. Cover. Cook approximately 1 1/2 hours. When the beans have cooked for 1 hour, add remaining ingredients. Puree half of this mixture in blender for 15 seconds and add back to the rest of the soup. Cook for additional 30 minutes over low heat. Yields 4 cups

Summertime Potato Soup

9 ounces potatoes, sliced

1 teaspoon chopped fresh dill

1 teaspoon peppermint (fresh, if available)

2 tablespoons sesame oil

3 ounces scallions, chopped

Boil potatoes for 15 minutes in 4 cups water. Transfer potatoes, cooking water, seasonings and oil to blender. Puree until smooth. Place on low heat for 10 to 15 minutes. Add scallions.
Yields 2 cups

Venice Rice Noodle Soup

5 tablespoons extra virgin olive oil

1/2 cup sliced zucchini

1/2 cup sliced potatoes

1/2 cup sliced celery

1 cup diced onions

1/4 cup sliced mushrooms

1/4 cup chopped fresh parsley

1/2 cup broccoli florets

1 teaspoon salt

1/4 teaspoon freshly ground black pepper

2 bay leaves

1/4 cup chopped fresh dill

6 cups water

2 cups uncooked rice noodles

4 cloves crushed garlic

In a large saucepan, heat oil over medium heat and sauté vegetables about 10 minutes. Add remaining ingredients, except rice noodles, and let simmer over medium-low heat for 25 to 35 minutes. Add the noodles 10 minutes before finishing.

Serves 2

Year-round Savory Creamy Potato Soup

1 cup peeled, cubed potatoes

1/4 cup sliced celery

1/2 cup diced onions

2 tablespoons canola oil

1/4 teaspoon salt

1/4 teaspoon cayenne

dash of freshly ground black pepper

1 1/2 cups of water

1 vegetable bouillon cube (Morga)

1 to 2 cups soy milk

In a large saucepan, sauté potatoes, celery and onions in the oil over medium heat for 10 minutes. Add remaining ingredients and cook, covered, over medium to low heat for 25 to 30 minutes.

Serves 3

39

Lunch and Dinner Entrees

■■■

Popeye's Pick-Me-Up

3 ounces spinach, chopped

3 ounces okra, sliced

3 ounces red pepper, chopped

3 ounces split peas, cooked

1 1/2 tablespoons sunflower oil

1/2 teaspoon soy sauce

1/2 teaspoon tarragon

1/2 teaspoon salt

3 ounces brown rice, cooked

Steam spinach, okra and pepper for 7 minutes or until tender. Puree split peas in the blender along with oil, soy sauce, tarragon, salt and 2 ounces water until mixture achieves sauce consistency. Pour split peas over vegetables and brown rice and serve warm.

Serves 2

Navy Bean Mushroom Sauté

3 ounces mushrooms, sliced

3 ounces onions, sliced

2 tablespoons safflower oil

1/2 teaspoon salt

1/2 teaspoon minced garlic

1/2 teaspoon chopped fresh parsley

3 ounces navy beans, cooked

3 ounces amaranth, cooked

Sauté mushrooms and onions in skillet with safflower oil until onions are translucent. Add salt, garlic and parsley. Combine with navy beans and amaranth. Mix well and serve warm.

Serves 2

Peanutty Butternut Squash

3 ounces butternut squash

1 1/2 ounces shallots, chopped fine

1 1/2 ounces peanuts

2 tablespoons sunflower oil

1 teaspoon chopped fresh dill

1/4 teaspoon thyme

1/2 teaspoon basil

1/2 teaspoon salt

3 ounces avocado, sliced

Preheat oven to 400 degrees. Lightly oil 4 ´ 8 baking pan with sunflower oil. Cut squash in half, remove seeds and discard. Place squash halves in a baking pan, cut side down, with 1/3 inch water. Bake for 40 minutes. Take squash out of oven, and lower heat to 350 degrees. When cool enough to handle, remove skin from squash and cut squash into 1-inch cubes. Combine the shallots with the squash and transfer to baking pan. In a blender, place peanuts, oil, dill, thyme, basil and salt. Puree until smooth. Pour over squash and shallots, and bake for 20 minutes. Top with avocado.

Serves 2

Sweet-and-Sour Bean Stew

3 ounces navy beans, cooked

3 ounces basmati rice, cooked

1 1/2 ounces butternut squash, cubed

1 1/2 ounces onion, chopped

1 1/2 ounces raisins

1 tablespoon safflower oil

1/2 teaspoon thyme

1/2 teaspoon minced garlic

1/2 teaspoon salt

Combine all ingredients in medium saucepan. Set on stove over medium heat for about 20 minutes or until thoroughly heated. Stir occasionally. Serve at room temperature.

Serves 1

Sweet Potato Patch

3-ounce sweet potato

3 ounces carrot, sliced

1 1/2 ounces pine nuts

1 ounce crushed pineapple (unsweetened in its own juice, if canned)

1/2 teaspoon cinnamon

3 ounces mung beans, cooked

Preheat oven to 400 degrees. Pierce sweet potato with fork and place in oven for 45 minutes. When potato cools, cut into 1/2-inch cubes. Steam carrots for 8 minutes. Combine potato and carrots. Add remaining ingredients and mix well. Serve cool or at room temperature.

Serves 1

Squashed Potato Casserole

3-ounce sweet potato

3 ounces yellow squash, cubed

1 ounce green pepper, chopped

2 tablespoons safflower oil

1/2 teaspoon thyme

1/2 teaspoon basil

1/2 teaspoon salt

3 ounces basmati rice, cooked

3 ounces amaranth, cooked

Preheat oven to 400 degrees. Pierce sweet potato with fork and place in oven for 45 minutes. When potato cools, cut into 1/2-inch cubes. Lower heat to 375 degrees. Steam squash and pepper until slightly tender. Lightly grease 4 ´ 8 casserole pan with safflower oil. Combine all ingredients and mix well. Transfer to casserole pan and place in oven for 15 minutes.
Serves 2.

Macro Rice and Beans

3 ounces black-eyed peas

3 ounces hijiki (1 ounce dry)

1 1/2 ounces kale, coarsely chopped

3 ounces diakon, cut into bite-size pieces

3 ounces parsnip, cut into bite-size pieces

1 teaspoon soy sauce

3 tablespoons safflower oil

1 teaspoon salt

3 ounces basmati rice, cooked

Soak peas overnight in water. In the morning, rinse them, pour into saucepan, and add 32 ounces of fresh water. Bring black-eyed peas to a boil and lower to medium heat. Cook for about 2 hours with the lid on. While peas are cooking, soak and rinse hijiki two or three times. When peas have cooked for 1 1/2 hours, add remaining ingredients, except rice. Continue cooking for additional 30 minutes on low heat until beans are tender. Serve with rice.
Serves 3

Split Pea Ratatouille

3 ounces eggplant, sliced 1/4-inch thick

3 ounces zucchini, sliced 1/4-inch thick

3 ounces onion, sliced

2 tablespoons sunflower oil

3 ounces split peas, cooked

3 ounces cashews, chopped

1 teaspoon minced garlic

1 teaspoon salt

1/2 teaspoon rosemary

Preheat oven to 350 degrees. Steam eggplant, zucchini and onion for about 8 minutes. Lightly grease 4 ´ 8 baking pan with oil. Place split peas in blender with 2 ounces water, half of cashews, and the remaining ingredients. Blend until mixture achieves sauce consistency. Place eggplant in baking pan and pour the split pea sauce on top. Sprinkle with remaining cashews. Put in oven and bake for 20 minutes.

Serves 2

Kidney Bean Bonanza

1 1/2 ounces filberts, chopped

2 tablespoons sunflower oil

1 tablespoon tarragon

3/4 teaspoon basil

1/2 teaspoon salt

1/3 teaspoon curry

3 ounces brown rice, cooked

3 ounces kidney beans, cooked

1 1/2 ounces cashew pieces

Preheat oven to 375 degrees. Lightly grease 4 ´ 8 baking dish with sunflower oil. Place filberts in blender with 2 ounces water, oil, tarragon, basil, salt, and curry. Blend until mixture achieves sauce consistency. Combine brown rice and beans. Transfer to baking dish. Top with filbert sauce. Sprinkle on cashews. Bake with cover for 15 minutes.

Serves 2

Sauté Florentine

3 ounces sunflower flour

2 teaspoons minced onions

1/3 teaspoon thyme

1/3 teaspoon oregano

1/2 teaspoon salt

1/2 teaspoon soy sauce

2 tablespoons sunflower oil

3 ounces spinach, coarsely chopped

3 ounces marinated artichoke hearts,
    chopped into bite-size pieces

3 ounces celery, chopped into bite-size pieces

3 ounces brown rice, cooked

Combine flour with onion, thyme, oregano, salt, soy sauce and oil. Mix well.
Sauté flour mixture with vegetables and sunflower oil in skillet or wok. Add rice
and sauté for 7 minutes.

Serves 2

Peter Pan Rice Casserole

1 1/2 ounces peanut butter

1 1/2 tablespoons sunflower oil

1/4 teaspoon thyme

1/2 teaspoon tarragon

1/2 teaspoon salt

3 ounces brown rice, cooked

1 1/2 ounces sunflower seeds

1 1/2 ounces shallots, chopped medium fine

Preheat oven to 325 degrees. Lightly grease 4 ´ 8 baking dish with sunflower
oil. In a blender, combine peanut butter, oil, thyme, tarragon, salt and 2 ounces
water. Blend until mixture achieves sauce consistency. Combine with rice, sunflower seeds and shallots. Mix well. Transfer to baking dish and bake for 20 minutes.

Serves 1

Mexican Medley

3 ounces asparagus, cut in 1/2-inch pieces

3 ounces cauliflower flowerets, in bite-size pieces

3 ounces celery, chopped

3 ounces kidney beans, cooked

1 1/2 ounces filberts, chopped medium fine

2 tablespoons sunflower oil

2/3 teaspoon chopped fresh dill

1/3 teaspoon chili powder

1/4 teaspoon basil

1/4 teaspoon celery seed

1/2 teaspoon minced garlic

1/2 teaspoon salt

Steam asparagus and cauliflower for approximately 10 minutes. Combine with celery. Set aside. In a blender, place beans, filberts and remaining ingredients. Puree until smooth. Pour this sauce over the asparagus mixture. Serve at room temperature.

Serves 2

Italian Rice

3 ounces celery, chopped

1 1/3 ounces shallots, chopped finely

3 ounces brown rice, cooked

2 tablespoons sunflower oil

1 1/2 teaspoons tarragon

1/4 teaspoon dill

3/4 teaspoon salt

1/4 teaspoon soy sauce

3 ounces alfalfa sprouts

1 1/2 ounces cashews, chopped

3 ounces cider vinegar

Sauté celery and shallots with brown rice in a skillet with sunflower oil for 5 minutes. Add herbs, salt and soy sauce. Transfer to bowl; add sprouts, cashews and cider vinegar. Mix well and serve at room temperature.

Serves 1

Three-Green Curry Casserole

3 ounces sunflower flour

3 ounces split peas, cooked

2 1/2 tablespoons sunflower oil

1/3 teaspoon curry

1/4 teaspoon minced garlic

1/4 teaspoon salt

1/4 teaspoon thyme

3 ounces spinach, coarsely chopped

3 ounces cauliflower, cut into bite-size pieces

3 ounces brown rice, cooked

3 ounces avocado, sliced

Preheat oven to 375 degrees. Lightly grease 4 x 8 baking pan with sunflower oil. In a blender, combine sunflower flour, split peas, oil, curry, garlic, salt, thyme and 2 ounces water. Separately, combine spinach, cauliflower and brown rice. Transfer to covered baking pan, add the flour and beans, and bake for 15 minutes. Place avocado slices on top for garnish.

Serves 2

Swiss Spaghetti Casserole

3-ounce spaghetti squash

3 ounces Swiss chard

3 ounces onion, chopped

3 ounces green pepper, chopped

1 1/2 ounces almonds, blanched and chopped

1 teaspoon minced garlic

2 teaspoons thyme

1/2 teaspoon salt

sesame oil

Preheat oven to 400 degrees. Lightly grease a 4 x 8 baking pan with sesame oil. Cut squash in half, remove the seeds and discard them. Place the squash in a baking pan cut side down, with 1/3 inch water. Bake for 40 minutes. Then lower oven to 375 degrees. When squash is cool enough to handle, cut into 1/2-inch cubes. Steam Swiss chard for 6 minutes. Combine all ingredients in a baking dish and bake for 15 minutes.

Serves 1

Brazilian Rice

3 ounces cauliflower florets, in bite-size pieces

2 tablespoons fresh chopped parsley

2 tablespoons sunflower oil

1/2 teaspoon soy sauce

1/2 teaspoon salt

3 ounces black beans, cooked

3 ounces brown rice, cooked

3 ounces avocado, sliced

Preheat oven to 375 degrees. Lightly grease a 4 x 8 baking pan with sunflower oil. Steam cauliflower for about 5 minutes. Combine all ingredients except for the avocado. Mix well. Transfer to baking pan and bake for 15 minutes. Garnish with avocado slices.

Serves 2

Green Barley Split

6 ounces split peas, cooked

6 ounces spinach, chopped coarsely

6 ounces barley, cooked

6 ounces asparagus, cut into 1-inch pieces

3 tablespoons sunflower oil

1/2 teaspoon minced garlic

1/2 teaspoon salt

Preheat oven to 375 degrees. Lightly grease 4 x 8 baking pan with sunflower oil. Combine all ingredients together. Toss and mix well. Transfer to baking pan and bake for 15 minutes or until thoroughly heated.
Serves 3

Vegetable Almondine Bake

3 ounces wheat flakes
3 ounces onion, chopped
3 ounces tomato, chopped
3 ounces green pepper, chopped
1 1/2 ounces scallions, chopped
1 1/2 ounces almonds, blanched and slivered
1/4 teaspoon thyme
1/4 teaspoon sage
1/4 teaspoon curry
1/2 teaspoon salt
2 tablespoons sesame oil

Preheat oven to 375 degrees. Lightly grease 4 x 8 baking dish with sesame oil. Cook wheat flakes in 12 ounces water for 10 to 12 minutes. Sauté vegetables, almonds, thyme, sage, curry and salt in a skillet with sesame oil for 5 minutes. Combine with wheat flakes and transfer to baking dish and bake for 15 minutes.
Serves 2

Mama's Make-Believe Spaghetti

3 ounces spaghetti squash
6 ounces tomato, chopped
3 ounces scallions, chopped
3 ounces green pepper, chopped
1 1/2 ounces onion, chopped
2 tablespoons olive oil
1/4 teaspoon basil
1 teaspoon salt

Preheat oven to 400 degrees. Cut squash in half; remove the seeds and discard them. Place the halves in a baking pan cut side down, with 1/3 inch water. Bake for 40 minutes. Sauté the tomato, scallions, green pepper, and onion in a skillet with olive oil for 5 minutes. Add the basil and salt. Remove the "spaghetti" from the squash and combine with the sautéed mixture. Toss gently. Serve hot. Serves 1

Halloween Spaghetti

6 ounces tomato, finely chopped

1 1/2 ounces scallions, finely chopped

1/2 teaspoon oregano

1/2 teaspoon basil

1/2 teaspoon salt

2 tablespoons olive oil

3 ounces rice pasta, cooked

1 1/2 ounces pumpkin seeds, roasted

Sauté tomato and scallions in a skillet with oregano, basil, salt and olive oil over low heat for 15 minutes. Combine with spaghetti and pumpkin seeds. Serve hot. Serves 1

Pyramid Pea Casserole

3 ounces chick peas, cooked

3 ounces barley, cooked

3 ounces turnip greens, chopped

1 1/2 ounces Brazil nuts, chopped

2 tablespoons soy oil

2 teaspoons chopped fresh chives

1/4 teaspoon thyme

1/2 teaspoon curry

1/2 teaspoon salt

Preheat oven to 375 degrees. Lightly grease a 4 x 8 baking pan with soy oil. Combine all ingredients and mix well. Transfer to baking pan and bake for 15 minutes.

Serves 2

Baked Rice Pasta Casserole

3 ounces potato

3 ounces rice pasta, cooked

3 ounces tomato, chopped medium fine

1 1/2 ounces scallions, chopped medium fine

1 1/2 ounces sesame seeds

1 1/2 tablespoons sesame oil

1/4 teaspoon thyme

1/4 teaspoon minced garlic

1/2 teaspoon salt

Preheat oven to 400 degrees. Lightly grease 4 x 8 baking pan with sesame oil. Bake potato for 40 minutes. When cooled, cut into 1/2-inch cubes. Combine all ingredients together. Lower heat to 375 degrees. Transfer to a baking pan and bake for 15 minutes.

Serves 2

Mushroom and Onion Rice Pasta

3 ounces mushrooms, sliced

3 ounces onions, sliced

3 ounces tomato, chopped

1/2 teaspoon basil

1/4 teaspoon oregano

1/2 teaspoon salt

2 tablespoons olive oil

6 ounces rice pasta, cooked

Sauté mushrooms, onions and tomato with basil, oregano and salt in olive oil for 5 minutes. Combine with rice pasta and toss gently. Serve warm.

Serves 2

Flavorful Beans with Mushrooms

3 ounces mushrooms, finely chopped

3 ounces scallions, finely chopped

3 ounces aduki beans cooked

2 tablespoons olive oil

1/2 teaspoon tarragon

1/4 teaspoon dill

1/2 teaspoon salt

Preheat oven to 300 degrees. Lightly grease a 4 x 8 baking dish with sesame oil. Combine all ingredients and place in the baking dish. Cover and bake for 25 minutes.

Serves 1

Mushroom Pepper Sauté

1 1/2 ounces triticale flour

1/2 teaspoon basil

1/2 teaspoon thyme

1/4 teaspoon salt

1/2 teaspoon soy sauce

1 tablespoon sesame oil

6 ounces mushrooms, sliced

1 1/2 ounces green pepper, chopped

1 1/2 ounces scallions, chopped

Preheat oven to 325 degrees. Lightly grease a 4 x 8 baking dish with sesame oil. Mix triticale flour with basil, thyme, salt, soy sauce and 2 ounces water. Sauté the vegetables, adding the triticale sauce, for 4 minutes. Transfer ingredients to a covered baking dish and bake for 20 minutes.

Serves 2

Little Italy Rice Spaghetti

3 ounces onion, chopped

1 1/2 tablespoons olive oil

1/2 teaspoon minced garlic

1/4 teaspoon basil

1/4 teaspoon oregano

1/2 teaspoon salt

6 ounces tomato, finely chopped

3 ounces mushrooms, finely chopped

3 ounces green pepper, finely chopped

2 ounces tomato paste

6 ounces rice spaghetti, cooked

Sauté onion in a sauce pan with olive oil until onions are translucent. Add garlic, basil, oregano and salt. Stir. Add vegetables and tomato paste. Continue to cook over medium heat, covered, for 15 minutes. Add rice spaghetti and toss. Serve hot.

Serves 2

Mushroom Millet Magic

3 ounces millet, cooked

3 ounces mushrooms, sliced

3 ounces green pepper, chopped

3 ounces onion, chopped

1 1/2 ounces pumpkin seeds

2 tablespoons olive oil

1/2 teaspoon salt

1/4 teaspoon cumin

1/4 teaspoon basil

1 1/2 ounces triticale flour

sesame oil

Preheat oven to 350 degrees. Lightly grease a 4 x 8 baking dish with sesame oil. Combine all ingredients together gradually stirring in tritcale flour. Transfer to covered baking dish and bake for 20 minutes.

Serves 1

Tantalizing Tempeh Dinner

1/2 ounce dulse, dry

3 ounces chick peas, cooked

3 ounces soybean sprouts

3 ounces broccoli florets, in bite-size pieces

3 ounces tempeh, cut into 1/2-inch cubes

2 tablespoons soy oil

1 teaspoon minced onion

1 teaspoon chopped fresh chives

1/4 teaspoon salt

Preheat oven to 350 degrees. Lightly grease a 4 x 8 baking pan with soy oil. Soak and rinse dulse 2 or 3 times in cold water. Combine with the remaining ingredients and mix well. Transfer to baking pan and bake for 20 minutes.
Serves 2

Vegetable Millet Delight

6 ounces millet, cooked

1/2 teaspoon coriander

1/2 teaspoon salt

3 tablespoons sesame oil

3 ounces mushrooms, chopped

3 ounces red and green pepper, chopped

3 ounces onion, chopped

Place cooked millet in blender with 16 ounces water, coriander, salt, and oil. Purée until smooth. Pour into saucepan over medium heat. Add chopped vegetables, and cook for 15 minutes or until vegetables are tender.
Serves 3

Brazilian Broccoli Beans

3 ounces broccoli florets, in bite-size pieces

3 ounces snap beans, cut into bite-size pieces

3 ounces kale, coarsely chopped

3 ounces soybeans, cooked

1 1/2 ounces Brazil nuts, chopped

1 1/2 tablespoons soy oil

1/2 teaspoon minced garlic

1 1/2 ounces fresh chives, minced

1/4 teaspoon tarragon

1/2 teaspoon salt

Steam broccoli, snap beans, and kale for 8 minutes or until tender. Combine with remaining ingredients and mix well. Serve hot or cold.

Serves 2

Island Lentil Dish

6 ounces lentils, cooked

6 ounces brown rice, cooked

6 ounces celery, chopped

6 ounces cauliflower florets, in bite-size pieces

3 tablespoons sunflower oil

1 teaspoon thyme

1/2 teaspoon salt

Preheat oven to 375 degrees. Lightly grease 4 x 8 baking pan with sunflower oil. Combine all ingredients. Toss and mix well. Transfer to baking dish and bake for 15 minutes.

Serves 3

Curried Chick Peas with Veggies

3 ounces turnips, sliced 1/4-inch think

3 ounces broccoli florets, in bite-size pieces

3 ounces chick peas, cooked

3 ounces barley, cooked

2 tablespoons minced fresh chives

2 tablespoons soy oil

1/2 teaspoon curry

juice of 1/2 lemon

Steam turnips and broccoli for 8 minutes. Combine with remaining ingredients. Mix well. Serve warm.

Serves 2

Crunchy Beans with Turnips

3 ounces turnips, sliced 1/4-inch thick

3 ounces lima beans, cooked

2 tablespoons minced chives

1 teaspoon curry

1 teaspoon soy sauce

1/2 teaspoon salt

2 tablespoons soy oil

1 1/2 ounces walnuts, chopped

3 ounces soybean sprouts

Preheat oven to 375 degrees. Lightly grease 4 x 8 baking pan with soy oil. Steam turnips. Combine lima beans, chives, curry, soy sauce, salt and soy oil in a blender with 2 ounces water. Purée until smooth. Combine all ingredients together and mix well. Transfer to baking pan and cook for 15 minutes.

Serves 2

Snappy Bean Bake

3 ounces broccoli florets, in bite-size pieces

3 ounces snap beans, cut into bite-size pieces

3 ounces tofu, cut in 1/2-inch cubes

3 ounces lima beans, cooked

1 1/2 ounces Brazil nuts, chopped

2 tablespoons soy oil

1 teaspoon mustard

2 teaspoons minced fresh chives

1 teaspoon chopped fresh parsley

1/2 teaspoon tarragon

1/2 teaspoon salt

Preheat oven to 350 degrees. Lightly grease 4 x 8 baking pan with soy oil. Combine all ingredients and bake for 20 minutes with a cover.
Serves 2

Aromatic Green Casserole

3 ounces snap beans, cut into bite-size pieces

3 ounces Brussels sprouts, cut into bite-size pieces

3 ounces broccoli, cut into bite-size pieces

1 1/2 ounces walnuts, chopped

2 tablespoons soy oil

1/2 teaspoon chopped fresh dill

1/4 teaspoon sage

1/2 teaspoon salt

juice of 1/2 lemon

pinch cayenne

Steam beans, Brussels sprouts, and broccoli for 8 minutes. Combine beans and walnuts with remaining ingredients and 2 ounces water. Transfer to blender and purée until smooth. Pour sauce over vegetables. Serve hot or cold.
Serves 2

Tantalizing Tofu

3 ounces tofu, cut into bite-size pieces

3 ounces broccoli, cut into bite-size pieces

3 ounces turnip greens, coarsely chopped

1 1/2 ounces walnuts, chopped

1/2 teaspoon basil

1/2 teaspoon salt

2 tablespoons soy oil

3 ounces romaine lettuce

Sauté all ingredients except for lettuce in soy oil for 3 to 4 minutes. Arrange on a bed of lettuce.

Serves 2

Tarragon Tempeh

3 ounces tempeh, cut into 1/2-inch pieces

1 1/2 ounces Brazil nuts, chopped

2 teaspoons fresh chives, minced

1 teaspoon tarragon

1/2 teaspoon salt

corn oil

Preheat oven to 350 degrees. Lightly grease baking sheet with corn oil. Sauté tempeh in corn oil for 3 minutes. Blend Brazil nuts in blender until finely ground. Mix nut meal with chives, tarragon, and salt, as well as 1 ounce water. Dip tempeh in this batter and place on baking sheet. Place in oven for 15 minutes.

Serves 1

Stuffed Potatoes with Kidney Beans and Soy Cheese

3 Idaho potatoes, baked, halved, with center taken out and skins set aside

2 tablespoons chopped sweet onion

2 tablespoons chopped fresh parsley

1 cup mashed kidney beans
1/4 teaspoon cayenne pepper
1/2 teaspoon paprika
1/2 teaspoon salt
1/2 teaspoon freshly ground black pepper
1 cup shredded soy cheese (optional)
2 to 3 tablespoons extra virgin olive oil

In a large bowl, combine all the ingredients in the order in which they are listed. Stuff the mixture back into the skins and bake in a preheated 425 degrees oven for 10 minutes.
Serves 2

Exotic Tofu Dip

2 cups silken tofu
2 tablespoons chopped fresh chives
4 tablespoons prepared mustard
1/2 cup soy mayonnaise
3 tablespoons balsamic vinegar
1 teaspoon freshly ground black pepper
2 tablespoons chopped fresh dill paprika for garnish

Process all the ingredients, except the paprika, in a food processor or blender until smooth. Sprinkle with paprika. Serve chilled with raw carrot and celery sticks and broccoli and cauliflower florets.
Yields 2 1/2 to 3 cups

Thai Aromatic Rice

5 teaspoons peanut oil
1/4 cup chopped zucchini
1 cup chopped yellow onions
1/2 teaspoon chopped shallots
1/4 cup chopped unsalted roasted peanuts
1/2 cup roasted macadamia nuts

3 cups cooked long grain brown rice

5 artichoke hearts

1/4 cup canned water chestnuts

3 teaspoons chopped garlic

4 1/2 teaspoons chopped fresh mint for garnish

Heat the peanut oil in a skillet or wok over high heat until hot but not smoking. Add the zucchini, onions and shallots, and sauté over medium heat for 5 minutes. Add the remaining ingredients one at a time, stirring after each addition, and cook until hot. Garnish with chopped mint.

Serves 4

Carmen Miranda Brazilian Rice

1 cup chopped onions

1 fresh tomato, chopped or 1/2 cup prepared tomato sauce

1 1/2 teaspoons drained, crushed capers

1/2 cup large pitted black olives

1/2 cup hearts of palm

1 bay leaf

4 tablespoons extra virgin olive oil

2 cups cooked basmati rice

2 tablespoons roasted sunflower seeds

2 tablespoons pumpkin seeds

1/4 teaspoon cayenne

1/4 teaspoon dried thyme

1/2 teaspoon freshly ground black pepper

1/4 teaspoon chili pepper

4 cloves crushed garlic

1 teaspoon sea salt

In a large sauce pan, sauté the onions, tomatoes, capers, olives and bay leaf in oil over medium heat until the onions are clear. Add the remaining ingredients and sauté another 4 minutes until hot. Serve with black beans.

Serves 4

Stewed Vegetable Medley

2 cups chopped red cabbage

2 cups chopped green cabbage

4 cups water

1 1/2 cups sliced onions

2 tablespoons caraway seeds

1 tablespoon turmeric

4 tablespoons curry powder

4 tablespoons extra virgin olive oil

1/4 teaspoon freshly ground black pepper

1 1/2 teaspoons sea salt

1 cup peeled chopped potatoes

1/2 cup frozen peas

1/4 cup frozen corn

1 tablespoon curry powder

In a large saucepan, combine all the ingredients and bring to a boil. Reduce heat to medium–low and cook for 30–35 minutes. Serve hot or cold.

Serves 4 to 6

Savory Stuffed Artichokes

2 artichokes

4 tablespoons orange juice

4 tablespoons plus 1 teaspoon lemon juice

2 cups water

1/2 cup chopped avocado

1/4 cup chopped fresh tomatoes

1/4 cup chopped black pitted olives

1/4 cup chopped onions

2 tablespoons extra virgin olive oil

1/2 cup chopped fresh basil

3 tablespoons toasted sesame seeds

1/2 cup roasted macadamia nuts

1 teaspoon salt

1 sliced lemon (for garnish)

Trim the thorns from the artichoke leaves with a pair of scissors and trim the bottoms so they will stand upright. In a medium-size saucepan, simmer the artichokes in the water and lemon juice over medium heat for about 50–60 minutes, until the leaves pull out easily. Remove the artichokes from the water and let them cool. Gently pull out the center leaves and scoop out the fuzzy choke with a spoon. Combine the remaining ingredients in a small mixing bowl and stir well. Spoon the stuffing mixture into the centers of the artichokes and garnish with lemon slices.

Serves 4

Southern Soul Dish

1 cup finely chopped kale, steamed 5 minutes
1 cup diced apples
4 1/2 teaspoons apple juice
1 cup sliced mushrooms
1/2 cup sliced fennel root
1 cup black-eyed peas, steamed 15 minutes
1/2 teaspoon cayenne
1 teaspoon sea salt
1 teaspoon freshly ground black pepper
2 tablespoons extra virgin olive oil
3 tablespoons chopped fresh parsley
3 teaspoons ground cinnamon
1 teaspoon ground nutmeg
1/2 cup toasted almonds

In a large saucepan, sauté the kale, apples, mushrooms, fennel, salt, pepper and cayenne in the oil over medium–high heat for 7 minutes. Add the remaining ingredients and cook an additional 10 minutes. Serve hot.

Serves 3 to 4

Sweet Basil Rice Pasta

2 cups chopped fresh tomatoes

1 cup sweet peas

1 cup chopped green beans

1 cup chopped yellow onions

4 tablespoons capers

1 cup diced yellow and red sweet peppers

2 1/2 cups chopped fresh basil

1/3 teaspoon sliced garlic

1/4 teaspoon dried oregano

1/4 cup extra virgin olive oil

4 cups cooked rice pasta

In a large saucepan, sauté all the ingredients, except the rice pasta, in the oil for 10 to 15 minutes. Serve hot as a sauce over the cooked spaghetti.

Serves 3 to 4

Thai Peanut Rice Noodles

1 cup diced yellow onions

1/2 cup sliced scallions

1/4 cup diced celery

7 tablespoons toasted sesame oil

1 cup stemmed and sliced shitake mushrooms

1 clove garlic

1/4 cup smooth peanut butter

1 teaspoon pure maple syrup

1 teaspoon fresh lime juice

1/3 cup plus 1 tablespoon water

2 drops hot chili oil or Tabasco sauce

gomasio (sesame salt) to taste

1/4 pound cooked rice noodles

Combine 1 tablespoon oil, garlic, peanut butter, maple syrup, lime juice, water and hot chili oil in a blender and mix until smooth, 2 to 3 minutes, and set aside. In a large saucepan, heat the oil over medium heat, then sauté the scallions and mushrooms for 8 to 10 minutes. Remove from the heat and stir in the gomasio and peanut sauce. Toss the rice noodles with the sauce in a large bowl until all the noodles are covered. Chill for an hour and a half and serve cold.

Serves 2 to 4

Japanese Rice Threads

4 cups stemmed and sliced shitake mushrooms

1 cup diced yellow onions

1 cup sliced scallions

1/4 cup toasted sesame oil

2 teaspoons grated fresh ginger

1/2 cup plus 1 tablespoon tamari

3 cups thinly sliced carrot matchsticks, steamed 10 minutes

2 cloves crushed garlic

2 tablespoons lemon juice

2 tablespoons orange juice

6 cups water

2 cups dry rice noodles

In a large saucepan, heat the oil over medium heat and sauté the mushrooms, scallions, onions, ginger and carrot sticks for 3 minutes. Add the tamari, noodles and water and cook for another 4 to 6 minutes.

Serves 3 to 4

Angel Hair with Radicchio

1 cup sliced mushrooms

1 cup sliced radicchio

1 cup fresh or frozen peas

1 tablespoon salt

1/2 cup soy milk

4 tablespoons capers

1 cup sliced black pitted olives

1 tablespoon sea salt
3/4 teaspoon freshly ground black pepper
1 cup soy Parmesan cheese (nondairy)
4 cups cooked angel hair rice pasta

In a large saucepan, heat the oil over medium heat and sauté the mushrooms and peas for 6 minutes or until tender. Add the capers, basil, fennel, salt, pepper and milk, cover and cook for another 2 minutes. Add the radicchio and cook for 1 additional minute. Remove from heat and toss with the cheese and rice pasta.
Serves 3 to 4

Sweet and Sour Tempeh

2 cups cubed tempeh
1 cup cubed pineapple
1/2 cup chopped peanuts
1 cup broccoli florets
2 tablespoons sliced scallions
2 tablespoons hot sesame oil
2 teaspoons crushed garlic
3 tablespoons tamari
1 cup chopped roasted macadamia nuts
1 cup sweet basil leaves
1/4 cup toasted sesame seeds

In a large saucepan, sauté all the ingredients in the oil over medium heat for 5 to 10 minutes, stirring constantly. Serve with brown rice.
Serves 2

Vietnamese Cabbage Rolls with Pears

1 1/2 cups chopped shitake mushrooms
1/2 cup diced carrots
1/4 cup chopped scallions
1/2 cup chopped zucchini

1/4 cup chopped fresh parsley

2 teaspoons tamari

1 cup cooked white beans

dash of freshly ground black pepper

5 tablespoons toasted sesame oil

1 1/2 cups brown rice

1/4 cup sesame seeds

2 cups sliced pears

1 cup apple juice

1/2 head or 10 leaves red cabbage, steamed 4 minutes

1 cup roasted cashews

1/2 cup chopped nuts

In a large saucepan, sauté the mushrooms, carrots, scallions, zucchini, parsley, tamari and pepper in the oil for 6–8 minutes over medium heat. Stir in the beans, rice and sesame seeds, and set aside. In a separate saucepan, cook the pears and juice over medium heat for 2 to 4 minutes or until tender, and set aside. Place 1 to 2 tablespoons of the vegetable stuffing on each cabbage leaf where the thick stem is. Fold the right side of the leaf over it, then the left, and roll it up. Place the stuffed leaves in a greased pan and top with the pear mixture and nuts. Cover and bake in a preheated oven at 375 degrees for 30 minutes.
Serves 2

Tempeh with Orange and Ginger

1 cup red and yellow sweet peppers

3 tablespoons toasted sesame oil

1 cup cubed tempeh

2 tablespoons sliced scallions

1 cup peeled diced seedless oranges

1/2 teaspoon grated fresh ginger

2 tablespoons soy sauce

1/4 teaspoon freshly ground black pepper

1/4 cup gomasio (sesame salt) for garnish

In a large saucepan, sauté all the ingredients, except for gomasio, over medium heat for 10 minutes. Add garnish and serve hot with brown rice.

Serves 3

Mediterranean String Beans

4 cups string beans, strings removed

1 1/2 cup chopped or sliced onions

6 cloves garlic, sliced

5 cups sliced mushrooms

1 cup chopped fresh basil

3 tablespoons chopped fresh parsley

1 teaspoon chopped fresh oregano

2 tablespoons peppercorns

1/2 teaspoon red pepper

1 teaspoon dill

3 cups chopped fresh tomatoes

1/4 cup extra virgin olive oil

1 cup grated soy Parmesan cheese (non-dairy)

In a large saucepan, sauté the string beans, onions, garlic, mushrooms, basil, parsley, oregano, peppercorns, red pepper, and dill in the oil over medium–high heat for 5 to 7 minutes. Add the tomatoes and cook another 15 to 20 minutes. Garnish with the cheese and serve with brown rice.

Yields 6 to 7 cups

Spicy Broccoli Stir-fry

2 tablespoons hot sesame oil

2 cups cubed baked tofu

2 cups broccoli florets

1 teaspoon cornstarch, dissolved in 1/2 cup water

2 tablespoons grated orange peel

2 tablespoons grated lemon peel

1 tablespoon chili pepper

2 tablespoons tamari
2 tablespoons fennel
1/4 teaspoon hot red pepper flakes (optional)
2 cloves garlic, minced
1 teaspoon grated fresh ginger

In a medium saucepan, sauté the tofu and broccoli in oil over medium heat for 3 minutes. Remove from the pan and place the mixture in a bowl. Combine the remaining ingredients in the pan. Cook on low–medium heat until simmering for one minute. Add the broccoli mixture, cover, and cook for 2 minutes. Stir well and serve with short-grain brown rice.
Serves 3 to 4

Stir-fry Garlic and Kombu

1 cup sweet peas
1 cup diced yellow and red sweet peppers
2 cups chopped bok choy
2 tablespoons mustard powder
5 cloves garlic, crushed
4 tablespoons toasted hot sesame oil
1 cup cubed firm tofu
4 tablespoons tamari
1/4 cup sun dried tomatoes
1 cup kombu, soaked and drained (see below)

In a large sauce pan, sauté the peas, peppers, bok choy, mustard powder and garlic in the oil over medium heat for 15 minutes. Add the tofu and cook an additional 2 to 3 minutes. Add the tamari and kombu, mix in lightly and serve with brown rice.
Serves 2

Note: Kombu leaves will disintegrate if stirred vigorously. Soak for 10 to 20 seconds, drain and use.

40

Desserts

■■■

Coconut Mango Pudding

6 ounces mango
3 ounces brown rice, cooked
1 1/2 ounces coconut, shredded (unsweetened)
1 1/2 ounces dates
10 ounces coconut milk
2 heaping teaspoons Egg Replacer
pinch of cinnamon

Combine all ingredients in blender and purée until smooth. Transfer to saucepan and cook over medium heat for 5 minutes, stirring frequently. Chill in refrigerator for 45 minutes.
Serves 2

Sunny Rice Pudding

3 ounces mango
3 ounces brown rice, cooked
5 teaspoons carob powder
1 1/2 ounces sunflower seeds
1 ounce date sugar
1 teaspoon vanilla
1 1/2 ounces dates
2 heaping teaspoons Egg Replacer

Combine all ingredients and purée until smooth. Transfer to saucepan and cook over medium heat for 5 minutes, stirring frequently. Chill in refrigerator for 45 minutes.

Serves 2

Cinnamon Papaya Pudding

3 ounces papaya
3 ounces oatmeal, cooked
6 ounces apple juice
3 tablespoons honey
2 heaping teaspoons Egg Replacer
pinch of cinnamon
3 ounces apples, cut into 1/2-inch cubes

Combine all ingredients in blender except apples. Purée until smooth. Transfer to saucepan and cook over medium heat for about 5 minutes. Add apples and stir. Chill in refrigerator for 45 minutes or until set.

Serves 2

Apple-Papaya Honey Pudding

6 ounces pineapple
6 ounces papaya juice
3 tablespoons honey
2 tablespoons Egg Replacer
pinch of cinnamon
4 1/2 ounces apples, chopped
1 1/2 ounces pecans, chopped

Combine all ingredients in blender except apples and pecans. Purée until smooth. Transfer to saucepan and cook over medium heat for 5 minutes. Add apples and nuts. Stir. Chill 45 minutes in refrigerator.

Serves 2

Kiwi Pudding

5 ounces strawberries

2 ounces kiwi

3 ounces millet, cooked

4 ounces maple syrup

6 ounces coconut milk

2 heaping teaspoons Egg Replacer

1 teaspoon vanilla

1 teaspoon fresh mint

1 teaspoon lemon juice

pinch of cinnamon

1 1/2 ounces slivered almonds

Place all ingredients in blender, except almonds. Purée until smooth. Transfer to saucepan and set over medium heat for 5 minutes, stirring constantly. Chill for 45 minutes in the refrigerator. Top with almonds when chilled.

Serves 3

Strawberry Orange Pudding

4 ounces strawberries

3 ounces orange sections

1 1/2 ounces plums

3 ounces maple syrup

6 ounces coconut milk

1 1/2 ounces slivered almonds

Combine all ingredients in blender, except for almonds. Purée until smooth. Transfer to saucepan and set over medium heat for 5 minutes, stirring constantly. Chill for 45 minutes in refrigerator. Top with almonds when chilled.

Serves 2

Carob Banana Tofu Pudding

6 ounces banana, mashed

3 ounces peaches, sliced

3 ounces tofu, cut into bite-size pieces

4 ounces barley malt

6 ounces peach juice

1/2 ounce carob powder

1 teaspoon vanilla

3 heaping teaspoons Egg Replacer

pinch of cinnamon

Combine all ingredients in blender. Purée until smooth. Transfer to saucepan and set over medium heat for 5 minutes, stirring frequently. Chill for 45 minutes in refrigerator.

Serves 2

Peach Julep Pudding

6 ounces peaches, sliced

3 ounces barley, cooked

8 ounces peach juice

4 ounces barley malt

1 1/2 ounces walnuts

1 teaspoon vanilla

2 teaspoons fresh mint

1 teaspoon lemon juice

Place all ingredients in blender, Purée until smooth. Transfer to saucepan and set over medium heat for 5 minutes, stirring frequently. Chill for 45 minutes in refrigerator.

Serves 2

Pear-Apple-Hazelnut Crisp

2 pears, core and sliced

2 apples, cored and diced

2 oranges, peeled and puréed

4 plums, peeled, pitted and sliced

3/4 teaspoon grated orange rind

2 tablespoons fresh lemon juice

2 tablespoons almond extract

1 tablespoon vanilla extract

TOPPING

1/4 cup coarsely chopped roasted hazelnuts

1/4 cup coarsely chopped roasted pecans

1/2 cup coarsely chopped macadamia nuts

1/4 cup canola oil

3/4 cup maple syrup

1/4 cup oat or barley flour

1 tablespoon brown cinnamon

In a large bowl, combine the pears, apples, oranges, plums, rind and extract. Pour into a square 9-inch baking dish. Combine the topping ingredients and sprinkle on top of the fruit mixture. Bake in a preheated 375 degrees oven for 25 to 35 minutes.

Serves 6 to 8

Banana Heavenly Delight

1 cup rice or soy milk

4 tablespoons Egg Replacer

4 teaspoons vanilla extract

2 teaspoons almond extract

1/4 cup pure maple syrup

1/2 teaspoon ground nutmeg

1 cup sliced bananas

1/2 teaspoon cinnamon

1/4 cup agar flakes

1/4 cup roasted pecans

In a medium saucepan, bring the milk, Egg Replacer, extracts, syrup and nutmeg to a simmer. Stir constantly with a whisk and use a tapered spoon to make sure the bottom doesn't burn. Once thickened, remove from the heat and stir in the banana slices, and chill for 2 to 4 hours. To serve, gently loosen the pudding from the sides of the dish by running a butter or small knife around the inside of the glass. Next, place a plate on top of the dish and invert the plate and dish. Serves 4

Pecan-Maple Custard

4 tablespoons apple juice
3 cups silken tofu
4 tablespoons vanilla extract
4 1/2 teaspoons almond extract
1 cup chopped roasted pecans
3 tablespoons chia seeds
1/4 cup agar flakes

In the blender or food processor, combine all the ingredients except the pecans, until smooth. Chill, top with pecans, and serve.
Serves 4

Poached Pears

4 pears peeled and quartered
2 cups apple juice
4 tablespoons orange rind and juice
1 tablespoon lemon extract
2 cups fresh or frozen raspberries
3/4 cup maple syrup
1/4 cup toasted macadamia nuts for garnish
4 fresh mint leaves for garnish

In a large saucepan, bring the pears, juices, and extract to a boil, reduce the heat to low, and cook for 5 minutes, covered. In a separate saucepan, combine the raspberries and maple syrup. Bring to a simmer and let cook for 2 minutes. Remove from the heat and serve over the drained pears. Add the garnish and serve with nondairy ice cream.

Serves 4

PART EIGHT

Testimonials

I wrote this book to give hope to people who otherwise might get the idea there isn't any hope that has their name on it. Throughout these pages, you've read about the ways and means to make yourself a happier and healthier person through nutritional approaches to a wide range of illnesses and pathologies. But the story isn't all told if you're getting the idea that it's just between you and what ails you and the ways you can be doing better. That is all important. But it isn't the whole story. The secret of our success is how we inspire one another, how we work together, how we benefit and learn from the experiences of others.

The big drug companies, with all their money, pay hundreds of millions to show the efficacy of the drugs they make their profits from. Because of their self-interest and the resulting biases, the fairness and accuracy of these studies are increasingly doubtful.

But where are the efficacy studies, the scientific studies, for nutritional approaches to illness? Where are the studies of nonproprietary vitamin supplements? They don't exist, because these are already in the public domain. They are inexpensive. So the pharmaceutical companies don't want us to know about them. Not only do they not generate the big profits, they compete with the products that do.

So what we're left with are the testimonials of people like us who have tried the alternative approaches. As assembled here, they serve as a reminder that these approaches work, and that you are not alone.

JEAN, 72 YEARS OLD

I am a lung cancer survivor. I had radiation, chemotherapy, and several body scans which left me anemic. I also developed osteoarthritis which incapacitated me. Walking was difficult and I needed help to board a bus. I used pain medication. My blood pressure was slightly elevated. Although I considered myself to be nutritionally aware, I used dairy products. My energy was quite low after cancer treatment. I joined a support group to rebuild my immune system. I wanted to be healthy.

The arthritis has diminished. I no longer require medication. I take walks and practice yoga. I am totally vegan, drink juices, and follow a Gary's protocol totally. Group homework assignments expanded my self-awareness and created new insights.

I am delighted with the results of each new blood test. I am cancer-free and optimistic. My work, in the wardrobe department of a theatrical company, is enjoyable, and I look forward to a good season with the crew again.

ROSE

I have been listening to health radio for many years and continuously learn and absorb even the little things and all the helpful information. When Gary announced that a new support group was forming, I decided to be courageous and attend.

I suffered from headaches and a runny nose, and from food allergies, so I was reticent about attending functions away from home. Because I am visually impaired, I needed behavior modification.

I am now vegan, use green powders, and follow a vegan protocol.

My health and energy have improved. No more headaches and runny nose. I have energy and vitality. I bravely embarked upon attending group meetings and found positive energies that motivated me. I am now deeply involved in tai chi twice weekly, alternating with two hours of yoga on the off weeks. These practices trained me to be self-assertive and gave me spontaneous courage to achieve changes in spite of my visual problem. I wrote homework assignments in class and hired a person to read them to me at home. Facing my inhibitions was detoxifying, challenging, and strengthening. I use public transportation, go to concerts without hesitation, and live an easier and more peaceful life.

NARLENE

I used to have menstrual cramps that were so painful that I was prescribed high doses of Motrin. Taking it made some of the pain go away. Since I started Gary's protocols, I have had no menstrual pain and a cyst in my breast is shrinking. I have firmer breasts, more energy, have lost weight, and now I am working on ridding myself of negative thought patterns.

JEAN

My husband and I began to notice our bodies were not in good condition. He was a meat and potatoes man and a very picky eater. Over the years, he was exposed to lead paint and cadmium on his job and developed nocturnal seizures, low energy, digestive discomfort, and memory loss. I handled stress badly and was often intolerant. I had a bad accident: my breasts were caught between two doors and throbbed for two years.

We started to follow a vegan protocol from a health book. We studied urine therapy and acupuncture, and began to use colonics and sprouting.

My husband has fewer seizures today, has more energy and enhanced memory, and enjoys his new diet. He is enthusiastic and looks forward to his seventy-fifth birthday. We are energetic and without intestinal problems, and we handle stress well because we are no longer toxic. My female organs function as well as they did in my younger years. Our naturopath told me I avoided fracturing a hip during a fall because my bones are well mineralized. We are vegan, eat raw vegetables, juice, and invent nutritious recipes using a dehydrator. I am involved in community affairs.

Our outlook is cheerful. We love spreading the word.

CHARLES

My journey toward improving my health began when I attended a health seminar. I worked in construction as an iron worker and had several accidents. During my younger years, I held several jobs at a time and developed hypertension. It was time to rebuild my physical system. I considered my energy to be adequate for an aging man.

I gradually investigated organic foods and vegeterian replacements for flesh foods. My health is maintained with supplements, using weights, gardening, and drinking power shakes with red and green powders. I still work in building and construction, and just built a playhouse for my grandchildren.

Listening to health programs on the radio gave me some information. Following today's healthier lifestyle and taking proper products supplies me with more energy than I have ever had. I bounce back easily from exhaustion. Except for a constant knee condition, I do not feel the consequences of having fallen off buildings. I do not have hypertension.

My family does not follow or cooperate with my food preparation. I prepare my meals separately and enjoy them. Hopefully, one day my grandchildren will be open to this healthy concept. I feel younger than my sixty-nine years and look forward to a happy future.

ALICE

I realized my stressful job caused adverse health conditions. I was in contact with negative situations. I began to lose my figure. I did not choose to continue this lifestyle. I respected Gary's radio show information and joined a support group.

The total change from accustomed foods that made me tired and bloated, to new fresh foods, was exciting. My entire physical system is cleaner. I quickly dropped thirteen pounds and noticed my digestion improved. No more acid reflux.

I prepare vegetable juices and powdered drinks with pure water. I am vegan and use appropriate supplements. I practice aerobics during the a.m. hours and yoga later in the day. I use an exercise bike, power walk, and run. The behavioral aspect of the program opened me up to self-analysis personally and objectively. Establishing goals over the years led to my very successful business in a health-related industry. I am trim, firm, look better as I age, and still read Gary's books.

ALSTON, 92 YEARS OLD

I retired from the merchant marines at age sixty-five. I have always been very active and considered myself to be healthy, but considered my future health. I heard Gary Null on the radio and began to read books on health and nutrition. I follow a vegetarian diet and juice. I use a rebounder every morning. I get on the train and travel to Manhattan to buy supplements.

I do not see many people my age these days. Most of them have caretakers and are dependent. I am totally self-sufficient: I care for my home, shop, wash my clothes, and even take my curtains down to wash and replace them alone. I do not need anyone to take care of me. I can accomplish my self-sustaining tasks alone.

I believe my diet and nutritional supplements are responsible for maintaining my health.

AMY

I was unhappy in my recessive role in personal relationships. I would grind my teeth during the night and was concerned about a double heartbeat. Medications would not heal my cystic skin condition.

I began a vegan protocol. Detoxing my system produced very positive results. The double heartbeat rarely occurs. The ganglian wrist cyst healed. Cystic acne cleared, and my skin is healthy. I no longer grind my teeth during sleep. The homework and lectures gave me much to consider. Today I take a stronger role in my relationships meeting my expectations, not only the other person's. Cleaning my life, body, and environment helped me develop my potential.

ANDREA

I considered orthopedic surgery to eliminate constant pain. I did not know options were open to me. I did not think a support group could help but, in desperation, I joined one and went to Paradise Gardens for a week. It was there, in Florida, with other people creating healthy and stress-free lives, that I understood change is available and in my hands.

I gained much-needed weight by following the protocol and choosing a healthy diet. Using chiropractic, acupuncture and neck traction reflexology, along with massage and Epsom salt baths, my pain began to subside. The homework and lectures opened my insights into my feelings of guilt and dissatisfaction. My home today is uncluttered, peaceful, and stress-free. Best of all, my family follows the protocol.

ANDREA

I was trapped inside the typical American diet with its false sense of security.

I weighed 300 pounds and was not diagnosed with illness.

My back ached, veins in my legs hurt, I felt ill after ingesting most foods—especially dairy—and yearned to wear normal-sized clothing.

I joined a support group as size 24 to 26. Applying myself to the protocol, feeling centered with a new sense of values, I soon said "no" easily and lost seventy-five pounds, to size 18. I am vegan today, use the protocol, and enjoy the world of real food, delicious tastes, and an athletic life in a healthy, attractive body. I volunteer in needy countries where my nursing skills help me help other people, bringing positive, vital energy.

ANGELO

I was 300 pounds. I had high cholesterol and blood pressure, high hemoconiosis (abnormal hemoconia count in blood), and hepatitis B. I had discoloration around my eyes, eczema, bleeding knuckles and elbows, hemorrhoids. I felt sluggish and fatigued, used an inhaler, and had pain with simple movements. I listened to Gary's radio show and joined a support group with my wife in 1999.

Now all the above-mentioned ailments are gone. I lost one hundred pounds. I have constant energy. I run, race walk, power walk, skate, do aerobics, and train in a gym. I've lost one width of a shoe size. Skin and hair improved, I need more frequent haircuts. I have no additional greying of hair.

I follow the protocol, including juices and using green and red powders. I create organic vegetarian menus with my wife. I find I easily complete tasks and am on a wild uncluttering spree. I do image consulting today. My children are slowly adopting my lifestyle.

ATHENA

I could not connect with people. I felt distant. I was dissatisfied with my job. Depression was exhausting. I could not handle more physical and emotional trauma. I entered a support group, "just in case I will learn something."

I learned the theory behind detoxifying the body and mind. After a short time juicing, eating vegan, and eliminating food allergies, my energy picked up. I no longer have PMS symptoms nor do I feel cysts in my breast. Depression lifted within six weeks. Eye floaters lessened. I notice new hair on my head grows in darker. As my body eliminated toxins, so did my relationships. I slowly allow new friends into my life and recently accepted a job I enjoy at a higher wage.

BARBARA

I read books on a holistic, vegan lifestyle and saw helpful programs on TV. I joined a support group in 1994.

I am not on pain medication. The pain is sporadic. I exercise in a rehab center for my disk problem. My major changes began two to three weeks into the protocol. I am an organic vegan and do not use coffee or sugar. Throwing up stopped when sensible eating and probiotics began. I am a vegeterian cook and intend to study vegetarian meal preparation.

I never saw life in the past as I experience it today.

BENJAMIN

I am a forty-four-year-old man diagnosed as a "worst case disability."

I was considered to be a healthy baby at birth. After I was vaccinated at three months of age, an eczema developed over my body. This was the beginning of being treated with medications throughout my life.

I became asthmatic at age nineteen and used various drugs including prednisone 20-30x. Diagnosed with "anxiety," I was tested for food, yeast allergies, and infections. At this point I was told I had a cerebral allergy. I could not concentrate in school, could not reach my potential, and learning was slow. Additional medications were prescribed. I was always uncomfortable and ill. The family diet at that time was "the typical American diet." Seldane and erythromycin cleared my skin but again made me nervous and anxious. Listening to Gary Null on the radio opened me to new possibilities. Would detoxing and following a new food plan change my life?

I am vegan, use organic foods, and eat vegetables and fruits. I discovered my allergy to wheat. With a clear mind, learning comes quickly to me now. I no longer harbor yeast infections. I work in a synagogue. My skin is clear, and the behavioral problems and anxieties which held me back ceased.

I use supplements, an air filter, antioxidants, and Vitamin C. I recently began walking as exercise to lose weight, a current problem.

BOB

I was a heroin addict and methadone user until 2001. I was depressed, physically weak with elevated blood pressure and glaucoma. My hair was thinning. It was time for a change. I did not attend a support group but booked a consultation with Luanne Pennessi at Metropolitan Wellness Center and began a series of drips under the care of a naturopathic physician. Green and red powders, supplements, and a vegan diet changed my body and returned me to my health.

My blood pressure is normal. I no longer have glaucoma. I consider Gary to be my teacher and follow the protocol. My hair is thicker and curly again. Using Gary's night cream reduced brown skin spots. My mercury fillings were removed in 2002. I'm living in the present today and working in a hospital drug and alcohol rehab center. Using heavenly aloe, powders, and supplements keeps me in excellent health and my outlook positive.

THOMAS, 70 YEARS OLD

I became aware of the importance of nutrition and studied various theories, but my physical problems continued. Parkinson's symptoms caused me shame in public. I could not write. I typed with two fingers. My hands trembled when I put food in my mouth. I was advised to take medications. Past experiences with drugs were unpleasant. I refused them. I went on Gary's protocol and learned the specifics of diet and organics, the biochemical necessity of green juices and grasses, the importance of attitude and beliefs.

It was when I combined supplements with my diet that things began to look up. I honor myself, unclutter my life of people and objects, and share this important knowledge with others. I am alert, without past negative influences. Green and red powders keep me going.

These are my happiest and proudest times. I intend to live another seventy years.

TERRY

I joined a support group in August 2000 and lost seven pounds quickly. I am an organic vegan, spiritual, with increased energy after eating vegetables. My hair is thicker, I sleep less, and handle the time between jobs as quality time in which to unclutter. Creating forgiveness letters helped me peel away the past to work on unresolved issues. The homework opened perspectives for my future. I am now attracted to people on a "cellular level." My asthma attacks are less frequent. I can identify their cause. Upper respiratory infections heal quickly.

I set secure boundaries, effectively avoiding toxic situations, like when my family calls me a health nut when I bring my food to family dinners. Exercising includes volleyball, weight lifting, eliptical machine, skating, and bike riding.

SCOTT

I was a construction worker. I felt I was slowly losing stamina and aging. I ate the typical American diet and felt unhealthy. I listened to Gary's Natural Living radio show and discussed the show with a friend.

Now I follow the protocol as best as I can. I juice, use organic foods only, and exercise. My physical endurance has increased. I am able to keep up with my twenty-five- to thirty-year-old coworkers.

Writing forgiveness letters motivated me to create new directions in life. I became self-aware. Today I am able to focus on myself and avoid all toxic situations.

SARA

My mother's illnesses—diabetes, high blood pressure, cardiac disease, and obesity—motivated me to join a group specifically to prevent future diseases in my system. I had severe PMS symptoms for fourteen years. My skin aged prematurely. Its texture was saggy, with pimples and cysts which caused scars. My digestive problems caused bloating. Now I am organic and vegan. I joined a support group and read Gary's book *Get Healthy Now!* My skin tightened with fewer lines. Pimples and discoloration from cysts are fading. Hair analysis indicated traces of copper toxicity and liver congestion which, I feel, cleared with the detox protocol. I have good energy. Working on my journals and writing letters empowered me. I am confident, fearless, and comfortable with issues in the past that once caused pain. I use a rebounder, ride a bicycle, and belly dance.

The men in my life today are quite different from those in my toxic relationships of the past.

RICK, 77 YEARS OLD

I've followed Gary Null's protocol for the past ten years. My health has been severely challenged during that time and I have survived each assault. I had surgery many years ago for a hiatic hernia. My diet of vegetables and juices controls this condition. My father and two sisters died from aortal abdominal aneurisms. My brother had one repaired successfully. I was diagnosed with this condition. Surgery was indicated. I prepared myself for six months with a specific protocol. This included good vitamin intakes, mental and attitudinal insights, and healthy food.

During that time I obtained a copy of the surgical procedure from a medical library and realized it was an extensive operation. My internal organs were going to be removed from ribs to the pubic bone. My aorta had a balloon type defect which would be opened and patched. My organs would then be replaced. I meditated on every organ in my body several times before surgery. I was relaxed before and after the procedure. I demanded of my body that it heal itself. My immune system was at its peak. I survived the surgery well, in excellent condition. I left intensive care in two days and took a bus home a few days later. My physicians were amazed. I explained that I obtained my strong immune system with diet, supplements, and respect for my body.

I am now in the process of creating the biggest project of my life: building the world's largest windfarm. Following the Gary Null protocol gave me the strength and energy I must call upon to complete this mission.

I encourage seniors to build your energies, both mental and physical, and to create new goals, exercise, build your immune system, study, and be a part of your environment.

RAY

I ate burgers, chicken, fried foods, and fried vegetables. I drank a lot of soda and on occasion had alcoholic beverages. Garlic bread, chocolate, and plain milk accompanied each meal. Even with that poor diet I felt healthy, but realized I was not at my peak energy level. I could feel my movements were below my potential. I had difficulty at times thinking through and solving daily problems.

Realizing people were reversing illness using various supplements, I began to drink green tea, and to use garlic and onions and a few vitamins. Still I felt sunken within myself. My higher energy level was not actualized. At that point I started listening to Gary on his radio show.

I was determined to give my body the elements it badly required. I took Gary's advice and studied his products. My diet and vitality improved 75 percent. I started to feel energetic. My power zoomed. Now I sleep less. I have increased endurance and have keener mental cognition. I tackle daily responsibilities in detail, think faster, and am patient with problems. I am emotionally positive. In short, I am healthy and confident.

PAUL

I am a Parkinson's patient. I joined several support groups, but did not complete them for the duration. I listened to Gary on Natural Living and read Gary Null books. I consumed chicken and wheat. I felt encouraged by other members of the support group. It was an uplifting experience. I wanted to learn how to improve my health.

Now my body feels more energetic. Parkinson's symptoms have lessened. I juice, use green powders, and eat organic produce. I work and feel stronger. My body movements are calmer today. I intend to remain on the protocol.

OWEN

I was a vegetarian who ate unhealthy foods: soda, sugar, dairy. I assumed I was healthy because I never was ill. I had listened to Natural Living since 1985 and felt I was ready to change with a program providing parameters. Now I have 3 percent body fat. I'm energetic. I sleep six hours a night, have thicker hair, and appear thinner. I uncluttered my apartment, discarding all nonfunctional items. I exercise five times a week and am considering using feng shui. I guide my behavior within the parameters of the protocol and spend two to four hours on class homework. It is the best way to deal with the past and plan the future. I am now an organic cook, aware of my reactions to toxic foods. I designed an efficient meal program and now juice two to three times a day.

MONTY

I was "semi-vegeterian" and slightly overweight. I ate dairy, had digestive problems, angered easily, and was a student of Chinese medicine and herbology. I studied German electro-acupuncture. I lived in Italy for many years and am a trained psychologist but have a defensive anger.

I joined a support group to learn the protocol for myself and my patients. My eating patterns have improved by being vegan and by juicing. I feel a stronger vitality. Boundaries are easily set. I will not tolerate abuse. I've developed insight into my former behavior and my tendency to get angry. The support group experience created the strength for self-empowerment.

MICHAEL, 62 YEARS OLD

In 1989, I attended a Gary Null retreat. I learned the benefits of Vegetarianism, juicing, supplements, and meditation. In 1994, I became disabled due to carbon monoxide poisoning. I am still in the process of recovery. I no longer work. I cannot look at computer screens. Surgery for two detached retinas affected my eyesight. My blood pressure was extremely high. My heartbeat accelerated to a dangerous level. I took several pharmaceutical drugs to control these conditions. A few years later, seizures began with Alzheimer-like symptoms. Abnormally severe edema in my legs incapacitated me. I was in a coma for sixty days. Nursing home care was considered.

My health took an upward turn on the Gary Null protocol. Juicing, stress management, and homework opened me to my potentials and purpose in life. I discovered the best of what works and realized I was not doing anything worthwhile.

Today I no longer need a compressor for leg edema. My leg size decreased 30 percent. I sleep less. I exercise with hand weights. I recently received a bowflex to build my upper body. I have lost twenty-three pounds. My blood pressure is lower. My brain speed seems to be faster. I feel like a teenager, just blossoming. I plan a future including research of natural life energies.

MICHAEL

I used medications for anxiety and depression. I wanted to discontinue medications. My hair was greying. My complexion was dry with bumpy skin. I had nervous twitches.

Now I am 99 percent vegan and organic. I juice and exercise. I don't use medications for colitis. Being aware of my mind-body connection has altered my behavior and created a change in my body chemistry. The psychological and emotional changes empowered me. I now understand the negative impact of toxic foods and people. I stopped fighting life and allowed life to support me.

I receive ozone therapy at Metropolitan Wellness. My twitching stopped. My hair is long and healthy. I left a toxic job and actualized a new career enabling people to self-empower their lives.

MARY

I was infertile, I did not ovulate. The orthodox treatment was ineffective and had bad side effects. My husband and I joined a health support group together in 2000. Four months into the program I ovulated and conceived during my third ovulation. I believe my hormonal system is stronger. I had a natural birth but experienced post-depression. I was labeled "clinically depressed" and was advised to discontinue nursing and take medication. I rejected the diagnosis and continued nursing without medication. My health returned six months post-partum with exercise and meditation. My family is vegan, juicing, organic, keeping to the protocol.

I research post-partum depression and reach out to women suffering with the condition. I am studying for a degree in technical communication and once I have my degree will process technical texts into lay language.

LARRY

I felt my diet was healthy and adequate most of my life. I was wheat and dairy free. I did not exercise and had allergies. I was diagnosed with a testicular mass. My physicians suggested removal in order to determine diagnosis. I would not have surgery and researched alternative medical options.

I listened to Gary on the radio and, although the information made sense, I followed the diet part only. Eventually I sought teachers of meditation and consulted with Luanne Pennesi. The impact of the total protocol was fantastic. Feeling healthier I totally devoted myself and my future to the protocol [the teacher] offered.

It took two years for the mass to reduce in size. Throughout this ordeal my bloodwork was normal. My tests are normal today even though the mass remains, but my life and objectives have changed.

Professional and family relationships improved. I understand myself and my family after reading *Who Are You Really*. I am a positive, healthy man.

LADANIA

I run a day care center for children. My grandson had a cancerous kidney removed at age two. At age four he was diagnosed with stage 4 lung cancer. My daughter and I desperately sought help for my grandson. We read many books with alternate approaches to combat cancer and wrote letters to many authors.

We never received answers. We contacted the Metropolitan Wellness Center in New York City. They were the only facility that responded. Luanne Pennesi requested my grandson's medical records. She felt the child's parents and I would learn and benefit from a Gary Null lecture. At that time my grandson's x-ray showed two frightening spots on his lungs.

We spoke to Gary. He suggested the boy take specific supplements, and emulsified cod liver oil. A month and a half later a new x-ray revealed clear lungs, no spots. Today my grandson is seven years old. He is home schooled. His health continues to be good. This experience changed many of our concepts. People have tools for health and healing. There is much to learn. The information is there. Appropriate resources are available.

I no longer serve the children in my day care center canned foods. I create delicious vegetable sandwiches on healthy bread. The children adapted to the taste of real food and love it. My grandson's health is perfect. Gary Null simplifies information. His protocol and suggestions are practical and easy to follow. My family and I continue our life enhancing lifestyle. Our hopes and goals did come together.

JUDY

I was the sole caretaker for my husband during his last years. I spent a great deal of time in hospitals totally involved in his illness. My diet at that time was not healthy. I drank sodas and coffee and was too exhausted to cook meals. I was low energy most of the time and felt awful: headaches, joint pain, and indigestion. My hair and skin were dull, no shine, no bounce or strength.

A week before my husband passed away I was diagnosed with stage 4 metastatic breast cancer. At that time my daughter-in-law attended a workshop in a natural cooking school. Gary visited that day and suggested I consult with Luanne Pennesi. The cancer spread to my cervix and liver. There was a tumor on my appendix. I was given two chemotherapy procedures. Luanne told me to stay on the chemo but to also begin Gary Null's protocol.

I started juicing, using protein shakes, and changing my diet. As I continued, I felt more awake; little by little more energy returned. My lifestyle began to change. When I looked at other cancer patients I realized the difference between us. I looked healthier, not dull and sallow. I changed physically. Today I am vegetarian, eat fresh fruit and vegetables, and exercise by walking and using a rebounder. I have a veggie kitchen—wheat-dairy-sugar free—and love my diet. There are so many substitutes for foods I used to crave. Also, I am free of the heaviness of overeating. I invent new recipes.

My children lost a wonderful father. I refused to let them lose their mother. Many people prayed for me. I am most grateful. My last body scan revealed that I am cancer free.

JOHN

I developed psoriatic arthritis thirty years ago and had surgery to fuse my right wrist. My knees and neck were deteriorating. I used heavy medications and over-the-counter analgesics. My physician advised me to change careers and my daughter motivated me to join a health support group.

Now I am vegan, no sugar or wheat. I was pain free within four weeks and do not take any medication. The swelling has subsided. My doctor commented that the condition of my knee joints are the best he has observed. My blood pressure is normal. I take long walks. I have reclaimed my life. My neighbors now follow the protocol. One couple, a diabetic and his wife with multiple sclerosis, report physical improvements. My cousin lost ten pounds in two weeks and no longer has heartburn.

JOB, 74 YEARS OLD

My mother introduced me to good diet and healthy living. Although I listened to Gary Null for twenty-three years, I did not actualize. I weighed 210 pounds, smoked three packs of cigarettes a day, drank alcohol, felt depressed, and had knee pains and upper respiratory infections. One day I looked at the very aged man in the mirror and was shocked.

Today I follow the protocol and use Gary's green, red, and protein powders. The shakes keep me feeling full and satisfied all day. I am no longer obese, drink "clean" water, use supplements, and feel terrific. I did not get a cold in five years, no more upper respiratory infections. I am organic and vegan, and do not take vaccines. My neighbors tell me I look forty-five years old. They admire my changes. I appreciate my healthy lifestyle. It makes me quite aware of the tremendous amount of obesity today. I am confident and pleased with my life.

WENDY

I was a long-time vegeterian, not organic. I was very emotional, angry, low energy, and self critical, with bladder infections, and I did not consider healthy food choices. The quality of my personal relationships was poor. I had fibroid surgery in 1985, which damaged organs, gave me hemorrhoids, and made my kidneys sluggish.

I joined a support group in April 2001 with my husband to renew our relationship. Now I follow the protocol and enjoy juices and powders. My energy is strong and I work out in a gym. I am organic and vegan. I study yoga and tai chi. I now focus on personal healing instead of changing my partner.

Forgiveness letters and introspective writings have motivated and made me self aware.

GLENROY, 68 YEARS OLD

I was diabetic and developed cellulitis serving in the military and had severe knee and lower disk back pain. I could not climb stairs and used crutches and a cane, and for two months was paralyzed in a wheelchair. My blood pressure and cholesterol were elevated. I ate the typical American diet: flesh foods, wheat, dairy. Underneath it all I wanted to be healthy.

My legs are no longer swollen from cellulitis. My backache has subsided. My circulation is normal. I can easily walk up three flights of steps to my apartment. I buy organic food and follow the protocol; I eat fish and use green and red powders and supplementation. My life is active. I am retired and work on a veteran's council. It is wonderful to babysit my granddaughter feeling lighter and more energetic. All past symptoms are gone. The homework we did in the support group caused me to focus on myself. I learned to be tolerant, less pushy, and humble. This teaching enhanced my body and life.

GLEN

The homework assignments and questions were painful at first but created a method of organizing problems and intelligently handling them. Letter writing caused a personal metamorphosis allowing me to forgive and understand, lifting burdens so I can ascertain repetitive patterns and be introspective.

ETTA

I had a hysterectomy for uterine cancer. The cancer returned. I went through chemotherapy and radiation. I had arthritis, psoriasis, and low energy, and was overweight and unhappy at work.

Now I am vegan, organic, and following protocol. My cancer seems to be in full remission. I've lost twenty-six pounds. My psoriasis is gone. My hair and skin are healthy and my immune system is strong. It was through class assignments and other workbook activities that I understood I was "hard" on myself and soon experienced the positive relief of forgiveness of self and others. I left a toxic job. I meditate twice daily, exercise, practice yoga, and lift weights.

ESTELLA, 85 YEARS OLD

Before, I had great fatigue and was anemic. My energy was low even though I practiced yoga. My blood pressure was elevated. Although most of my food was vegetarian, I was not happy about the way I felt. I decided to change.

Since I began to follow the protocol I need less sleep and just "feel good." My blood pressure is lower. My skin looks great. That makes me very happy.

I have increased my yoga schedule. I am totally vegetarian—lots of salad and steamed greens, tofu. Look at me with all this vitality, feeling positive. This support group has changed my life and health. I'm very pleased with the results.

DIANE

I was a New York City paramedic diagnosed with occupational asthma. I inhaled a mixture of bleach and ammonia during a medical pick-up and developed a condition called osteopenia from prednisone. My vision diminished, my hair began to turn gray, and my skin peeled as if it was ash. I was stressed, had insomnia and sinusitis, and slept three hours a night. I retired from the fire department because of the accident and joined a support group.

Today I am vegetarian, organic, and juicing, and am no longer suffering with sinusitis, hypertension, or asthma. My black hair is returning, my skin is lovely, and my vision has improved. I sleep six hours a night and am calm and happy. My family has joined a food coop. My vitality and energy have zoomed up.

I work out in an adult ballet class, study flamenco, and will perform in a recital. I also roller blade, spin cycle, and study toward a rabbinical career.

DAVID

My wife and I listened to health programs on the radio for two years. At that time I did feel the effects of middle age: body fat, cynicism, low energy. I looked "old." We ate the typical American diet. I became acutely dissatisfied with myself. Stress, fear of high cholesterol from alcoholic beverages and fast foods, loss of energy, and thoughts of physical illnesses weighed me down, and all the time we neglected to use the good information on Gary's radio show, Natural Living.

Finally, the logic of health and science brought us to a support group. Our insights from lectures and homework, the release we felt as our bodies detoxified, and the energy we developed created health, self-esteem, and optimism.

I am less critical. I accept myself. No more alcohol. We attended Gary's health retreat and read self-empowerment books. I was not old. I was drowning in internal pollutants.

CONNIE, 65 YEARS OLD

My positive changes began in a health support group. I simply changed my diet, began juicing, and did homework assignments. Although not familiar with exercise, I tried power walking. Within weeks I realized I had more energy, I no longer felt sluggish each afternoon. I lost twenty pounds, look younger, and my hair and nails grew.

Physically, life is happier without aches and pains. Emotionally, I handle what were once overwhelming family issues with acceptance. Vegetarian food is delicious.

CLARA

I had four children—three Caesarians—and felt old and unhealthy. I wore a size 20. My blood pressure elevated at times. I lived a fast and stressful life on an organic farm the city wanted to confiscate for "open land." My brother died of cancer and I was aware of the increase of that disease.

I've lost weight and wear a size 13. My family is organic and uses green and red powders, no sugar or dairy. My daughter had one asthma attack that did not repeat after eliminating sugar and dairy.

I am energetic and focused, and I exercise four to six times a week. The homework exposed my weak areas and increased my determination to strengthen them. I now think before doing and always unclutter.

RALPH, A SENIOR

I assumed I was healthy most of my life. A couple of years ago I began to feel ill and was diagnosed with a cardiac condition. Triple bypass was suggested. I refused the surgery. Medications and wheelchair dependency added to my discomfort. I traveled to California seeking options. When I returned to New York I joined a health support group. The protocol was sensible and fellow group participants improved their lives and health. I was motivated.

Today, grateful for the experience, I attend meetings and share my information with others. I follow the lifestyle and became a runner. My future seems exciting. I plan to begin a support group in Chicago.

CHERYL

I had severe allergies and upper respiratory infections. I wanted to develop tools for a healthy life because I was angry, anxious, and uncomfortable in my temper and disposition. I wanted freedom from temper and stress.

Now I have no more upper respiratory infections. I am vegetarian and organic, and I juice. Meditation helps me understand my family with compassion. They do not occupy my mind. I am no longer consumed with anger. I am detached from those that caused me anxieties.

The process of uncluttering objects and toxic people had the effect of uncluttering me emotionally. I am rid of unnecessary objects at home. Writing forgiveness letters to my mother calmed my anger and helped me articulate my feelings. I no longer dwell on the past.

I am happy in my new career as a freelance editor and satisfied with my clients. It is a pleasure not to be in a toxic office. I am active in political causes, especially legislation to stop violence against women and creation of hotlines and shelters.

CHARLES, 64 YEARS OLD

I ate the typical American diet of meat, dairy, and sugars. I thought my primary health concern was gaining weight.

I began to listen to Gary's radio show. Researchers presented valid research. People spoke about their experiences in health support groups. They sounded energetic and happy as if they had created new, free lives. Many of these speakers were my age or older. Their testimonials influenced me to change my life.

Now I follow a protocol on my own, one I found in a book. I use green, red and protein powders. I no longer put poison in my system from meat. Mine is a natural way of eating. I walk six to eight miles a day and use supplements.

Gary's radio show is my classroom on the air. I gather information daily and put it to use. My health is better today than it was in my younger years.

BRIAN

I was a cardiac patient in 1996 using prescribed medication. I joined a health support group. Today, in 2007, I am vigorous and quite pleased with the lifestyle I still enjoy. Following the protocol and not straying, I am athletic and ski with my family.

I do not use any flesh food. My weight was 230 pounds in 1996. Today I am 180 pounds. I am a runner and engage in as many sports as I have time for. I feel happier, lighter.

ANNA

My skin was flaky. I overslept yet felt exhausted and napped during the afternoon. I had sinus problems and migraine headaches. Seasonal upper respiratory infections hit me each change of season. I ate the typical American diet and socialized with problematic people.

Following Gary's protocol changed my health and outlook. Today I am 90 percent vegan aiming for 100. My skin is 70 percent improved. I need less sleep, feel alert, and do not need midday rest periods. Energy is liberating. I walk all over the city without a need for "recovery time." Although I cannot purchase all the supplements required at one time, I have seen my health and life turn around. I rarely get a cold and use echinacea and golden seal, vitamin C, and coenzyme Q10 to prevent these infections. I traded negative, toxic people for an interesting, ever-learning life without obstacles.

TOM

Since I've become conscious of the benefit of organic foods, getting out into the sunlight, using prayer and thinking positively, my life has improved. I am a more confident, stronger man.

EDUARDO

I cannot afford all the required supplements, yet even so I am vigilant about my organic food intake. I juice organic fruits and vegetables. My vegan lifestyle supplies me with constant energy throughout the day. I remember the times I crashed with exhaustion in the past around midday. Instead of being home with upper respiratory infections, today they are mild annoyances. My healthy body recuperates easily without absences from work.

MONICA JACKSON

My husband and I were introduced to a physical and emotional lifestyle change at Gary's health retreat. We are not totally vegan, but are aiming to be. We no longer smoke. We increased our exercise schedule, take trips to the shore for clean air, and eat more fish. We both noticed our skin lesions clear completely; the lesions and blotches on our legs are disappearing and our sleep has improved. We look forward to another retreat. Our bodies are healthier and toned as we pursue lifestyle improvements.

JACKLYN MORGAN

I was in a bad place emotionally when a close friend died. Stuck in depression, being alone, reflecting on memories of yesterdays, I needed a jump start to regain my life. It was at a vegan health lecture that I understood relationship toxicity. I began the jump start by juicing vegetables and fruits. I am vegan and go on fasts using green and red powders. I lost weight and feel liberated and healthy.

PEDRO

I began to run again when I changed my diet. I felt great within a month, unbelievable! I mix green and red powder into a drink before each run and I outrun professionals. At one point I lost too much weight, but I keep to the program and rarely go off it. No sugars. I enjoy milk-free chocolate and the recommended supplements. The diet and the exercise built me up and I'm enjoying my life and body.

JOSEPH

I attended a 2004 support group with good results. I was able to eliminate asthma medication. I felt stronger and in a better mindset without the usual anxiety while I used green and other vegetable juices and followed Gary's protocol. I eat fish most of the time and feel healthy today.

My personal behavior improved during my time in the group. I am with it 80 percent today and plan to reactivate my juicing and healthy lifestyle.

HARRY

Following Gary's food protocols brought valuable changes to me and to other people in my support group. I had a negative medical diagnosis. Family problems left me low in enthusiasm. I required long hours of sleep to rest from daily stress.

Following the program, exercising, juicing, and using supplements, green powders, red powders, and vitamin C, I lost weight and gained a new vitality. I sleep less. Although I am handling an acute family crisis today, my energy allows me to meet my responsibilities and make long distance trips. I look forward to my next support group. It's time to continue progress.

LEONARD, 62 YEARS OLD

I changed my life after attending a vegan health retreat several years ago. I continue to follow a vegan protocol and lifestyle teaching. I am organic and vegan and feel terrific.

No longer dependent on blood pressure medication, I use red yeast rice, lecithin, red and green powders, fish oil, vitamins, garlic supplements, organically grown produce, and pure water. Food never tasted better. Exercise strengthens my body and mind. A clean, pure diet made these years pleasurable emotionally and physically.

LUIS

I listened to Gary's radio show and read Gary's books to get a jump start before entering a support group in November 1999. I was a musician who weighed 155 pounds.

Now I weigh 145 pounds. I am organic, juicing, and using pure water. My hair and eyebrows are thicker, the best it's been in my life. My energy is terrific, my blood pressure is lowered, and my cholesterol is normal. My memory has improved and my complexion is fantastic. I can read without glasses.

As a very careful vegan, I eat my last meal before 6:00 p.m., experiencing new tastes and trying new teas. People compliment me daily and want to understand the reasons my health improved.

I plan to hold home-based meetings to introduce people interested in life changes to a vegan protocol.

JIM, 71 YEARS OLD

My wife had to convince me to attend a support group and challenge myself. I was a workaholic. My temper and attitude caused family dissatisfaction. For a guy who thought he knew it all, I sure learned a new lifestyle.

With the help of my family, I attended a support group and became vegan. Flesh foods, gluten, and high carbs affected my attitude. I soon realized why I fell asleep several times a day. Learning the rationale of this new lifestyle and following the common sense of pure food and exercise created wonderful changes. I felt free and clean. I developed not only into a champion runner and businessman, having created a successful restaurant that expanded five times, I was voted the 2006 Long Island Handicapped Employer of the Year. I received the Goldman Sachs Handicapped Entrepreneur of the Year award, and the 2006 Achilles Athlete of the Year award. I have finished first, second, and fourth place in four of the twenty-four road runner races, and I came in second in the cross country challenge. I've competed in seven New York City Marathons in seven years. My wife and I work seventeen hours a day. Our healthy diet and respect for life make me realize these changes came with personal respect. How one feels about oneself, putting fears aside, and disregarding society's opinions are the keys. If you are healthy, you can rebuild at any age.

Appendices

Appendix A

Resources

■■■

Much of the information in this book comes from interviews and consultations with experts in the field. For further inquiry into the topics discussed, we have compiled a resource list of practitioners. You will also find in this appendix a sampling of relevant scientific research summaries, article citations, books, and websites. Please note that this material is provided for informational purposes only, and should not be viewed as individual recommendations or endorsements.

Biographies and Addresses of Practitioners

DR. RICHARD ASH, M.D., went to the Medical College of Pennsylvania in Philadelphia. He has been in private practice since then, specializing in internal medicine, and alternative and complementary therapies. He also founded the Ash Center for Comprehensive Medicine. He has a radio show every Sunday in New York.

Ash Center for Comprehensive Medicine
800A Fifth Avenue
New York NY 10021
Tel: (212) 758-3200
DrAsh@ashmd.com

ROBERT C. ATKINS, M.D., graduated from Cornell University Medical College and had hospital affiliations with both Columbia and Rochester Universities. He was the founder and executive medical director of the Atkins Centers for Complementary Medicine, and president of the Foundation for the Advancement of Innovative Medicine. He specialized in treating a wide variety of disorders, including asthma, cancer, chronic fatigue, hypoglycemia, and immune system disorders. He passed away in 2003.

www.atkinscenter.com

SIDNEY M. BAKER, M.D., is a practicing physician with an interest in nutritional, biochemical, and environmental aspects of chronic illness in adults and children. He is the co-founder of the Autism Research Institute's DAN! (Defeat Autism Now!) project.

FRED BAUGHMAN, JR., M.D., is a pediatric neurologist in La Mesa, California, a medical advisor for the National Right to Read Foundation, and a fellow of the American Academy of Neurology. He is the author of *The ADHD Fraud: How Psychiatry Make "Patients" Out of Normal Children.*

www.adhdfraud.com

SYD BAUMEL, a medical writer, is the author of *Serotonin: How to Naturally Harness the Power Behind Prozac and Phen/Fen*, and *Natural Antidepressants*.

www.mts.net/~baumel

ROBERT BERNSTEIN is an educational therapist with a private practice in Dobbs Ferry, New York. He has a master's degree in special education from Teacher's College of Columbia University. He goes to schools and other institutions to give presentations on education, and is a consultant to the Putnam New York chapter of the National Council on Alcohol and other Drug Dependencies.

191 Woodlands Avenue
White Plains NY 10607
Tel: (914) 478-4868
RobEDU@aol.com

MARY ANN BLOCK, M.D., an osteopathic physician, founded the Block Center in Dallas, Texas, and has written several books on health and nutrition.

1750 Norwood Drive
Hurst Texas 76054
Tel: (817) 280-9933
www.blockcenter.com

NEIL BLOCK, M.D., is a board-certified specialist in family practice, preventive nutrition, and orthomolecular body-brain imbalances. He has certificates in homeopathy, naturopathy, herbal medicine, Bach flower remedies, and sports performance, and training. His special interests include fatigue syndrome, endocrine disturbances, holistic healing, ADD, sleep-mood disorders, and respiratory diseases.

60 Dutch Hill Road
Orangeburg NY 10962
Tel: (845) 359-3300

PETER R. BREGGIN, M.D., graduated from Harvard College and attended Case Western Reserve School of Medicine. He has been in full-time private practice with individuals, families, and children, with a focus on the adverse effects of psychiatric treatments and medical-legal issues. He is the founder and former director of the International Center for the Study of Psychiatry and Psychology, which publishes a peer-reviewed journal and a newsletter and holds national conferences. He is the author of many articles and books, including the most recent *The Ritalin Fact Book* and *The Antidepressant Fact Book*

101 E. State St., #112
Ithaca NY 14850
Tel: (607) 272-5328
www.breggin.com

JENNIFER BRETT, M.D., is a naturopathic doctor at the Wilton Naturopathic Center in Stratford, Connecticut.

998 Nichols Avenue
Stratford CT 06614
Tel: (203) 576-4122
herb-dr@msn.com

HAROLD BUTTRAM, M.D., specializes in family practice, environmental medicine, nutrition-based modalities, and the treatment of allergies.

5724 Clymer Road
Quakertown PA 18951
Tel: (215) 536-1890
www.woodmed.com

CHRISTOPHER CALAPAI, M.D., is an osteopathic physician board certified in family practice. He specializes in a variety of treatment modalities, including the use of intravenous vitamin therapy, chelation therapy, and reconstructive nerve therapy.

1900 Hempstead Turnpike
East Meadow NY 11554
Tel: (516) 794-0404
or
18 E. 53rd Street, 3rd Floor
New York NY 10022
Tel: (212) 838-9100
www.drcalapai.net

DR. PAULA CAPLAN, PH.D., is a Radcliffe-Harvard graduate and affiliated scholar at Brown University's Pembroke Center. She is the author of ten books, including *They Say You're Crazy: How the World's Most Powerful Psychiatrists Decide Who's Normal*; *Don't Blame Mother: Mending the Mother-Daughter Relationship*; and *The Myth of Women's Masochism*.

Pembroke Center
Brown University
Box 1958
Providence RI 02912
paulajcaplan.net

CATHERINE CARRIGAN, a graduate of Brown University, is the author of *Healing Depression: A Holistic Guide*. She has years of training and experience in fitness, nutrition, and healing.

1951 Northside Drive
Atlanta GA 30318
Tel: (404) 350-8581
catherine@totalfitness.net

HYLA CASS, M.D., is a holistic psychiatrist who integrates psychotherapy and nutritional medicine in her Santa Monica-based practice. In addition to being a media and corporate consultant, speaker, and seminar leader, she is an assistant clinical professor of psychiatry at UCLA School of Medicine.

2730 Wilshire Boulevard, #301
Santa Monica CA 90403
Tel: (310) 459-9866

www.cassmd.com

ALAN COHEN, M.D., graduated from SUNY Stonybrook School of Medicine, and is board-certified in family practice, acupuncture, and homeopathy. He has a private practice, where he treats entire families, from newborns to seniors, by integrating both conventional and alternative approaches. He is the author of *Misdiagnosis:A Physician's Triumph Over His Thirty-Year Battle With Depression.*

67 Cherry Street
Milford CT 06460
Tel: (203) 877-1936

TY COLBERT, PH.D., a licensed clinical psychologist, is the president of the Center for Psychological Alternatives to Biopsychiatry, a publishing and website venture for practitioners and patients looking for information and resources. He is an active member of the National Association for Rights, Protection and Advocacy and is on the advisory council for the Center for the Study of Psychiatry.

DrTy@2excel.net
Tyco33@aol.com

GABRIEL COUSENS, M.D., is a holistic medical doctor, psychiatrist, family therapist, and a licensed homeopathic physician in the state of Arizona. He is founder and director of the Tree of Life Foundation and Tree of Life Rejuvenation Center in Patagonia, Arizona.

Tree of Life Rejuvenation Center
686 Harshaw Road
Padagonia AZ 85624
Tel: (520) 394-2520
www.treeoflife.nu

WILLIAM CROOK, M.D., received his medical education and training at the University of Virginia, the Pennsylvania Hospital, Vanderbilt, and John Hopkins. He was the author of numerous articles in medical and lay literature and fourteen books. He passed away in 2002.

www.yeastconnection.com

DR. JOSEPH DEBE is a chiropractor with board certification in nutrition. He is a licensed dietitian-nutritionist, as well as a certified chiropractic sports practitioner.

North Shore Fitness
38 Great Neck Road
Great Neck NY 11021
Tel: (516) 829-1515
www.drdebe.com

JERRY DORSMAN is a certified addiction counselor working in Maryland.

P.O. Box 71
Elk Mills, MD 21920
Tel: (410) 392-9685
www.self-renewal.com

JOHN EADES holds a doctorate in counseling psychology and has worked for more than twenty years in hospital settings with alcohol- and drug-addicted people.

DR. SAMUEL DUNKELL is director of the Insomnia Medical Services in New York City, former director of Payne Whitney's Insomnia Clinic, and assistant professor of psychiatry at Cornell University Medical College.

1065 Lexington Avenue
New York NY 10021
Tel: (212) 628-2236

EVA EDELMAN, N.D., has worked for three decades in the field of natural health, specializing in mental health. She works as a nutritional consultant at SAFE, a drop-in center run by and for people with mental disorders.

3762 W. 11th Avenue
Eugene OR 97402
Tel: (541) 683-8720
edelman@boragebooks.com

LEANDER T. ELLIS, M.D., is a board-certified psychiatrist who has 30 years of experience studying the effect of allergies, infections, nutrition, and other physical factors on emotional conditions such as anxiety, depression, autism, and autoimmune diseases.

LYNNE FREEMAN, PH.D., has her doctorate in counseling and psychology and is the director of the Open Doors Institute in Los Angeles, California.

12932 La Maida Street
Sherman Oaks CA 91423
Tel: (818) 754-1575
opendoorsinstitute.com

KENDALL GERDES, M.D., is board certified in both internal medicine and allergy/immunology. He was an early student of Theron Randolph, the father of environmental medicine. Dr. Gerdes is a past president of the American Academy of Environmental Medicine. He has been in private practice since 1979.

1617 Vine Street
Denver CO 80206
Tel: (303) 377-8837

WILLIAM J. GOLDWAG, M.D., is the medical director of the Center for Preventive/Holistic Medicine in Southern California, and is on the board of directors of the American Holistic Medical Association. He has been one of the pioneers in the use of chelation therapy and other nutritional and complementary medical therapies for the treatment of chronic health disorders.

7499 Cerritos Avenue
Stanton CA 90680
Tel: (714) 827-5180

JAMES S. GORDON, M.D., a graduate of the Harvard Medical School, was a research psychiatrist at the National Institute of Mental Health for ten years. Founder and director of the Center for Mind-Body Medicine, he is also a clinical professor in the departments of psychiatry and family medicine at the Georgetown University School of Medicine. Dr. Gordon served as the first chairman of the Program Advisory Council of the National Institutes of Health's Office of Alternative Medicine. He integrates relaxation therapies, hypnosis, meditation, acupuncture, nutrition, herbalism, musculoskeletal manipulation, dance, yoga, and physical exercise in his own practice of medicine and psychiatry.

Center for Mind-Body Medicine
5225 Connecticut Avenue, NW, Suite 414
Washington DC 20015
Tel: (202) 966-7338
www.cmbm.org
www.jamesgordonmd.com

JAN GAGNON, M.D., is a naturopathic physician in Seattle, Washington. She spent many years working at the Tufts Mental Health Center in Massachusetts and the Virginia Mason Hospital in Seattle, and regularly integrates mind-body healing into her practice.

JANE GUILTINAN, N.D., studied naturopathic medicine at Bastyr University in Seattle, Washington. She is currently director of the Bastyr Center for Women's Wellness, clinical professor at Bastyr Center for Natural Health, member of the board of trustees at Harborview Medical Center and in private practice.

1307 North 45th Street, Suite 300
Seattle WA 98103

LETHA HADADY, D.AC., received her diplomate of Acupuncture from the Tri-State Institute for Traditional Chinese Medicine and also did special studies in China. Besides being in private practice for years, she also consults and holds rejuvenation workshops. She teaches doctors at the Botanical Medicine in Modern Clinical Practice Conference at Columbia's Rosenthal Center. She is adjunct faculty for the New York Botanical Garden.

PHILIP JAY HODES, ED.D., has spent three decades learning about holistic health, detoxification, and orthomolecular nutritional therapies. He is a researcher, writer, speaker, and educator, as well as a health care practitioner.

144 Keer Avenue
Newark NJ 07112

ABRAM HOFFER, M.D., PH.D., received his Ph.D. from the University of Minnesota and his M.D. from the University of Toronto. He was director of psychiatric research for the Province of Saskatchewan from 1950 to 1967. In private practice since 1967, specializing in the treatment of schizophrenia and cancer, he helped introduce orthomolecular medicine, in which vitamins are used as a primary treatment modality.

2727 Quadra Street, Suite 3-A
Victoria BC V8T 4E5 Canada
Tel: (250) 386-8756

DHARMA SINGH KHALSA, M.D., is a graduate of Creighton University of Medicine in Omaha, Nebraska, and was trained at the University of California and Harvard Medical School. Since 1981, he has been an American Sikh. He is the president and medical director of the Alzheimer's Research and Prevention Foundation, and was recently named associate fellow of the University of Pennsylvania Medical School, Center for Spirituality and the Mind.

6300 E. El Dorado Plaza, Suite 400
Tuscon AZ 85715
Tel: (520) 749-8374
www.drdharma.com

PARRIS KIDD, PH.D., is a nutrition educator and dietary supplement developer. He received his Ph.D. in cell biology from the University of California at Berkeley. Dr. Kidd is internationally recognized for his expertise in brain nutraceuticals.

www.dockidd.com

RICHARD A. KUNIN, M.D., is a founder and past president of the Orthomolecular Medical Society. He is in private practice, specializing in orthomolecular ecology medicine, in San Francisco.

2698 Pacific Avenue
San Francisco CA 94115
Tel: (415) 346-2500

STEPHEN LANGER, M.D., practices preventive medicine in Berkeley, California, specializing in the treatment of chronic fatigue, among other illnesses.

3031 Telegraph Avenue, #230
Berkeley CA 94705
Tel: (510) 548-7384

MICHAEL LAPCHICK is the author *of The Label Reader's Pocket Dictionary of Food Additives*. He is a Philadelphia-based health and nutrition writer.

Tel: (215) 533 0598

WARREN M. LEVIN, M.D., is an orthomolecular physician who is board certified in family practice, environmental medicine, and chelation therapy.

407 Church Street, NE, Suite E
Vienna VA 22180
Tel: (703) 255-0313
warrenmlevinmd.net

JOAN MATTHEWS-LARSON, PH.D., holds a doctorate in nutrition and is the founder and executive director of the Health Recovery Center in Minneapolis. She writes and speaks on psychobiological approaches to treating addiction.

www.healthrecovery.com

JAY LOMBARD, M.D., is clinical assistant professor of neurology at Cornell University Medical College. Board certified in neurology, he is in private practice in New York City. Dr. Lombard has published in several peer-reviewed journals and is the author of *The Brain Wellness Plan*.

Tel: (718) 597-6925

MICHAEL NORDEN, M.D., is a psychiatrist and clinical associate professor at the University of Washington.

JAMES PEARL, PH.D., is a member of the Sleep Panel at the Presbyterian St. Luke Medical Center in Denver, Colorado, and is in private practice as a psychologist.

DORIS J. RAPP, M.D., is a board-certified pediatric allergist and specialist in environmental medicine. She has written and presented her videos of children's responses to treatment to physicians and the public in many countries. Videotapes of patients' responses to treatment can be obtained by calling 1-800-787-8780.

1421 Colvin Boulevard
Buffalo NY 14223
Tel: (716) 875-0398
www.drrapp.com

JUDYTH REICHENBERG-ULLMAN is a board-certified diplomate of the Homeopathic Academy of Naturopathic Physicians. She is a graduate of Bastyr University in Seattle, Washington, and received her master's degree in psychiatric social work from the University of Washington. She has had more than two decades of clinical experience as a naturopathic and homeopathic physician.

The Northwest Center for Homeopathic Medicine
131 Third Avenue
N. Edmonds WA 98020
Tel: (425) 774-5599
www.healthyhomeopathy.com

JOEL ROBERTSON, M.D., is the director of the Robertson Research Institute, which provides neurochemical evaluations and treatment techniques.

www.robertsonresearchinstitute.org

SHERRY ROGERS, M.D., is a diplomate of the American Board of Family Practice, a fellow of the American College of Allergy and Immunology, and a diplomate of the American Academy of Environmental Medicine. She is the author of *Depression: Cured at Last* and other books on health.

Tel: (941) 349-7127

JUDITH SACHS has taught stress management at the College of New Jersey and conducts workshops on stress, mid-life, and menopause and sexuality, throughout the New York tristate area.

404 Burd Street
Pennington NJ 08534
Tel: (609) 737-8310

RAY SAHELIAN, M.D., obtained a B.Sc. in nutrition from Drexel University and completed his training at Thomas Jefferson Medical School, both in Philadelphia. He is certified by the American Board of Family Practice, and is the author of books on leading edge nutrients and hormones.

www.raysahelian.com

MICHAEL B. SCHACHTER, M.D., is a graduate of Columbia University's College of Physicians and Surgeons and a board-certified psychiatrist. He has been practicing orthomolecular medicine and psychiatry since 1974. Dr. Schachter directs a health care facility in Suffern, New York, using nutritional medicine, chelation therapy, homeopathy, and other complementary treatment methods.

2 Executive Boulevard, Suite 202
Suffern NY 10901
Tel: (845) 368-4700
www.mbschachter.com

ALEXANDER SCHAUSS, PH.D., is a research psychologist and mental health therapist, and holds associate professorships at colleges of naturopathic medicine in Oregon and Arizona. He is the research director of the life sciences division at the American Institute for Biosocial Research, and is the author of *The Health Benefits of Cat's Claw: Its Role in Treating Cancer, Arthritis, Prostate Problems, Asthma, and Many Other Chronic Conditions.*

Tel: (206) 922-0448

PRISCILLA ANNE SLAGLE, M.D., has a private practice in Palm Springs, California. Specializing in nutritional medicine and psychiatry, she treats most illnesses from the perspective of diet change, nutritional supplementation, and natural hormones as needed.

Tel: (800) 289-8497
www.theweayup.com

LENDON H. SMITH, M.D., a graduate of the University of Oregon Medical School, specialized in nutrition-based therapies since 1975. He passed away in 2001.

ALLAN N. SPREEN, M.D., is a general practitioner in Jacksonville, Florida, with a specialization in nutrition-based medicine.

WALT STOLL, M.D., A.B.F.P., is a board-certified family practitioner with more than thirty years of experience, the last seventeen of which were spent as a holistic physician. During those seventeen years he has combined his traditional Western (allopathic) training with fifteen other healing philosophies, practiced by trained professionals in his Holistic Medical Centre in Lexington, Kentucky. On November 17, 1994, after fourteen years of harassment by the Kentucky Medical Licensing Board, his license to practice medicine was revoked.

415 South Bonita Avenue
Panama City FL 32401-3963
Tel: (850) 747-8669
www.askwaltstollmd.com

RICARDO B. TAN, M.D., practices holistic and preventive medicine, including nutrition-based modalities, chelation therapy, acupuncture, sclerotherapy, and homeopathy.

3220 North Freeway
Fort Worth TX 76111
Tel: (817) 626-1993

JACOB TEITELBAUM, M.D., is the author of *From Fatigued to Fantastic*. He received his medical degree at Ohio State University, where he lost a year when he contracted chronic fatigue syndrome. He has spent many years working with chronic fatigue and fibromyalgia patients.

66 Forelands Road
Annapolis MD 21401
Tel: (410) 573-5389
www.vitality101.com

LINDA TOTH, PH.D., received a doctorate in communications from UCLA. She is a senior staff writer for the *Journal of Longevity Research* and the author of *Why Can't I Remember?*

Tel: (310) 475-3139

JOSEPH TRACHTMAN, M.D., received his doctorate of optometry degree from Pennsylvania College of Optometry, a masters in education from Johns Hopkins University, and a masters in vision science from State University in New York. He also has a Ph.D. in experimental psychology from Yeshiva University. During the past twenty-five years, Dr. Trachtman has developed instruments and computer software to improve vision disorders using biofeedback techniques.

Tel: (718) 852-0625

GARRY M. VICKAR, M.D., F.R.C.P. (C.), is a psychiatrist who specializes in acutely ill patients. With an active full-time private practice, Dr. Vickar is board certified by the Royal College of Physicians and Surgeons of Canada and the American Board of Psychiatry and Neurology. He is the chairman of the department of psychiatry at Christian Hospital Northeast, where he is the medical director of the schizophrenia treatment and education programs. He is a fellow of the American Psychiatric Association.

1245 Graham Road, Suite 506
St. Louis MO 63031
Tel: (314) 837-4900

BRUCE WEISMAN, national president of the Citizens' Commission on Human Rights, holds a graduate degree from California State University, San Jose. A former chairman of the department of history at John F. Kennedy University, he has been a human rights advocate and an outspoken critic of damaging psychiatric abuses for more than twenty-five years.

Citizens Committee on Human Rights
6362 Hollywood Boulevard, Suite B
Los Angeles CA 90028
Tel: (727) 723-2176

AUBREY M. WORRELL, JR., M.D., is a board-certified allergist/immunologist with special interests in clinical ecology, environmental medicine, and nutrition.

RAY C. WUNDERLICH, JR., M.D., is a graduate of Columbia University's College of Physicians and Surgeons. He practices nutritional and preventive medicine.

8821 MLK Street North
St. Petersburg FL
Tel: (727) 822-3612

JOSÉ A. YARYURA-TOBIAS, M.D., is the medical director at the Institute for Bio-Behavioral Therapy and Research. He has worked extensively on OCD and schizophrenia, and is a visiting professor at the University of Cuyo in Argentina.

935 Northern Boulevard
Great Neck NY 11021
Tel: (516) 487-7116

ALFRED V. ZAMM, M.D., is a diplomate of both the American Board of Dermatology and the American Board of Environmental Medicine. In addition to his private practice based in Kingston, New York, he is a consultant to five hospitals in the Hudson Valley.

111 Maiden Lane
Kingston NY 12401-4597
Tel: (914) 338-7766

MARCIA ZIMMERMAN is a certified nutritionist, specializing in ADHD. She has been in practice for twenty-five years.

Appendix B

Clinical Studies

■■■

Scientific Article Summaries, by Subject

The following are capsule descriptions of just some of the recent scientific articles that demonstrate the connection between nutritional factors and mental illness. The articles are from respected peer-reviewed journals. Physicians reading this book will want to use this appendix as a resource guide. It will lead them to the original scientific research, which in turn will bolster and substantiate the ideas and clinical strategies expounded in this book. I encourage you to follow this lead and request reprints of individual articles that address your area of specialization directly from the medical journals themselves. You may find yourself more open to the practice of orthomolecular psychiatry than you ever expected. For the general reader, you too will find that just reading the short summaries of some of the articles listed below will help strengthen your resolve. There is solid medical research to support many of the claims our contributing physicians have made throughout this book.

Addictions

Effects of Melatonin on Oxidative Stress and Spatial Memory Impairment Induced by Acute Ethanol Treatment in Rats. Gönenç S; Uysal N; et al. *Physiological Research*, 2005, 54(3):341-348.

The researchers determined that melatonin influences ethanol-induced oxidative stress and spatial memory impairment.

■■■

Review Article: Nutritional Therapy in Alcoholic Liver Disease. Stickel F; Hoehn B; et al. *Alimentary Pharmacology & Therapeutics*, 2003 August 15, 18(4):357-373.

Among the nutritional therapies that benefit alcoholic patients are thiamine and folate supplements, branched-chain amino acids, metadoxine and S-adenosyl-L-methionine (SAMe).

■■■

S-Adenosyl-L-Methionine: Its Role in the Treatment of Liver Disorders. Lieber CS. *American Journal of Clinical Nutrition*, 2002 November, 76(5):1183S-1187S.

S-Adenosyl-L-methionine (SAMe), a supernutrient that helps protect the liver, acts as a precursor for cysteine, and opposes the toxicity of free radicals generated by alcohol and other pathogens that cause oxidative stress.

■ ■ ■

S-Adenosyl-L-Methionine and Alcoholic Liver Disease in Animal Models: Implications for Early Intervention in Human Beings. Lieber CS. *Alcohol*, 2002 July, 27(3):173-177.

Using animal models, the researchers determined that S-Adenosyl-L-methionine (SAMe) is depleted considerably in the early development of alcoholic liver disease, and that supplementation with the nutrient can be used to treat associated liver lesions and mitochondrial injury.

■ ■ ■

Effect of Ethanol on Brain Metallothionein in Transgenic Mice. Suzuki Y; Cherian MG. *Alcoholism: Clinical and Experimental Research*, 2000 March, 24(3):315-321.

Free radical generation is believed to cause cell injury following ethanol administration. Metallothionein may be linked with oxidative stress and can protect against ethanol toxicity.

■ ■ ■

The Use of an Infusion of St. John's Wort in the Combined Treatment of Alcoholics with Peptic Ulcer and Chronic Gastritis. Krylov AA; Ibatov AN. *Vrach Delo*, 1993 February-March, (2-3):146-148.

In this study, hypericum herbal infusion was used in combination with psychotherapy in 57 outpatients with alcoholism and concomitant diseases of digestive organs. Results indicated that two months of daily intake proved to be effective.

■■■

Vitamin A Status of Alcoholics Upon Admission and After Two Weeks of Hospitalization. Chapman KM; Prabhudesai M; Erdman JW Jr. *Journal of the American College of Nutrition*, 1993 February, 12(1):77-83.

Elevated bilirubin levels seen in alcoholics may indicate low vitamin A levels. Caution in levels of vitamin A therapy in these cases is advised, and consideration should instead be given to beta-carotene supplementation.

Aggression

Improved Mood and Behavior During Treatment With a Mineral-Vitamin Supplement: An Open-Label Case Series of Children. Kaplan BJ; Fisher JE; et al. *Journal of Child and Adolescent Psychopharmacology*, 2004 Spring, 14(1):115-122.

A nutrient supplement was found to be effective in children with aggression, depression and mood swings.

■■■

Treatment of Mood Lability and Explosive Rage with Minerals and Vitamins: Two Case Studies in Children. Kaplan BJ; Crawford SG. *Journal of Child and Adolescent Psychopharmacology* 2002 Fall, 12(3):205-219.

Two nonmedicated boys with mood lability and explosive rage demonstrated reduced symptoms while taking a micronutrient supplement. When the nutrient was stopped temporarily, the symptoms returned. Both boys were followed and determined to be stable on the medication for more than two years.

■■■

Laboratory-measured Aggressive Behavior of Women: Acute Tryptophan Depletion and Augmentation. Marsh DM; Dougherty DM; et al. *Neuropsychopharmacology*, 2002 May, 26(5):660-671.

This study assessed laboratory-induced aggression in 12 women. The researchers determined that plasma L-tryptophan can influence aggressive behavior, and that certain women may be more vulnerable to serotonin manipulation.

■■■

Tryptophan Depletion Increases Aggression in Women During the Premenstrual Phase. Bond AJ; Wingrove J; et al. *Psychopharmacology*. 2001 August, 156(4):477-480.

Healthy women received an amino acid drink either depleted or with a balanced amount of tryptophan. Those who had the depleted drink showed more aggression in response to provocation.

■■■

The Effect of Vitamin-Mineral Supplementation on Juvenile Delinquency Among American Schoolchildren: A Randomized, Double-Blind Placebo-Controlled Trial. Schoenthaler SJ; Bier ID. *Journal of Alternative and Complementary Medicine*, 2000 February, 6(1):7-17.

According to this study, adequate nutrition lowers institutional violence and antisocial behavior by almost half.

■■■

Differential Behavioral Effects of Plasma Tryptophan Depletion and Loading in Aggressive and Nonaggressive Men. Bjork JM; Dougherty DM; et al. *Neuropsychopharmacology*, 2000 April, 22(4):357-369.

The findings from this study correlate with previous data indicating that men who are aggressive may be affected by alterations in plasma tryptophan.

Alzheimer's Disease

The Spice Sage and its Active Ingredient Rosmarinic Acid Protect PC12 Cells From Amyloid-Beta Peptide-Induced Neurotoxicity. Iuvone T; De Filippis D; et al. *Journal of Pharmacology and Experimental Therapeutics*, 2006 June, 317(3):1143-1149.

A standardized extract from the culinary herb sage and its active ingredient rosmarinic acid provided protection against Alzheimer amyloid-beta peptide (Abeta)-induced toxicity in cultured rat cells.

■ ■ ■

Neuroprotective Effects of Green and Black Teas and Their Catechin Gallate Esters Against Beta-Amyloid-Induced Toxicity. Bastianetto S; Yao ZX; et al. *European Journal of Neuroscience*, 2006 January, 23(1):55-64.

The findings support the hypothesis that black as well as green teas may be beneficial against Alzheimer's disease and other age-related neurodegenerative conditions.

■ ■ ■

Carnosine and Carnosine-related Antioxidants: A Review. Guiotto A; Calderan A; et al. *Current Medicinal Chemistry*, 2005, 12(20):2293-2315.

Recent studies have revealed that the naturally occurring dipeptide carnosine can act against neurodegenerative disorders such as Alzheimer's disease, cardiovascular ischemic damage and inflammatory diseases.

■ ■ ■

Curcumin Inhibits Formation of Amyloid Beta Oligomers and Fibrils, Binds Plaques and Reduces Amyloid In Vivo. Yang F; et al. *Journal of Biological Chemistry*. 2005 February, 280:5892-5901.

Curcumin, the yellow curry pigment, has antiinflammatory and antioxidant properties, and can protect against oxidative damage, inflammation, cognitive deficits and amyloid accumulation. Results from this study support the use of curcumin in clinical trials aimed at preventing or treating Alzheimer's disease.

■ ■ ■

Relation of the Tocopherol Forms to Incident Alzheimer Disease and to Cognitive Change. Morris, MC; et al. *American Journal of Clinical Nutrition*, 2005 February, 81(2): 508-514.

Various forms of tocopherol (vitamin E) may yield protective benefits in people with Alzheimer's disease.

■ ■ ■

Pharmacotherapeutic Approaches to the Prevention of Alzheimer's Disease. *American Journal of Geriatric Pharmacotherapy*, 2004 June, 2(2):119-132.

Preventive interventions for Alzheimer's disease include vitamins, nonsteroidal anti-inflammatory drugs and agents that protect the endothelium.

■ ■ ■

Alzheimer's Disease, Oxidative Injury, and Cytokines. Summers WK. *Journal of Alzheimer's Disease*, 2004 December, 6(6):651-657.

Antioxidant therapy plays an important role in the prevention or reversal of Alzheimer's disease.

■ ■ ■

Docosahexaenoic Acid Protects from Dendritic Pathology in an Alzheimer's Disease Mouse Model. Calon F; et al. *Neuron*, 2004 September 2, 43(5):633-

6   4   5   .

This study demonstrated the positive effects of docosahexaenoic acid (DHA), an essential omega-3 polyunsaturated fatty acid, in treatment of mice with neurodegenerative diseases.

■■■

Pharmacological Studies Supporting the Therapeutic Use of Ginkgo Biloba Extract for Alzheimer's Disease. Ahlemeyer B; Krieglstein J. *Pharmacopsychiatry*, 2003 June, 36 (Suppl. 1):S8-S14.

The researchers cited experimental evidence for a neuroprotective effect of ginkgo biloba extract in patients with mild and moderate Alzheimer's disease.

■■■

Clinical Efficacy and Safety of Huperzine Alpha in Treatment of Mild to Moderate Alzheimer Disease, A Placebo-Controlled, Double-Blind, Randomized Trial. Zang Z; et al. *Zhonghua Yi Xue Za Zhi.* 2002 July 25, 82(14):941-944.

This study of 202 patients concluded that huperzine alpha is a safe and effective treatment that "remarkably improves" the behavior, mood and cognitive status of people with mild to moderate Alzheimer's disease.

■■■

Neuroprotective Effect of Garlic Compounds in Amyloid-Beta Peptide-Induced Apoptosis in Vitro. Peng Q; Buz'Zard AR; et al. *Medical Science Monitor*, 2002 August, 8(8):BR328-BR337.

The researchers found beneficial effects of aged garlic extract (AGE) and S-allyl cysteine (SAC) on Abeta-induced apoptosis and reactive oxygen species (ROS) generation in a rat cell line.

■■■

The Green Tea Polyphenol (-)-Epigallocatechin Gallate Attenuates Beta-Amyloid-Induced Neurotoxicity in Cultured Hippocampal Neurons. Choi YT; Jung CH. *Life Sciences*, 2001 December, 21:70(5):603-614.

Green tea polyphenols have protective effects against betaA-induced neuronal apoptosis, which may be beneficial for the prevention of Alzheimer's disease.

■■■

Oxidative Stress and Alzheimer Disease. *American Journal of Clinical Nutrition*, 2000, 71(2):621S-629S.

Among the substances that have demonstrated anti-Alzheimer effects are free vitamin E, deprenyl, ginkgo biloba extract, desferrioxamine (an iron-chelating agent) and estrogens.

■■■

Vitamin E and Alzheimer Disease. *American Journal Of Clinical Nutrition*, 2000, 71(2): 630S-636S.

Vitamin E administered in doses of 2000 IU/day may slow the rate of functional deterioration in patients with moderately advanced Alzheimer's disease.

■■■

Serum Dehydroepiandrosterone (DHEA) and DHEA-sulfate (DHEA-S) in Alzheimer's Disease and in Cerebrovascular Dementia. Yanase T; et al. *Endocrinology Journal*, 1996 February, 43(1):119-123.

Results of this study found significantly lower levels of serum DHEA-S in elderly Japanese patients suffering from Alzheimer's and/or cerebrovascular dementia relative to age-matched healthy controls.

■■■

Clinical and Neurochemical Effects of Acetyl-L-carnitine in Alzheimer's Disease. Pettegrew JW; et al. *Neurobiology of Aging*, 1995 January-February, 16(1):1-4.

Results of this double-bind, placebo-controlled study found that patients treated with acetyl-L-carnitine experienced significantly less deterioration in mental status than controls.

Anxiety Disorders

Long-term Goals in the Management of Acute and Chronic Anxiety Disorder. Kjernisted KD; Bleau P. *Canadian Journal of Psychiatry*, 2004 March, 49(3 Suppl. 1):51S-63S.

This article describes, among other things, the significant benefits of cognitive-behavioral therapy in the management of anxiety disorders.

■■■

Kava Treatment in Patients with Anxiety. Geier FP; Konstantinowicz T. *Phytotherapy Research*, 2004 April,18(4):297-300.

This placebo-controlled double-blind study was designed to examine the dosage range and efficacy of kava special extract WS 1490 in patients with nonpsychotic anxiety. Results indicated that 150 mg per day was well tolerated with no adverse effects.

■■■

Kava-Kava Extract LI 150 is As Effective As Opipramol and Buspirone in Generalised Anxiety Disorder—An 8-week Randomized, Double-blind Multi-centre Clinical Trial in 129 Out-patients. Boerner RJ; Sommer H; et al. *Phytomedicine*, 2003, 10 (Suppl. 4):38-49.

This double-blind study determined that kava-kava extract LI 150 is well tolerated and as effective as psychopharmaceuticals in the acute treatment of generalized anxiety disorder.

■■■

Double-blind, Controlled, Crossover Trial of Inositol Versus Fluvoxamine for the Treatment of Panic Disorder. Palatnik A; Frolov K; et al. *Journal of Clinical Psychopharmacology*, 2001 June, 21(3):335-339.

Patients receiving inositol experienced a reduction in the number of panic attacks per week by 4.0, compared with a reduction of 2.4 in patients who took fluvoxamine.

■■■

The Influence of Phosphatidylserine Supplementation on Mood and Heart Rate When Faced with an Acute Stressor. Benton D; et al. *Nutritional Neuroscience*, 2001, 4(3):169-178.

Young, healthy adults with higher than average neuroticism scores reported feeling less stressed when asked to perform a difficult mental arithmetic task after taking 300 mg of phosphatidylserine daily.

■■■

Kava Extract for Anxiety. *Journal of Clinical Psychopharmacology*, 2000, 20:1, 84-89.

A literature review and expert analysis revealed that kava extract is superior to placebo as a symptomatic treatment for anxiety.

■■■

Inositol Treatment of Obsessive-Compulsive Disorder. Fux M; et al. *American Journal of Psychiatry*, 1996 September, 153(9):1219-21.

Results of this double-blind, placebo-controlled, crossover study found that the administration of 18 g per day of inositol for six weeks had significant beneficial effects in patients suffering from obsessive compulsive disorder.

■ ■ ■

Stress-induced 5-HT1A Receptor Desensitization: Protective Effects of Ginkgo Biloba Extract (EGB 761). Bolanos-Jimenez F; et al. *Fundamentals of Clinical Pharmacology*, 1995, 9(2):169-174.

This study examined the effects of subchronic cold stress on hippocampal 5-HT1A receptors functioning and potential protective effects of ginkgo biloba extract in old isolated rats. Results showed that the extract prevented the stress-induced desensitization of 5-HT1A.

■ ■ ■

Double-blind, Placebo-controlled, Crossover Trial of Inositol Treatment for Panic Disorder. Benjamin J; et al. *American Journal of Psychiatry*, 1995 July, 152(7):1084-1086.

In this double-blind, placebo-controlled study, panic disorder patients with or without agoraphobia received 12 g of inositol per day. Results showed a significant decline in the frequency and severity of panic attacks and agoraphobia relative to controls.

Attention Deficit Hyperactivity Disorder (ADHD)

Omega-3 Fatty Acids in ADHD and Related Neurodevelopmental Disorders. Richardson AJ. *International Review of Psychiatry*, 2006 April, 18(2):155-172.

This review article explores the role of omega-3s in complementing conventional treatments for ADHD, as well as dyslexia, developmental coordination disorder (DCD) and autism. The authors report that dietary supplementation with fish oils may reduce ADHD-related symptoms in some children.

■ ■ ■

Double-blind, Placebo-Controlled Study of Zinc Sulfate in the Treatment of Attention Deficit Hyperactivity Disorder. Bilici M; Yildirim F; et al. *Progress in Neuro-Psychopharmacology & Biological Psychiatry*, 2004 January, 28(1):181-190.

In patients with ADHD, zinc proved to be more effective than placebo in reducing symptoms of hyperactivity, impulsivity and impaired socialization.

■ ■ ■

The Effects of a Double Blind, Placebo Controlled, Artificial Food Colourings and Benzoate Preservative Challenge on Hyperactivity in a General Population Sample of Preschool Children. Bateman B; Warner JO; et al. *Archive of Diseases in Childhood*, 2004 June, 89(6):506-511.

This sample of 1873 children revealed that artificial food coloring and benzoate preservatives adversely affect the behavior of 3 year olds according to parent reports but not a simple clinic assessment.

■ ■ ■

EFA Supplementation in Children with Inattention, Hyperactivity, and Other Disruptive Behaviors. Stevens L,; Zhang W; et al. *Lipids*, 2003 October, 38(10):1007-1021.

This pilot study suggests that EFA supplements may be beneficial in children with behavioral disorders.

■ ■ ■

Does Zinc Moderate Essential Fatty Acid and Amphetamine Treatment of Attention-Deficit/Hyperactivity Disorder? Arnold LE; Pinkham SM; et al. *Journal of Child and Adolescent Psychopharmacology*, 2000 Summer, 10(2):111-117.

Zinc nutrition may be important for treatment of ADHD even in those treated with pharmacotherapy.

■ ■ ■

The Potential Role of Fatty Acids in Attention-Deficit/Hyperactivity Disorder. Richardson AJ; Puri BK. *Prostaglandins Leukotrienes and Essential Fatty Acids.* 2000 July-August, 63(1-2):79-87.

The authors contend that a functional deficiency of certain long-chain polyunsaturated fatty acids may contribute to ADHD. They propose a treatment protocol with this in mind.

Autism Spectrum Disorders

Children with Autism: Effect of Iron Supplementation on Sleep and Ferritin. Dosman CF; Brian JA; et al. *Pediatric Neurology*, 2007 March, 36(3):152-158.

An 8-week open-label trial with oral iron supplementation was conducted to assess the link between low serum ferritin and sleep disturbance in children with autism spectrum disorder. Iron therapy was associated with considerable reduction in restless sleep.

■ ■ ■

Improvement of Neurobehavioral Disorders in Children Supplemented with Magnesium Vitamin B6. II. Pervasive Developmental Disorder-Autism. Mousain-Bosc M; Roche M; et al. *Magnesium Research*, 2006 March, 19(1):53-62.

This study concluded that behavioral improvement was achieved in PDD-Autism with the combination vitamin B6-magnesium.

■ ■ ■

Magnesium Profile in Autism. Strambi M; Longini M; et al. *Biological Trace Element Research*, 2006 February, 109(2):97-104.

The researchers found that children with autistic spectrum disorders had lower plasma concentrations of magnesium than normal subjects, leading them to conclude that dietary management is crucial.

■■■

Developmental Neurotoxicity of Industrial Chemicals. Grandjean, P; Landrigan, PJ. *The Lancet*, 2006, 368:2167-2178

Autism and other neurodevelopmental disorders may be caused by exposure to industrial chemicals such as lead, methylmercury, polychlorinated biphenyls, arsenic and toluene. An additional 200 chemicals are known to have adverse neurological effects in adults. The authors state that new approaches for testing and control of chemicals that take into account the developing brain are needed.

■■■

Pilot Study of a Moderate Dose Multivitamin/Mineral Supplement for Children with Autistic Spectrum Disorder. Adams JB; Holloway C. *Journal of Alternative and Complementary Medicine*, 2004 December, 10(6):1033-1039.

The results of this study may explain the functional need for high-dose vitamin B6 supplementation in people with autism.

■■■

Effects of Tryptophan Depletion in Drug-Free Adults with Autistic Disorder. McDougle CJ; Naylor ST; et al. *Archive of General Psychiatry*, 1996 November, 53(11):993-1000.

Results from this double-blind, placebo-controlled study indicated that short-term reduction of serotonin precursor availability may worsen some symptoms of autism.

■■■

Vitamin B6 Versus Fenfluramine: A Case-study in Medical Bias. Rimland B. *Journal of Nutrition and Medicine*, 1991, 2(3):321-322.

Vitamin B6 and magnesium—as opposed to the drug fenfluramine—constitute the first-choice treatment in the treatment of autistic children and adults.

Behavioral and Learning Disorders

Maternal Consumption of a Docosahexaenoic Acid-Containing Functional Food During Pregnancy: Benefit for Infant Performance on Problem-Solving but not on Recognition Memory Tasks at Age 9 Months. Judge MP; Harel O; et al. *American Journal of Clinical Nutrition*, 2007 June, 85(6):1572-1577.

Infants whose mothers consumed a DHA-containing functional food during pregnancy were found at age 9 months to have advantages in problem solving but not recognition memory.

■■■

Effects of N-3 Long Chain Polyunsaturated Fatty Acid Supplementation on Visual and Cognitive Development Throughout Childhood: A Review of Human Studies. Eilander A; Hundscheid DC; et al. *Prostaglandins, Leukotrines & Essential Fatty Acids*. 2007 April, 76(4):189-203.

The researchers detected cognitive benefits to infants and children from maternal n-3 long chain polyunsaturated fatty acid supplementation during pregnancy and lactation.

■■■

Melatonin Improves Learning and Memory Performances Impaired by Hyperhomocysteinemia in Rats. Baydas G; Ozer M; et al. *Brain Research*, 2005 June 7, 1046(1-2):187-194.

Homocysteine causes behavioral deficits, and melatonin may protect against homocysteine toxicity.

■ ■ ■

The Effect of Vitamin-Mineral Supplementation on the Intelligence of American Schoolchildren: A Randomized, Double-Blind Placebo-Controlled Trial. Schoenthaler SJ; Bier ID; et al. *Journal of Alternative and Complementary Medicine*, 2000 February, 6(1):19-29.

Vitamin-mineral supplementation significantly increased the nonverbal intelligence of a minority of American schoolchildren. Parents of children with low academic performance should obtain a full nutritional assessment.

■ ■ ■

Randomized Study of Cognitive Effects of Iron Supplementation in Non-anaemic Iron-deficient Adolescent Girls. Bruner AB; et al. *Lancet*, 1996 October 12, 348(9033):992-996.

This double-blind, placebo-controlled study examined the effects of 13 mg per day of supplemental iron for 8 weeks on cognitive function in adolescent girls with non-anemic iron deficiency. Results showed that girls receiving iron scored higher on verbal learning and memory tests relative to controls.

■ ■ ■

Aged Garlic Extract Prolongs Longevity and Improves Spatial Memory Deficit in Senescence-Accelerated Mouse. Moriguchi T; et al. *Biological and Pharmaceutical Bulletin*, 1996 February, 19(2):305-307.

Results of this study showed that the chronic dietary administration of aged garlic extract improved spatial learning in senescence-accelerated mice.

■ ■ ■

Ginseng Root Prevents Learning Disability and Neuronal Loss in Gerbils with 5-minute Forebrain Ischemia. Wen TC; et al. *Acta Neuropathologica*, 1996, 91(1):15-22.

This study examined the neuroprotective effects of ginseng roots in 5-minute ischemic gerbils. Red ginseng powder, crude ginseng saponin, crude ginseng non-saponin, and pure ginsenosides Rb1, Rg1 and Ro were administered 7 days prior to ischemia. Results showed that red ginseng and crude ginseng saponin prevented delayed neuronal death.

■■■

An Herbal Prescription, S-113m, Consisting of Biota, Ginseng, and Schizandra, Improves Learning Performance in Senescence Accelerated Mouse. Nishiyama N; et al. *Biological and Pharmaceutical Bulletin*, 1996 March, 19(3):388-393.

Ginseng containing herbal prescription improved memory retention disorder in the senescence accelerated mouse on a passive avoidance test and increased conditioned avoidance rate in a lever press test.

■■■

Panax Ginseng Extract Improves the Performance of Aged Fischer 344 Rats in Radial Maze Task but Not in Operant Brightness Discrimination Task. Nitta H; et al. *Biological and Pharmaceutical Bulletin*, 1995 September, 18(9):1286-1288.

Administration of 8g/kg per day of a Panax ginseng extract over a period of 12 to 33 days reduced impairment of learning performance on a radial maze task in rats.

■■■

Effects of Chinese Ginseng Root and Stem-leaf Saponins on Learning, Memory, and Biogenic Monoamines of Brain in Rats. Wang A; et al. *Chung Kuo Chung Yao Tsa Chih*, 1995 August, 20(8):493-495.

This study found that 50 mg/kg x 7d of ginseng root saponins enhanced the memory and learning of male rats. The same dosage of ginseng stem-leaf saponins had even stronger effects on antielectroconvulsive shock-induced memory impairment.

Bipolar Disorder

Pronounced Cognitive Deficits Following an Intravenous L-Tryptophan Challenge in First-Degree Relatives of Bipolar Patients Compared to Healthy Controls. Sobczak S; Honig; et al. *Neuropharmacology*, 2003 April, 28(4):711-719.

The researchers investigated the effects of an intravenous tryptophan challenge and placebo on cognitive performance in 30 healthy first-degree relatives of bipolar patients.

■ ■ ■

Effects of a Branched-Chain Amino Acid Drink in Mania. Scarna A; Gijsman HJ; et al. *British Journal of Psychiatry*, 2003 March,182:210-213.

The researchers found that administration of a complex tyrosine-free amino acid drink led to a reduction in manic symptoms.

■ ■ ■

Effects of Acute Tryptophan Depletion on Mood and Cortisol Release in First-Degree Relatives of Type I and Type II Bipolar Patients and Healthy Matched Controls. Sobczak S; Honig A; et al. *Neuropsychopharmacology*, 2002 November, 27(5):834-842.

The researchers investigated the effects of acute tryptophan depletion in healthy first-degree relatives of bipolar patients, and determined that serotonergic vulnerability affected mood and cortisol release.

■ ■ ■

Cognition Following Acute Tryptophan Depletion: Difference Between First-Degree Relatives of Bipolar Disorder Patients and Matched Healthy Control Volunteers. Sobczak S; Riedel WJ; et al. *Psychological Medicine*, 2002 April, 32(3):503-515.

This study analyzed the effects of acute tryptophan depletion on cognition in healthy first-degree relatives of bipolar patients, and determined that serotonin may be involved in speed of information processing, verbal and visual memory, and learning processes.

■■■

Antidopaminergic Effects of Dietary Tyrosine Depletion in Healthy Subjects and Patients with Manic Illness. McTavish SF; McPherson MH; et al. *British Journal of Psychiatry*, 2001 October,179:356-360.

Tyrosine depletion causes adverse increases in dopamine neurotransmission following methamphetamine administration in patients with mania.

■■■

Effective Mood Stabilization with a Chelated Mineral Supplement: An Open-label Trial in Bipolar Disorder. Kaplan BJ; et al. *Journal of Clinical Psychiatry*, 2001, 62:936-944.

The purpose of this study was to ascertain the benefits of a nutritional supplement for bipolar disorder. Eleven participants aged 19 to 46 years with a diagnosis of bipolar disorder received high doses of a broad-based supplement of dietary nutrients, primarily chelated trace minerals and vitamins. After six months, symptom reduction ranged from 55 percent to 66 percent, and the need for psychotropic medications decreased by more than 50 percent.

Brain Aging

The Effects and Mechanisms of Mitochondrial Nutrient Alpha-Lipoic Acid on Improving Age-Associated Mitochondrial and Cognitive Dysfunction: An Overview. Liu J. *Neurochemical Research*, 2007 June 29.

Alpha-lipoic acid in combination with other mitochondrial nutrients such as acetyl-L-carnitine and coenzyme Q10 has been shown to improve mitochondrial and cognitive decline in older adults.

■ ■ ■

Long-term Effects of Cognitive Training on Everyday Functional Outcomes in Older Adults Willis, SJ; et al. *Journal of the American Medical Association*, 2006, 296:2805-2814.

This large study concluded that cognitive training resulted in improved cognitive abilities in elderly patients.

■ ■ ■

Coenzyme Q10 Modulates Cognitive Impairment Against Intracerebroventricular Injection of Streptozotocin in Rats. Ishrat T; Khan MB; et al. *Behavioural Brain Research*, 2006 July 15, 71(1):9-16.

Results indicated that coenzyme Q10 (CoQ10) study has a neuroprotective effect against cognitive impairments and oxidative damage in the hippocampus and cerebral cortex of rats infused with streptozotocin.

■ ■ ■

The Psychopharmacology of European Herbs with Cognition-Enhancing Properties. Kennedy DO; Scholey AB. *Current Pharmaceutical Design*, 2006,12(35):4613-4623.

Among the plant-derived and traditional herbal remedies that have been deemed effective against cognitive decline are ginkgo biloba, sage and lemon balm, all of which are described in this article.

■ ■ ■

Concurrent Administration of Coenzyme Q10 and Alpha-Tocopherol Improves Learning in Aged Mice. McDonald SR; Sohal RS; et al. Forster MJ. *Free Radical Biology & Medicine*, 2005 March 15, 38(6):729-736.

Administering alpha-tocopherol and coenzyme Q10 (CoQ10) simultaneously appears to be more beneficial against age-related learning difficulties than administration of either substance alone.

■ ■ ■

Roles of Unsaturated Fatty Acids (Especially Omega-3 Fatty Acids) in the Brain at Various Ages and During Ageing. Bourre JM. *Journal of Nutrition, Health & Aging*, 2004, 8(3):163-174.

This article describes the fatty acids that are essential for brain functioning, as well as the consequences of deficiency on brain aging.

■ ■ ■

Effect of Alpha Lipoic Acid on Intracerebroventricular Streptozotocin Model of Cognitive Impairment in Rats. Sharma M; Gupta YK. *European Neuropsychopharmacology*, 2003 August, 13(4):241-247.

This study concluded that alpha lipoic acid in effective in preventing cognitive impairment and oxidative stress.

■ ■ ■

Ginkgo Biloba Extract Egb 761 in Dementia: Intent-To-Treat Analyses of a 24-Week, Multi-Center, Double-Blind, Placebo-Controlled, Randomized Trial. Kanowski S; Hoerr R. *Pharmacopsychiatry*, 2003 November, 36(6):297-303.

This study corroborated previous findings that ginkgo biloba extract EGb 761 improves cognitive function in patients with dementia.

■■■

Natural Extracts as Possible Protective Agents of Brain Aging. Bastianetto S; Quirion R. *Neurobiology of Aging*, 2002 September-October, 23(5):891-897.

The findings suggested that ginkgo biloba extract EGb 761 and red wine-derived constituents may protect against cell death produced by beta-amyloid (Abeta) peptides and oxidative stress.

■■■

Oral Administration of Soybean Lecithin Transphosphatidylated Phosphatidylserine Improves Memory Impairment in Aged Rats. Suzuki S, et al. *Journal of Nutrition*, 2001 November, 131(11):2951-2956.

This study found that phosphatidylserine significantly improved a rat's ability to escape a water maze. It also increased acetylcholine release and synaptic activity.

■■■

An Open Trial of Plant-Source Derived Phosphatidylserine for Treatment of Age-Related Cognitive Decline. Schreiber S, et al. *Israel Journal of Psychiatry and Related Sciences*, 2000, 37(4):302-307.

In this study of 15 healthy older adults with age-related memory impairment, the authors determined that 300 milligrams per day of plant-source derived phosphatidylserine improved memory after 12 weeks.

■■■

Pharmacological Effects of Phosphatidylserine Enzymatically Synthesized from Soybean Lecithin on Brain Functions in Rodents. Sakai M; et al. *Journal of Nutritional Science and Vitaminology*, 1996 February, 42(1):47-54.

Results of this study indicated that the oral administration of 300 mg per day of soybean transphosphatidylated phosphatidylserine can improve and/or prevent senile dementia.

■■■

The Potent Free Radical Scavenger Alpha-lipoic Acid Improves Memory in Aged Mice. Stoll S; et al. *Pharmacology Biochemistry and Behavior*, 1995 October-December, 111(4): 6-8.

Results of this study showed that alpha-lipoic acid improved memory in aged mice.

■■■

Memory-improving Effect of Aqueous Extract of Astragalus Membranaceus (Fisch.) Bge. Hong GX; et al. *Chung Kuo Chung Yap Tsa Chih*, 1994 November, 19(11):687-688.

Results of this study found that an aqueous Astragalus membranaceus extract improved anisodine-induced impairment on memory acquisition and alcohol-induced memory retrieval deficit in step-down behavior of mice.

■■■

Cognitive Decline in the Elderly: A Double-blind, Placebo-controlled Multi-center Study on Efficacy of Phosphatidylserine Administration. Cenacchi T; et al. *Aging*, 1993 April, 5(2):123-133.

This double-blind, placebo-controlled study examined the effects of 300 mg per day of phosphatidylserine in cognitive impaired geriatric patients. Results showed the treatment had significant positive cognitive and behavioral effects relative to controls.

Candida

Antioxidant, Antimalarial and Antimicrobial Activities of Tannin-Rich Fractions, Ellagitannins and Phenolic Acids from Punica Granatum L. Reddy MK; Gupta SK; et al. *Planta Medica*, 2007 May, 73(5):461-467.

Punica granatum L. (pomegranate) by-product POMx and pomegranate juice may be useful in bolstering immunity and fighting various infections including Candida.

■■■

Prevalence of Candida Species in Turkish Children: Relationship Between Dietary Intake and Carriage. Kadir T; Uygun B; et al. *Archives of Oral Biology*, 2005 January, 50(1):33-37.

In exploring the prevalence and intensity of Candida species in 300 healthy Turkish children, the researchers determined that candidal carriage was 18.5 percent in children who were fed with both breast milk and bottle milk or other fluids, as compared with 0 percent in children fed only with breast milk.

■■■

Effect of Oral Zinc Supplementation on Agents of Oropharyngeal Infection in Patients Receiving Radiotherapy for Head and Neck Cancer. Ertekin MV; Uslu H; et al. *Journal of International Medical Research*, 2003 July-August, 31(4):253-266.

Zinc or placebo was administered to 30 patients who were receiving radiotherapy for head and neck cancer. Findings suggested that some infections with Candida species and staphylococci were prevented by zinc supplementation.

■■■

Effect of Calcium Ion Uptake on Candida Albicans Morphology. Holmes AR; Cannon RD; Shepherd MG. *Fems Microbiology Letters*, 1991 January 15, 61(2-3):187-193.

Calcium was shown to inhibit the growth of Candida albicans yeast cells.

■■■

Inhibition of Candida adhesion to buccal epithelial cells by an aqueous extract of Allium sativum (garlic). Ghannoum MA. *Journal of Applied Bacteriology*, 1990 February, 68(2):163-169.

Garlic extract inhibits the adhesion of Candida cells to human cells taken from the inside of the cheek.

■■■

Respiratory Burst and Candidacidal Activity of Peritoneal Macrophages are Impaired in Copper-Deficient Rats. Babu U; Failla ML. *Journal of Nutrition*, 1990 December, 120(12):1692-1699.

In rats, a copper-deficient diet resulted in reduced resistance to Candida cells. Rats fed a diet with adequate copper, by contrast, had better systemic defenses against Candida.

Chronic Fatigue

Erythrocyte Oxidative Damage in Chronic Fatigue Syndrome. Richards RS; et al. *Archives of Medical Research*, 2007 January, 38(1):94-98.

Previous studies have determined that there is a connection between erythrocyte morphology and erythrocyte oxidative damage in chronic fatigue syndrome (CFS). This research found an increase in erythrocyte antioxidant activity that is probably linked to the presence of stomatocytes. According to the authors, the results provide additional support for the role of free radicals in the pathogenesis of CFS.

■■■

High Cocoa Polyphenol Rich Chocolate Improves the Symptoms of Chronic Fatigue. Sathyapalan T; et al. *Endocrine Abstracts*, 2006,12:68.

In this double-blind, placebo-controlled study, patients who received high cocoa polyphenol rich chocolate, 15 g three times a day, showed improved scores on the Chandler Fatigue Scale and improved residual function as measured by the London Handicap Scale. In addition, two patients were able to go back to work after suffering with CFS for two years.

Depression

A Meta-Analytic Review of Double-Blind, Placebo-Controlled Trials of Antidepressant Efficacy of Omega-3 Fatty Acids. Lin PY; Su KP. *Journal of Clinical Psychiatry*, 2007 July, 68(7):1056-1061.

In their review of recent literature, the authors determined that omega-3 polyunsaturated fatty acids (PUFAs) can significantly improve depression in patients with clearly defined depression and bipolar disorder.

■■■

Effects of Omega-3 Polyunsaturated Fatty Acids on Depression. Severus WE. *Herz*, 2006 December, 31 (Suppl. 3):69-74.

Recent epidemiological and clinical research has indicated that omega-3 polyunsaturated fatty acids "may well represent a major advance in the treatment of depression."

■■■

Treatment of Depression: Time to Consider Folic Acid and Vitamin B12. Coppen A; Bolander-Gouaille C. *Journal of Psychopharmacology*, 2005 January, 19(1):59-65.

This study suggested that both folic acid (800 microg daily) and vitamin B12 (1 mg daily) should be included in the treatment of depression.

■■■

A Double-blind, Placebo-controlled, Exploratory Trial of Chromium Picolinate in Atypical Depression: Effect on Carbohydrate Craving. Docherty JP; Sack DA; et al. *Journal of Psychiatric Practice*, 2005 September,11(5):302-314.

Chromium picolinate may be beneficial for patients with atypical depression who also have severe carbohydrate craving.

■■■

Neural and Behavioral Responses to Tryptophan Depletion in Unmedicated Patients with Remitted Major Depressive Disorder and Controls. Neumeister A; Nugent AC; et al. *Archives of General Psychiatry*, 2004 August, 61(8):765-773.

In patients with remitted major depressive disorder, tryptophan depletion caused a temporary return of depression. The authors concluded that depletion of tryptophan may be related to serotonin dysfunction.

■■■

Effectiveness of Chromium in Atypical Depression: A Placebo-Controlled Trial. Davidson JR; Abraham K; et al. *Biological Psychiatry*, 2003 February 1, 53(3):261-264.

The researchers concluded that chromium picolinate is effective in treating atypical depression.

■■■

S-Adenosyl-Methionine in Depression: A Comprehensive Review of the Literature. Papakostas GI; Alpert JE; et al. *Current Psychiatry Reports*, 2003 December, 5(6):460-466.

SAMe is a natural supplement that is backed by 30 years of research regarding its effectiveness against depression.

■■■

A Double-blind, Randomized Parallel-group, Efficacy and Safety Study of Intramuscular S-Adenosyl-L-Methionine 1,4-Butanedisulphonate (SAMe) Versus Imipramine in Patients with Major Depressive Disorder. Pancheri P; Scapicchio P; et al. *International Journal of Neuropsychopharmacology*, 2002 December, 5(4):287-294.

The researchers found that 400 mg/d i.m SAMe is better tolerated than 150 mg/d oral imipramine and just as effective in reducing depression.

■■■

Role of S-adenosyl- L-methionine in the Treatment of Depression: A Review of the Evidence. Mischoulon D; Fava M. *American Journal of Clinical Nutrition*, 2002 November, 76(5):1158S-1161S.

This review article reported recent findings regarding the use of S-adenosyl-L-methionine (SAMe) to treat depression: a small number of clinical trials have determined that doses of 200 to1600 mg/d of SAMe are better than placebo and as effective as tricyclic antidepressants; SAMe may have a faster onset of action than conventional antidepressants; SAMe may potentiate the effect of tricyclic antidepressants; SAMe may protect against the adverse effects of Alzheimer's disease. In addition, although some cases of mania have been reported in bipolar patients, SAMe is well tolerated and only rarely associated with side effects.

■■■

Dehydroepiandrosterone (DHEA) Treatment of Depression. Wolkowitz OM; et al. *Biological Psychiatry*, 1997 February 1, 41(3):311-318.

In this study, 30 to 90 mg of DHEA per day was administered to six middle-aged and elderly patients over a period of four weeks. Results showed significant improvements in symptoms of depression and memory performance.

■ ■ ■

St. John's Wort for Depression—An Overview and Meta-analysis of Randomized Clinical Trials. Linde K; et al. *British Medical Journal*, 1996 August 3, 313(7052):253-258.

Results of this meta-analysis involving 23 randomized studies, 15 of which were placebo-controlled, found that hypericum extracts proved significantly effective in the treatment of patients suffering from moderate to mildly severe depression.

■ ■ ■

Cimicifuga for Depression. Frances D. *Medical Herbalism*, 1995 Spring/Summer, 7(1-2):1-2.

This article reports on the successful use of black cohosh in tincture form as a treatment for depression in three different case studies.

■ ■ ■

Treatment of Depressive Symptoms with a High Concentration Hypericum Preparation. A Multicenter Placebo-controlled Double-blind Study. Witte B; et al. *Fortschritte der Medizin*. 1995 October 10, 404-408.

Results of this double-blind, placebo-controlled study involving 97 depression outpatients showed that 100 to 120 mg of hypericum extract led to noticeable improvement in 70 percent of the patients.

■■■

Antidepressant Principles of Valerian Fauriei Roots. Oshima Y; et al. *Chemical and Pharmaceutical Bulletin*, 1995 January, 43(1):169-170.

Results of this study showed that a methanol extract of the roots of Valerian fauriei exhibited antidepressant activity in mice.

■■■

Rapidity of Onset of the Antidepressant Effect of Parenteral S-adenosyl-L-methionine. Fava M; et al. *Psychiatry Research*, 1995 April 28, 56(3):295-297.

Results of this study found that the parental administration of 400 mg of SAMe over a period of 15 days remitted depressive symptoms in patients suffering from depression.

Depression and Other Mental Disorders in Older Adults

Effect of a Qigong Exercise Programme on Elderly with Depression. Tsang HWH; et al. *International Journal of Geriatric Psychiatry*, 2006 September, 21(9): 890-897.

This study determined that qigong, an ancient Chinese practice involving breathing exercises, meditation and body movements, alleviated depression in older adults. When compared with a control group, 41 depressed people over age 65 who practiced qigong three times a week for 16 weeks reported improved mood, self-confidence, self-esteem, personal wellbeing and physical health.

■■■

The Role of Daily Positive Emotions During Conjugal Bereavement. Ong AD; et al. *The Journals of Gerontology Series B: Psychological Sciences and Social Sciences*, 2004 July, 59(4):168-176.

Researchers concluded that daily positive emotions, including humor coping skills, were critical in reducing stress after conjugal loss.

■ ■ ■

Hypericum Treatment of Mild Depression with Somatic Symptoms. Hubner WD; et al. *Journal of Geriatric Psychiatry and Neurology*, 1994 October, 7(Suppl):1-S12-14.

In this randomized, double-blind study, placebo-controlled study, 300 mg of the hyperium extract LI 160 was administered to depression patients three times daily for four weeks. The treatment group showed significant improvement compared to controls, with 70 percent showing no symptoms after four weeks.

■ ■ ■

Placebo-controlled Double-blind Study Examining the Effectiveness of an Hypericum Preparation in 105 Mildly Depressed Patients. Sommer H; Harrer G. *Journal of Geriatric Psychiatry and Neurology*, 1994 October, 7(Suppl. 1):S9-11.

Results of this double-blind, placebo-controlled study showed that 3 x 300 mg of hypericum extract over a period of four weeks led to significant improvements in depression outpatients relative to controls.

■ ■ ■

Benefits and Risks of the Hypericum Extract LI 160: Drug Monitoring Study with 3250 Patients. Woelk H; et al. *Journal of Geriatric Psychiatry and Neurology*, 1994 October, 7(Suppl 1): S34-S38.

This study evaluated the effects of a four-week treatment program with hypericum extract in 3,250 patients suffering from various levels of depression. Results showed that 30 percent of the patients experienced improvement while receiving the therapy.

■ ■ ■

Hypericum in the Treatment of Seasonal Affective Disorder. Martinez B; et al. *Journal of Geriatric Psychiatry and Neurology*, 1994 October, 7(Suppl .1):S29-S33.

Results of this study showed that treatment with 900 mg per day of hypericum coupled with two hours of daily light therapy significantly reduced symptoms of depression in patients suffering from seasonal affective disorder.

■ ■ ■

Multicenter Double-Blind Study Examining the Antidepressant Effectiveness of the Hypericum Extract LI 160. Hansgen KD; et al. *Journal of Geriatric Psychiatry and Neurology*, 1994 October, 7(Suppl. 1):S15-18.

Results of this double-blind, placebo-controlled study showed that treatment with hypericum extract over a period of four weeks led to significant improvements in patients suffering from depression.

Eating Disorders

How Does Zinc Supplementation Benefit Anorexia Nervosa? Birmingham CL; Gritzner S. *Eating and Weight Disorders*, 2006 December, 11(4):109-111.

Zinc supplements offer protection against neurotransmitter dysfunction in people with anorexia. The authors of this article suggested routine oral administration of 14 mg of elemental zinc daily for 2 months in all patients with the disorders.

■ ■ ■

Plasma Tryptophan During Weight Restoration in Patients with Anorexia Nervosa. Attia E; Wolk S; et al. *Biological Psychiatry*, 2005 March 15, 57(6):674-678.

The purpose of this study was to measure plasma tryptophan (TRP), the amino acid important in serotonin production, during the course of refeeding in patients with anorexia.

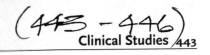

Effects of Acute Tryptophan Depletion on Mood in Bulimia Nervosa. Kaye WH; Gendall KA; et al. *Biological Psychiatry*, 2000 January 15, 47(2):151-157.

The moods of women with and without bulimia nervosa were compared after drinking a control mix of essential amino acids (100 g + 4.6 g tryptophan) on one day and a tryptophan deficient mix (100 g - 4.6 g tryptophan) on the other. Those with bulimia experienced more mood-lowering effects of the tryptophan depleted drink.

■ ■ ■

Zinc Deficiency and Childhood-Onset Anorexia Nervosa. Lask B; Fosson A; et al. *Journal of Clinical Psychiatry*, 1993 February, 54(2):63-66.

Zinc deficiency was found to be common in childhood-onset anorexia nervosa.

■ ■ ■

Zinc Status Before and After Zinc Supplementation of Eating Disorder Patients. McClain CJ; Stuart MA; et al. *Journal of the American College of Nutrition*, 1992 December, 11(6):694-700.

Since reduced food intake results from zinc deficiency, the acquired zinc deficiency of eating disorder patients may act as a sustaining factor for their abnormal eating behavior. Hospitalized bulimics and anorexics were shown to be deficient in the mineral, and to benefit from supplementation.

Insomnia

Scientific Evidence for a Fixed Extract Combination (Ze 91019) from Valerian and Hops Traditionally Used as a Sleep-inducing Aid. Brattström A. *Wiener Medizinische Wochenschrift*, 2007 July, 157(13-14):367-370.

The authors explained scientifically the mechanism of action of a valerian and hops combination in patients with sleep disorders.

■■■

A Randomized, Double Blind, Placebo-controlled, Prospective Clinical Study to Demonstrate Clinical Efficacy of a Fixed Valerian Hops Extract Combination (Ze 91019) in Patients Suffering from Non-Organic Sleep Disorder. Koetter U; Schrader E; et al. *Phytotherapy Research.* 2007 May 8.

A fixed valerian hops extract combination was found to be more effective than placebo in reducing sleep latency in people with insomnia. A single valerian extract did not achieve the same results, indicating that the addition of hops is important.

■■■

Clinical Efficacy of Kava Extract WS 1490 in Sleep Disturbances Associated with Anxiety Disorders. Results of a Multicenter, Randomized, Placebo-Controlled, Double-blind Clinical Trial. Lehrl S. *Journal of Affective Disorders*, 2004 February, 78(2):101-110.

The researchers concluded that kava special extract WS 1490 was safe and effective in treating people with sleep disturbances associated with nonpsychotic anxiety, tension and restlessness.

■■■

Critical Evaluation of the Effect of Valerian Extract on Sleep Structure and Sleep Quality. Donath F; Quispe S; et al. *Pharmacopsychiatry*, 2000 March, 33(2):47-53.

This double-blind, placebo-controlled study found that a herbal extract of radix valerianae benefited patients with mild psychophysiological insomnia.

■■■

Melatonin Replacement Corrects Sleep Disturbances in a Child with Pineal Tumor. Etzioni A; et al. *Neurology*, 1996 January, 46(1):261-263.

This article reports on the case of a child with a germ cell tumor involving the pineal region experiencing a melatonin secretion suppression associated with severe insomnia. Supplementation with 3 mg per night for two weeks of normalized sleep.

■■■

Sleep-inducing Effects of Low Doses of Melatonin Ingested in the Evening. Zhdanova IV; et al. *Clinical Pharmacology and Therapy*, 1995, 57(5):552-558.

In this double-blind, placebo-controlled study, healthy volunteers received either 0.3 or 1.0 mg of melatonin at 6, 8, or 9 P.M. Results showed that either doses given at either time reduced sleep onset latency.

■■■

Improvement of Sleep Quality in Elderly People by Controlled-release Melatonin. Garfinkel D; et al. *Lancet*, 1995 August 26, 346(8974):541-544.

Results of this double-blind, placebo-controlled study showed that 2 mg per night of controlled-release melatonin for three weeks significantly improved sleep quality in elderly subjects.

■■■

Melatonin Replacement Therapy of Elderly Insomniacs. Haimov I; et al. *Sleep*, 1995 September, 18(7):598-603.

This double-blind, placebo-controlled study examined the effects of melatonin replacement therapy on melatonin-deficient elderly insomniacs. Results showed that one-week treatment with 2 mg sustained-release melatonin was effective for sleep maintenance, while sleep initiation was improved by the fast-release melatonin. Such effects were increased following the two-month 1-mg sustained-release melatonin treatment.

■■■

L-dopa-responsive Dystonia: 2 Familial Cases of Adult Onset with Sleep Disorders. El Alaoui-Faris M; et al. *Revista de Neurologia*, 1995 May, 151(5):347-349.

This article reports on the cases of a woman and her son with progressive dystonia and chronic insomnia. Treatment with low dose L-dopa had significantly beneficial effects over a period of five years with respect to dystonia and insomnia without dyskinesia.

■■■

The Treatment of Sleep Disorders with Melatonin. Jan JE; et al. *Neurobiology*, 1994 February, 36(2):97-107.

In this study, 15 disabled children with severe, chronic sleep disorders received 2 to 10 mg of oral melatonin. Results showed significant positive effects.

Premenstrual Syndrome (PMS)

Value of Standardized Ginkgo Biloba Extract (Egb 761) in the Management of Congestive Symptoms of Premenstrual Syndrome. Tamborini A; Taurelle R. *Revue française de gynécologie et d'obstétrique*, 1993 July-September, 88(7-9):447-457.

This double-blind, placebo-controlled study examined the effects of Ginkgo biloba extract on congestive symptoms of PMS in a group of 165 women. Results showed that the extract proved to be effective in relieving symptoms, particularly those associated with the breasts.

■■■

Effect of a Nutritional Supplement on Premenstrual Symptomatology in Women with Premenstrual Syndrome: A Double-Blind Longitudinal Study. London RS; Bradley L; Chiamori NY. *Journal of the American College of Nutrition*, 1991 October, 10(5):494-499.

Nutritional supplements proved more effective than a placebo in relieving premenstrual syndrome.

■■■

Oral Magnesium Successfully Relieves Premenstrual Mood Changes. Facchinetti F; Borella P; Sances G; Fioroni L; Nappi RE; Genazzani AR. *Obstetrics and Gynecology*, 1991 August, 78(2):177-181.

Magnesium supplementation, when compared with a placebo, was effective in relieving premenstrual mood changes.

■■■

Premenstrual and Menstrual Symptom Clusters and Response to Calcium Treatment. Alvir JM; Thys-Jacobs S. *Psychopharmacology Bulletin*, 1991, 27(2):145-148.

Calcium supplementation was shown to alleviate three premenstrual symptoms—mood changes, water retention, and pain—and to relieve menstrual pain.

Schizophrenia

Membrane Phospholipid Composition, Alterations in Neurotransmitter Systems and Schizophrenia. du Bois TM; Deng C; et al. *Progress in Neuro-Psychopharmacology & Biological Psychiatry*, 2005 July, 29(6):878-888.

Supplementation with polyunsaturated omega-3 fatty acids (PUFA) can improve mental health rating scores in people with schizophrenia. Altered PUFA levels may contribute to the abnormalities in neurotransmission seen in the disorder.

■ ■ ■

Can Perinatal Supplementation of Long-Chain Polyunsaturated Fatty Acids Prevent Schizophrenia in Adult Life? Das UN. *Medical Science Monitor*, 2004 December, 10(12):HY33-HY37.

This author hypothesized that schizophrenia could be a low-grade systemic inflammatory disease originating in the perinatal period, and suggested that perinatal supplementation with long-chain polyunsaturated fatty acids may help prevent subsequent development of the disorder.

■ ■ ■

High-dose Glycine Added to Olanzapine and Risperidone for the Treatment of Schizophrenia. Heresco-Levy U; et al. *Biological Psychiatry*, 2004 January, 55(2):165-171.

This double-blind, placebo-controlled, six-week crossover treatment trial determined that .8 g/kg per day of glycine added to patients' ongoing antipsychotic medication resulted in a significant 23 percent reduction in negative symptoms.

■ ■ ■

Lipid Abnormalities in Schizophrenia—Current Knowledge. [Article in Polish] Michalak G. *Psychaitr Pol*, 2003 November-December, 37(6):965-976.

The author describes the research showing that lipid abnormalities are involved in the pathogenesis of schizophrenia. Included are assessments of essential fatty acids, the niacin flush test and treatment trials using supplementation with eicosapentaenoic acid.

■ ■ ■

Supplementation with a Combination of Omega-3 Fatty Acids and Antioxidants (Vitamins E and C) Improves the Outcome of Schizophrenia. Arvindakshan M; Ghate M; et al. *Schizophrenia Research*, 2003 August 1, 62(3):195-204.

Oral supplementation with a mixture of eicosapentaenoic acid (EPA)/docosahexaenoic acid (DHA) and antioxidants (vitamin E/C) over a four-month period proved beneficial to schizophrenic patients.

■■■

Amelioration of Negative Symptoms in Schizophrenia by Glycine. Javitt DC; et al. *American Journal of Psychiatry*, 1994 August, 151(8):1234-1236.

Results of this double-blind, placebo-controlled study involving 14 chronic schizophrenics on medication found that the administration of glycine led to significant improvements in symptoms associated with the disease.

■■■

Vitamin C in the Treatment of Schizophrenia. Sandyk R; Kanofsky JD. *International Journal of Neuroscience*, 1993 January, 68(1-2):67-71.

This paper reports on a single case of 37-year-old schizophrenic who was observed to have benefited from ascorbic acid supplementation to his ongoing neuroleptic medication.

■■■

Vitamin C Status in Chronic Schizophrenia. Suboticanec K; Folnegovic-Smalc V; Korbar M; Mestrovic B; Buzina R. *Biological Psychiatry*, 1990 December, 28(11):959-966.

Schizophrenic patients on the same hospital diet as control group patients showed lower levels of vitamin C in their blood, and even when they were supplemented to normalize their blood levels of the vitamin, levels excreted in their urine remained lower than those of the control group. The results support the view that schizophrenic patients need more vitamin C than the suggested requirement for healthy people.

Tardive Dyskinesia

Disrupted Antioxidant Enzyme Activity and Elevated Lipid Peroxidation Products in Schizophrenic Patients with Tardive Dyskinesia. Zhang XY; Tan YL; et al. *Journal of Clinical Psychiatry*, 2007 May, 68(5):754-760.

Findings revealed that oxidative stress is involved in the onset and progression of tardive dyskinesia, and there is a connection between oxidative stress and the severity of the disorder.

■ ■ ■

Branched Chain Amino Acid Treatment of Tardive Dyskinesia in Children and Adolescents. Richardson MA; Small AM; et al. *Journal of Clinical Psychiatry*, 2004 January, 65(1):92-96.

Treatment with branched chain amino acids (BCAA) significantly decreased tardive dyskinesia symptoms in children and adolescents.

■ ■ ■

The Effect of Vitamin E Treatment on Tardive Dyskinesia and Blood Superoxide Dismutase: A Double-blind Placebo-controlled Trial. Zhang XY; Zhou DF; et al. *Journal of Clinical Psychopharmacology*, 2004 February, 24(1):83-86.

The findings of this study confirmed previous research indicating that vitamin E is safe and effective in the treatment of tardive dyskinesia.

■ ■ ■

Efficacy of the Branched-Chain Amino Acids in the Treatment of Tardive Dyskinesia in Men. Richardson MA; Bevans ML; et al. *American Journal of Psychiatry*, 2003 June, 160(6):1117-1124.

Branched chain amino acids (BCAA) significantly decreased tardive dyskinesia symptoms in men.

■■■

Severe Tardive Dyskinesia in Affective Disorders: Treatment with Vitamin E and C. Michaela N; et al. *Neuropsychobiology*, 2002, 46 (Suppl. 1):28-30.

This study concluded that combining vitamin C and E in patients with affective disorders and tardive dyskinesia resulted in a reduction in symptoms with no adverse effects.

■■■

Treatment for Tardive Dyskinesia: A Double-blind, Placebo-controlled, Crossover Study. Shamir E; Barak Y; et al. *Archives of General Psychiatry*, 2001 November, 58(11):1049-1052.

In this double-blind, placebo-controlled study, 22 patients with schizophrenia and tardive dyskinesia received 10 mg/d of melatonin for six weeks. The results were favorable when compared with a control group.

■■■

Vitamin B6 in the Treatment of Tardive Dyskinesia: A Double-blind, Placebo-controlled, Crossover Study. Lerner V; et al. *American Journal of Psychiatry*, 2001, 158(9):1511-1514.

Fifteen patients with schizophrenia and tardive dyskinesia received either vitamin B6 or placebo for four weeks. Dosages were 100 mg of B6 per day, increasing by 100 mg per week to 400 mg daily by the fourth week. Significant improvements were noted in various movement scores with no adverse effects.

■■■

Melatonin Treatment for Tardive Dyskinesia. Shamir E; et al. *Archives of General Psychiatry*, 2001, 58:1049-1052.

The researchers used a double-blind, placebo-controlled, crossover model to assess the effectiveness of 10 mg per day of melatonin for six weeks in 22 patients with schizophrenia and tardive dyskinesia. Beneficial effects were found, as measured by the Abnormal Involuntary Movement Scale (AIMS).

Thyroid Disorders

Late-onset Bipolar Disorder due to Hyperthyroidism Nath J; Safar R. *Acta Psychiatrica Scandinavica*, 2001, 104:72-75.

The researchers determined that thyroid disorder could mimic late-onset bipolar disorder.

Appendix C

Environmental Causes of Mental Disease— A Bibliography

...

Arnold, L. E, et al. "Does Zinc Moderate Essential Fatty Acid and Amphetamine Treatment of Attention-Deficit/Hyperactivity Disorder?" *Journal of Child and Adolescent Psychopharmacology* 10 (2000): 111-117.

Arnold, L. E. "Alternative Treatments for Adults with Attention-deficit Hyperactivity Disorder (ADHD)." In: Wasserstein, J., Wolfe, L E, Lefever, F. F., eds. *Adult Attention Deficit Disorders: Brain Mechanisms and Life Outcomes.* New York: New York Academy of Sciences, 2001.

Aschengau, A.; Ziegler, S. and Cohen, A. "Quality of Community Drinking Water and the Occurrence of Late Adverse Pregnancy Outcomes." *Archives of Environmental Health* 48 (1993): 105-113.

Aschner, M. and Kimelberg, M., eds. *The Role of Glia in Neurotoxicity.* Boca Raton: CRC Press, 1996.

Bailey, A.J.; Sargent, J.D.; Goodman, D.C.; Freeman, J. and Brown, M.J. "Poisoned Landscapes: The Epidemiology of Environmental Lead Exposure in Massachusetts Children 1990-1991." *Social Science Medicine* 39 (1994): 757-776.

Bellinger D. et al. "Pre- and Postnatal Lead Exposure and Behavior Problems in School-Aged Children." *Environmental Research* 66, no. 1 (July 1994): 12-30.

Benton, D. "Micro-nutrient Supplementation and the Intelligence of Children." *Neuroscience and Biobehavioral Reviews* 125 (2001): 297-309.

Brockel, Becky A. and Cory-Slechta, Deborah A. "Lead, Attention, and Impulsive Behavior: Changes in a Fixed-Ratio Waiting-for-Reward Paradigm." *Pharmacology Biochemistry and Behavior* 60, no. 2 (June 1998): 545-552.

Bottiglieri, T. "S-Adenosyl-L-methionine (SAMe): From the Bench to the Bedside—Molecular Basis of a Pleiotrophic Molecule." *American Journal of Clinical Nutrition* 76, No. 5 (November 2002): 1151S-1157S.

Bottiglieri, T., et al. "Homocysteine, Folate, Methylation, and Monoamine Metabolism in Depression." *Journal of Neurology, Neurosurgery and Psychiatry* 69, No. 2 (August 2000): 228-232.

Bryce-Smith, D. "Environmental Chemical Influences on Behaviour and Mentation." *Chemical Society Review* 15 (1986): 93-123.

Chengappa, K. N, et al. "Inositol as an Add-on Treatment for Bipolar Depression." *Bipolar Disorder* 2 (2000): 47-55.

Cook, E. H., Jr., et al. "Association of Attention Deficit disorder and the Dopamine Transporter Gene." *American Journal of Human Genetics* 56 (1995).

Delle Chiaie R, et al. "Efficacy and Tolerability of Oral and Intra-muscular S-adenosyl-L-methionine 1,4- butanedisulfonate (SAMe) in the Treatment of Major Depression: Comparison with Imipramine in 2 Multicenter Studies." *American Journal of Clinical Nutrition* 76, No. 5 (November 2002): 1172S-1176S.

Gazzaniga, Michael, Ivry, Richard B. and Mangun, George R. *Cognitive Neuroscience*. New York: W. W. Norton, 1998.

Kahn, CA., Kelly, PC., Walker, WO. 1995. "Lead screening in children with attention deficit hyperactivity disorder and developmental delay." *Clinical Pediatrics* 34, no.9 (Sept 1995): 498-501.

Kaplan, B. J., et al. Effective Mood Stabilization with a Chelated Mineral Supplement: An Open-label Trial in Bipolar Disorder." *Journal of Clinical Psychiatry* 62 (2001): 936-944.

Kiecolt-Glaser, J. K., et al. "Emotions, Morbidity, and Mortality: New Perspectives from Psychoneuroimmunology." *Annual Review of Psychology* 53 (2002): 83-107.

Kiecolt-Glaser, J. K., et al. "Psychoneuroimmunology and Psychosomatic Medicine: Back to the Future." *Psychosomatic Medicine*, 64 (January-February 2002): 15-28.

Kiecolt-Glaser, J. K., et al. "Psychoneuroimmunology: Psychological Influences on Immune Function and Health." *Journal of Consulting and Clinical Psychology* 70, No. 3 (June 2002): 537-547.

Levy, N. A. and Janicak, P. G. "Calcium Channel Antagonists for the Treatment of Bipolar Disorder." *Bipolar Disorder* 2 (2000):108-119.

Levitt, Miriam. "Toxic Metals, Preconception, and Early Childhood Development." *Social Science Information* 38 (1999): 179-201.

Lieber, C. S. and Packer L. "S-Adenosylmethionine: Molecular, Biological, and Clinical Aspects—An Introduction." *American Journal of Clinical Nutrition* 76, No. 5 (November 2002): 1148S-1150S.

Manuzza, S., et al. "Adult Psychiatric Status of Hyperactive Boys Grown Up." *American Journal of Psychiatry* 155 (1998): 493-498.

Manuzza, S., et al. "Hyperactive Boys Almost Grown Up." *Archives of General Psychiatry* 46 (1989): 1073-1079.

Masters, Roger D. and Coplan, Myron. J. "Water Treatment with Silicofluorides and Lead Toxicity." *International Journal of Environmental Studies* 56 (1999a): 435-449.

Masters, Roger D. and Coplan, Myron J. "A Dynamic, Multifactorial Model of Alcohol, Drug Abuse, and Crime: Linking Neuroscience and Behavior to Toxicology." *Social Science Information* (1999b).

Masters, Roger D.; Coplan, Myron J. and Hone, Brian T. "Silicofluoride Usage, Tooth Decay, and Children's Blood Lead." Poster Presentation, Environmental Influences on Children: Brain, Development, and Behavior, *Conference at New York Academy of Medicine*, New York, NY, May 24-25, 1999.

Masters, Roger D.; Coplan, Myron J. and Hone, Brian T. "Heavy Metal Toxicity, Development, and Behavior." Poster Presentation, *17th International Neurotoxicology Conference*, Doubletree Hotel, Little Rock, AR, October 17-20, 1999.

Masters, Roger D.; Hone, Brian T. and Doshi, Anil. "Environmental Pollution, Neurotoxicity, and Criminal Violence." J. Rose, ed. *Environmental Toxicology*. London: Gordon and Breach, 1998. 13-48.

McLeod, M. N. and Golden, R. N. "Chromium Treatment of Depression." *International Journal of Neuropsychopharmacology* 3 (2000): 311-314.

Mendelsohn, Alan L.; Dreyer, Benard P.; Fierman, Arthur H.; Rosen, Carolyn M.; Legano, Lori A.; Kruger, Hillary A.; Limß, Sylvia W. and Courtlandt, Cheryl D. 1998. "Low-Level Lead Exposure and Behavior in Early Childhood." *Pediatrics* 101, No. 3 (March 1998): e10.

Mielke, H. "Lead in the Inner Cities." *American Scientist* 87 (1998): 62-73.

Minder, Barbara; Das-Smaal, Edith A.; Brand, Eddy F. J. M. and Orlebeke, Jacob F. "Exposure to Lead and Specific Attentional Problems in Schoolchildren." *Journal of Learning Disabilities* 27, no. 6 (June/July 1994): 393-398.

Muniyappa, R., et al. "Dehydroepiandrosterone (DHEA) Secretion in Healthy Older Men and Women: Effects of Testosterone and Growth Hormone Administration in Older Men. *Journal of Clinical Endocrinology and Metabolism* (August 22, 2006).

Needleman, Herbert L., ed. *Human Lead Exposure*. Boca Raton: CRC Press, 1991.

Needleman, Herbert L., et al. "Bone Lead Levels and Delinquent Behavior." *JAMA* 275 (1996): 363-69.

Needleman, Herbert L. "Environmental Neurotoxins and Attention Deficit Disorder." Presentation at Conference on Environmental Neurotoxins and Developmental Disability, *Academy of Medicine*, New York (May 24-25, 1999).

Papakostas, G. I., et al. "Serum Folate, Vitamin B12, and Homocysteine in Major Depressive Disorder, Part 2: Predictors of Relapse During the Continuation Phase of Pharmacotherapy." *Journal of Clinical Psychiatry* 65, No. 8 (August 2004): 1096-1098.

Rohr, U. D. "The Impact of Testosterone Imbalance on Depression and Women's Health." *Maturitas* 41 Supplement (April 2002): S25-S46.

Shaldubina, A., et al. "The Mechanism of Lithium Action: State of the Art, Ten Years Later." *Progress in Neuropsychopharmacology and Biological Psychiatry* 25 (2001): 855-866.

Tiemeier, H., et al. "Vitamin B12, Folate, and Homocysteine in Depression: The Rotterdam Study." *American Journal of Psychiatry* 159, No. 12 (December 2002): 2099-2101.

Tuthill, R. W. "Head Lead Levels Related to Children's Classroom Attention-Deficit Behavior." *Archives of Environmental Health* 51 (1996): 214-220.

Van der Does, A. J. "The Effects of Tryptophan Depletion on Mood and Psychiatric Symptoms." *Journal of Affective Disorders* 64 (2001): 107-119.

Useful Books

Richard Ash, DHEA: *Unlocking the Secrets to the Fountain of Youth* (contributor), Detroit Lakes: BL Publications, 1997.

Sidney M. Baker, *The Circadian Prescription* (with Karen Baar), New York: Penguin Putnam, 2000.

——*Detoxification and Healing: The Key to Optimal Health*, New Canaan: Keats, 1997.

——*Child Behavior: The Classic Childcare Manual from the Gesell Institute of Human Development* (contributor), New York: Harper Perennial, 1992.

Syd Baumel, *Natural Antidepressants*, Los Angeles: Keats Publishing, 1998.

——*Dealing with Depression Naturally*, Los Angeles: Keats Publishing, 1995.

Dr. Mary Ann Block, *No More Antibiotics: Preventing and Treating Ear and Respiratory Infections the Natural Way*, Kensington Publishing Corp., 2000.

——*No More Ritalin: Treating ADHD Without Drugs*, New York: Kensington Publishing Corp., 1996.

E. Braverman, *The Healing Nutrients Within*, 2nd ed. New Canaan, CT: Keats Publishing, 2003.

Peter Breggin, *The War Against Children of Color: Psychiatry Target Inner-City Youth* (with Ginger Ross Breggin), Monroe: Common Courage Press, 1998.

——*Talking Back to Ritalin: What Doctors Aren't Telling You About Stimulants for Children*, Monroe: Common Courage Press, 1998.

——*Talking Back to Prozac: What Doctors Aren't Telling You About Today's Most Controversial Drug*, New York: Tor Books, 1994.

Paula Caplan, *They Say You're Crazy: How the World's Most Powerful Psychiatrists Decide Who's Normal*, Reading: Addison-Wesley Publishing Co., 1995.

——*You're Smarter Than They Make You Feel: How the Experts Intimidate Us and What We Can Do About It*, New York: The Free Press, 1994.

Catharine Carrigan, *Healing Depression: A Holistic Guide*, New York: Marlowe & Co., 1999.

Dr. H. Richard Casdorph and Dr. Morton Walker, *Toxic Metal Syndrome*, Wayne: Avery Publishing, 1995.

Dr. Hyla Cass, *All About St. John's Wort*, Wayne: Avery Publishing, 1999.

——*Kava: Nature's Answer to Stress, Anxiety & Insomnia*, Rocklin: Prima Communications, Inc., 1998.

——*St. John's Wort: Nature's Blues Buster*, Wayne: Avery Publishing, 1998.

Ty Colbert, *Broken Brains or Wounded Hearts: What Causes Mental Illness*, Santa Ana: Kevco, 1996.

——*Depression & Mania: Friends or Foes*, Santa Ana: Kevco, 1995.

Dr. William Crook, *Healing Depression: A Holistic Guide*, New York: Marlowe and Company, 1999.

——*Help For The Hyperactive Child: A Practical Guide Offering Parents of Attention Deficit Disorder Alternatives to Ritalin*, New York: Professional Books, 1991.

Dr. Gabriel Cousens, *Depression-Free for Life: An All-Natural 5 Step Plan to Reclaim Your Zest for Living*, New York: William Morrow & Co., 2000.

——*Conscious Eating*, Santa Rosa: Vision Books, 1998.

Dr. Helen A. Derosis, *Women and Anxiety: A Step by Step Program for Managing Anxiety and Depression*, New York: Hatherleigh Co., Ltd., 1998.

Jerry Dorsman, *How to Quit Drugs for Good*, New York: Prima Communications, 1999.

——*How to Quit Drinking Without AA*, Rocklin: Prima Communications, 1997.

Dr. Samuel Dunkell, *Goodbye Insomnia, Hello Sleep*, New York: Dell Publishing Co., Inc., 1996.

Dr. John Eades, *The Seventh Floor Ain't Too High For Angels To Fly*, Deerfield Beach: Health Communications, Inc., 1995.

Eva Edelman, *Natural Healing for Schizophrenia and Other Common Mental Disorders*, Eugene: Borage Books, 1998.

Norman Ford, *Sleep RX, 75 Proven Ways to Get a Good Night's Sleep*, Saddle River: Prentice Hall, 1994.

Dr. Lynne Freeman, *Panic Free: Eliminate Anxiety and Panic Attacks Without Drugs and Take Control of Your Life*, Denver: Arden Books, 1999.

Dr. James Gordon, *Manifesto For A New Medicine: Your Guide to Healing Partnerships and the Wise Use of Alternative Therapies*, Reading: Addison Wesley Longman, Inc., 1996.

Letha Hadady, *Asian Health Secrets: The Complete Guide to Asian Herbal Medicine*, New York: Crown Publishing Group, 1996.

Dr. Abram Hoffer and Dr. Morton Walker, *Smart Nutrients: A Guide to Nutrients That Can Prevent and Reverse Senility*, Wayne: Avery Publishing, 1994.

S. F. Hotze, *Hormones, Health, and Happiness*. Houston, TX: Forrest Publishing, 2005.

Dharma Singh Khalsa, *Brain Longevity: The Breakthrough Medical Program That Improves Your Mind and Memory*, New York: Warner Books, 1997.

Michael Lapchick, *The Label Reader's Pocket Dictionary of Food Additives: A Comprehensive Quick Reference Guide to More Than 250 of Today's Most Common Food Additives*, New York: John Wiley & Sons, 1993.

M. Lesser and C. Kapklein, *The Brain Chemistry Diet*. New York: G.P. Putnam's Sons, 2002.

Jay Lombard, *The Brain Wellness Plan: Breakthrough Medical, Nutritional and Immune-Boosting Therapies*, New York: Kensington Publishing Corp., 1998.

Joan Matthews-Larson et al, *Seven Weeks to Emotional Healing: Proven Natural Formulas for Eliminating Anxiety, Depression, Anger, and Fatigue from Your Life*, New York: Ballantine Publishing Group, 1999.

——*Seven Weeks to Sobriety*, New York: Ballantine, 1992.

Michael Norden, *Beyond Prozac: Brain-Toxic Lifestyles, Natural Antidotes & New Generation Antidepressants*, New York: Regan Books, 1995.

James Pearl, *Sleep Right in Five Nights*, New York: Quill, 1996.

Dr. Alan Pressman, *Integrative Medicine: The Patient's Essential Guide to Conventional and Complementary Treatments for More Than 300 Common Disorders*, New York: St. Martin's Press, 2000.

——*Ginkgo: Nature's Brain Booster*, New York: Avon, 1999.

——*The Complete Idiot's Guide to Alternative Medicine*, editor, New York: Alpha Books, 1999.

——*Glutathione: The Ultimate Antioxidant*, New York: St. Martin's Press, 1998.

——*The GSH Phenomenon: Nature's Most Powerful Antioxidant and Healing Agent*, New York: St. Martin's Press, 1997.

Peggy Ramunda, *You Mean I'm Not Lazy, Stupid or Crazy?!: A Self-Help Book for Adults With Attention Deficit Disorder*, New York: Scribner, 1995.

Valerie Davis Raskin, *When Words Are Not Enough: The Woman's Prescription for Depression and Anxiety*, New York: Broadway Books, 1997.

Dr. Judyth Reichenberg-Ullman, Prozac-Free: *Homeopathic Medicine for Depression, Anxiety, and Other Mental and Emotional Problems*, Rocklin: Prima Pub, 1999.

——*Ritalin Free Kids: Safe and Effective Homeopathic Medicine for ADD and Other Behavioral and Learning Problems* (with Robert Ullman and Edward Chapman), Rocklin: Prima, 1996.

Joel Robertson, *Natural Prozac: Learning to Release your Body's Own Anti-Depressants*, New York: Harper Collins, 1997.

Sherry Rogers, *Depression: Cured at Last!*, Sarasota: SK Publishing, 1997.

Ethan Russo, ed., *Handbook of Psychotropic Herbs: A Scientific Analysis of Herbal Remedies for Psychiatric Conditions, with Case Studies*, Binghamton: Haworth Herbal Press, 2000.

Dr. Judith Sachs, *Break the Stress Cycle!: 10 Steps to Reducing Stress for Women*, Holbrook: Adams Media, 1998.

——*Nature's Prozac: Natural Therapies and Techniques to Rid Yourself of Anxiety, Depression, Panic and Stress*, Englewood Cliffs: Prentice Hall, 1997.

Ray Sahelian, *New Memory Boosters: Natural Supplements That Enhance Mind, Memory and Mood*, Thomas Dunne Books, 2000.

——*5-HTP: Nature's Serotonin Solution*, Garden City Park: Avery, 1998.

——*Kava: The Miracle Anti-Anxiety Herb*, New York: St. Martin's, 1998.

——*Pregnenolone: Nature's Feel Good Hormone*, Garden City Park: Avery, 1997.

——*DHEA: A Practical Guide*, Garden City Park: Avery, 1996.

Alexander Schauss, *Anorexia and Bulimia: A Natural Approach to the Deadly Eating Disorders*, New Canaan: Keats, 1997.

Karyn Seroussi and Bernard Rimland, Ph.D., *Unraveling the Mystery of Autism and Pervasive Developmental Disorder: A Mother's Story of Research and Recovery*, New York: Simon and Schuster, 2000.

Dr. Lendon Smith, *Feed Your Body Right*, New York: M. Evans & Co., 1995.

——*Feed Yourself Right*, New York: McGraw-Hill, c1983.

——*Feed Your Kids Right*, New York: McGraw-Hill, c1979.

James & Nancy Strohecker, eds. *Natural Healing For Depression: Solutions From the World's Great Health Traditions and Practitioners*, New York: Perigee Books, 1999.

Dr. Jacob Teitelbaum, *From Fatigued To Fantastic*, New York: Avery Pub., 1996.

Dr. Lynda Toth, *Why Can't I Remember?: Reversing Normal Memory Loss*, New York: Avery Pub., 1999.

Dr. Melvyn R. Werbach, *Nutritional Influences on Illness: A Sourcebook of Clinical Research*, 2nd ed., Tarzana: Third Line Press, 1993.

Bruce Wiseman, *Psychiatry: The Ultimate Betrayal*, Los Angeles: Freedom Pub., 1995.

G. D. Young, *Pregnenolone: A Radical New Approach to Health, Longevity, and Emotional Well-Being.* Salem, UT: Essential Science Publishing, 2001.

Dr. Jonathan Zeuss, *The Wisdom of Depression: A Guide to Understanding and Curing Depression Using Natural Medicine*, New York: Harmony Books, 1998.

——*The Natural Prozac Program: How to Use St. John's Wort, the Antidepressant Herb*, New York: Three Rivers Press, 1997.

Marcia Zimmerman, *The ADD Nutrition Solution: A Drug-Free Thirty-Day Plan*, New York: Holt, 1999.

Suggested Websites

www.garynull.com (news, reports, documents, activism, resources)

www.thenutritionreporter.com

www.healthy.net

www.healthfinder.gov (government portal)

www.noaw.com (Living with Schizophrenia)

www.naturopathic.org

lpi.oregonstate.edu (Linus Pauling Institute)

www.orthomed.org

www.ceri.com (Cognitive Enhancement Research Institute)

www.latitudes.org

www.holisticmed.com (information, chats, Q&As, listed by disorders)

www.futurehealth.org

www.somethingfishy.org (Eating Disorders Shared Awareness)

www.healthyideas.com

www.alternativementalhealth.com

www.healthyplace.com

www.recoverforever.com

www.helpguide.org/mental

exchange.healthwell.com

www.dorway.com

www.immunesupport.com

www.townsendletter.com

www.positivehealth.com

www.holisticonline.com

www.newsinferno.com

Appendix D

Autism and Vaccinations

■■■

Autism: Recent News and Opinion Pieces

Arthur Allen, "In Autism-Vaccine Case, RNA and a Prayer," *The Huffington Post*, June 18, 2007 http://www.huffingtonpost.com/arthur-allen/in-autismvaccine-case-r_b_52408.html

In Autism-Vaccine Case, RNA and a Prayer
by Arthur Allen

After the first week of a hearing into the claims of nearly 5,000 autistic children, the case of a tragically ill Arizona girl seemed to hinge on the legitimacy of an Irish laboratory's findings of measles virus fragments in the girl's GI tract.

Michelle Cedillo's complaint was framed, at the start, as a test case for the theory that two kinds of vaccines, one containing a weakened measles virus and the other the mercury-based preservative thimerosal, combined to cause autism in a subset of the thousands of children whose cases have been brought before the court.

The defense did not present a single expert on autism. On Monday, an experienced heavy metals toxicologist named H. Vasken Aposhian presented a theory of how thimerosal could have damaged the girl's immune system in a way that set her up for autism.

But none of Cedillo's other witnesses had much specialized knowledge in mercury or other metals, and the focus quickly shifted to the theory that the attenuated measles virus had created a persistent infection in her gut, causing a severe inflammation that resulted in brain damage and other injuries.

In order to win their case, it seems likely that Cedillos will have to convince the three special masters—the judges, in effect, in the special "vaccine court" at the U.S. Court of Claims—of the reliability of the witnesses' account that measles RNA was detected in her bowel and cerebrospinal fluid.

A biopsy from Cedillo's GI tract was sent in 2003 to Unigenetics, an Irish laboratory headed by Dr. John O'Leary, which reported finding the RNA. O'Leary and his colleagues had published a paper a year earlier that disclosed the discovery of measles RNA in the guts of several autistic children. (Measles virus and autism. O'Leary JJ, Uhlmann V, Wakefield AJ., Lancet. 2000 Aug 26;356(9231):772.)

The lab also was said to have found evidence of measles in spinal taps of autistic children, but those results were never published. Last year, two journal articles reported an inability to replicate the O'Leary lab's findings. There was also a negative turn of events for the MMR/vaccine damage claimants in the British vaccine court. In that court, the government pays for families to sue, but will only continue the funding when it believes the chance of success is greater than 50 percent. After an expert report commissioned by the British court found problems in Unigenetics' testing of the samples, all but two of the British cases were defunded.

In testimony that followed Aposhian this past week, five additional witnesses for Cedillo expressed full support for the Unigenetics findings. Those witnesses were gastroenterologist Arthur Krigsman, molecular biologist Karin Hepner, immunologist Vera Byers, virus immunologist Ronald C. Kennedy and Marcel Kinsbourne, a pediatric neurologist who has testified in vaccine court hundreds of times.

The defendant (called the respondent in vaccine court) in this case is the Department of Health and Human Services, which for the past 18 years has assumed responsibility for compensating the families of children damaged by vaccines. The Department of Justice represents HHS in the courtroom.

The Justice lawyers picked at the expertise of the witnesses and their source articles. They pointed out discrepancies in Dr. Byers' resume and problems Dr. Krigsman has had with the Texas medical board. However, they made little effort to refute Unigenetics' findings. It seemed clear, however, that that job would be left to some of the 12 respondent witnesses who are scheduled to testify next week.

The Cedillo family's argument for how vaccines hurt their child was presented most efficiently by Kennedy, a virus immunologist at Texas Tech University. He posited that the 112.5 millionths of a gram of thimerosal contained in six vaccines administered to Michelle during her first seven months of life had damaged her immune system. When she received an MMR vaccine at 16 months, shortly before Christmas 1995, the weakened vaccine virus lodged in her gut, causing an inflamed bowel and eventually damaging her brain.

Michelle is very ill. In addition to her autism she suffers from inflammatory bowel disease, a seizure disorder and chronic eye inflammations that have left her 90 percent blind. She was pushed into the courtroom in a wheelchair because arthritis has left her unsteady on her feet, her mother testified.

But the theory that vaccines caused all this pain and suffering is shaping up as a very hard sell. According to testimony in the trial, Michelle was a healthy baby prior to receiving the MMR vaccine. If the thimerosal she received had damaged her immune system prior to that, there were no manifestations of it. Michelle's parents first brought the case, in 1998, with a theory of damage from MMR. Thimerosal was tacked onto the claim, one of her attorneys said, after news accounts in 1999 of the Centers for Disease Control's request that the drug industry stop selling vaccines containing the preservative.

Perhaps one in 500,000 children who receives the MMR vaccination suffers a severe brain inflammation that can lead to lifelong mental disability—presumably including autism. The vaccine court has awarded several dozen such children over the past two decades. Michelle's parents might have brought their claim under this theory; according to her mother's testimony and medical records, she suffered an intermittent high fever, up to 106 degrees, and severe diarrhea following the shot.

However, before it agrees to compensate children for a so-called MMR encephalopathy, the court generally requires evidence that the child lost consciousness for an extended period following the shot. Michelle does not seem to have had a seizure or loss of consciousness. Though concerned about the fever, her mother did not bring Michelle to the doctor until 10 days after it first spiked.

According to Mrs. Cedillo's testimony, her daughter became less responsive and stopped talking during that acute illness. In a heartbreaking home video shot in mid-February 1996 that was projected in the courtroom, Michelle is seen sitting in a toy caboose, flapping her arms. She ignores the entreaties of her mother and grandfather. A year later, she was diagnosed with autism.

Aposhian, who has more than 100 publications on heavy metal poisoning to his name, is hard of hearing and was obstreperous at times during his cross-examination on Monday. For example, he insisted that in vitro studies were nearly always reproducible in animals, and that animal studies were nearly always reliable models for human effects. This is not a belief to which most toxicologists would subscribe.

Also under cross-examination, Aposhian said that he was not an immunologist and that he had composed his theory of thimerosal-induced immunological damage "three or four weeks ago."

When Matanoski tried to get Aposhian to acknowledge that most if not all cases of clinical mercury poisoning in the past had involved doses hundreds or thousands of times higher than what was administered to children in vaccines, Aposhian insisted that dose was not necessarily important.

"[Toxicologists] no longer believe that the dose makes the poison," he said. Far more important was the developmental stage of the child when the mercury was administered, and his or her genetic susceptibility.

During the mid- to late-1990s, some children received nearly three times as much thimerosal in their vaccinations than did children a generation earlier. The cumulative amount surpassed EPA guidelines, according to some interpretations.

Interestingly, though, because she received some of her immunizations in combined shots, the total thimerosal injected into Michelle Cedillo was only about 40 millionths of a gram more than a child would have received 30 years ago, well before the supposed "autism epidemic" began.

The findings of half a dozen epidemiological studies that have showed no link between thimerosal administration and autism diagnosis do not necessarily count for much in this courtroom. Nor do data that show autism diagnoses continue to grow in California in cohorts of children who got little or not thimerosal in their vaccines.

But Aposhian's theory of harm, based largely on in vitro and animal studies of mercury, seems very thin. Next week's panel of experts, which includes two autism doctors, two pediatric neurologists and experts in all the other relevant fields, will certainly have much to say about it.

Clare Dyer, "American court to hear case on MMR vaccine," *The Guardian*,   June   9,   2007
http://society.guardian.co.uk/health/story/0,,2099016,00.html

American court to hear case on MMR vaccine
by Clare Dyer, legal editor

Michelle Cedillo, a 12-year-old girl with autism from Arizona, will make legal history on Monday when her case becomes the first to go before a court to consider whether the MMR vaccine can cause the condition. The case before the US federal court of claims in Washington will reignite the controversy over the triple vaccine for measles, mumps and rubella.

Andrew Wakefield, a British gastroenterologist, caused an international scare over the vaccine in 1998 when, at a press conference in London to publicize his research on links between the measles virus, autism and bowel disease, he called for the MMR vaccine to be replaced by single vaccines.

Hundreds of parents of autistic children in the UK have been trying for 15 years to bring a group action over the vaccine to trial but their hopes of compensation were dealt a final blow yesterday, when a high court judge disbanded the action. Their case had been fatally wounded when the legal services commission withdrew legal aid funding in 2004 after spending £15m. To add to their chagrin, this week Mr. Justice Keith ruled at the high court that scientific reports obtained by the drug companies who were fighting their claims could be released to the US government, which is defending the cases there.

In the US, 4,800 claims have been brought against the government under its scheme for vaccine damage compensation. In three test cases, lawyers for the parents will put forward three theories: that autism was caused either by the MMR vaccine, or by other childhood vaccines containing the mercury preservative thimerosol, or by a combination of thimerosol and MMR.

Sherri Tenpenny, "Vaccinations and the Right to Refuse," NewsWith-Views.com, September 14, 2005. http://www.newswithviews.com/Ten-penny/sherri1.htm

Vaccinations and the Right to Refuse
by Dr. Sherri Tenpenny, DO

By way of introduction, I like to tell people I'm a physician by training and a compulsive researcher by inclination. To be specific, I've invested more than seven-thousand hours investigating the under-reported health hazards associated with vaccinations, along with the attendant ethical and legal issues.

What started as a fairly modest research exercise has turned into a second full-time career. I've discussed vaccination hazards on more than 50 radio and television programs, addressed hundreds of professional, political, and trade groups, produced two informational DVDs, and authored numerous articles for both print publications and Internet sites. In addition, I'm scheduled to produce two books relating to the subject over the next year.

The risk of vaccination must be considered as important—and potentially more serious—than the risk of a childhood disease. Years of experience and thousands of hours of research have lead to conclusions that are not uniformly accepted: the importance of legally ensuring vaccine exemptions in each State and the right to refuse Nationally mandated vaccinations.

Vaccination is a procedure and vaccines are medications. . . . and both have risks and side effects which are often ignored by the media and, worse, by many in the medical profession. As a population, we are against being forcibly medicated. We value our right to choose what is done to our bodies.

Humans are intrinsically healthy and tend to remain so if they are given nutritious, non-GMO foods, fresh air, and clean water. We have been blessed with God-given protective barriers against infectious diseases, including our skin and immune system.

Knowing that these facts are true for all members of the human species, how did we come to embrace the idea that injecting solutions of chemically-treated, inactivated viruses, parts of bacteria, traces of animal tissue and heavy metals, such as mercury and aluminum, was a reasonable strategy for keeping human beings—babies, children and adults—healthy?

If a "dirty bomb" exposed a large segment of US citizens simultaneously to Hepatitis B, Hepatitis A, tetanus, pertussis, diphtheria, Haemophilus influenza B, three strains of polio viruses, 3 strains of influenza viruses, measles, mumps, and rubella viruses, the chickenpox virus, and 7 strains of Streptococcus bacteria, we would declare a national emergency. We would call it an "extreme act of BIOTERRORISM." The public outcry would be immense and our government would act accordingly.

And yet, those are the very organisms that we inject through vaccines into our babies and our small children, with immature, underdeveloped immune systems. Many are given all at the same time. But instead of bioterrorism, we call it "protection." Reflect a moment on that irony.

Vaccine injuries are reported to be "rare," but only because very few reactions are "accepted" by the Centers for Disease Control (CDC), the Institutes of Medicine (IOM) and the Food and Drug Administration (FDA) as being caused by vaccines. I have frequently said that when a vaccine is given, and a bad reaction occurs, "ANYTHING BUT" the vaccine is "blamed" for the reaction. Here is a direct quote from the 6th edition of Epidemiology & Prevention of Vaccine-Preventable Diseases called "The Pink Book," published by the CDC:

> There is no distinct syndrome from vaccine administration, and therefore, many *temporally associated* adverse events probably represent background illness rather than illness caused by the vaccine…The DTaP may stimulate or precipitate inevitable symptoms of underlying CNS disorder, such as seizures, infantile spasms, epilepsy or SIDS. By chance alone, some of these cases will seem to be temporally related to DTaP.

I have to admit, the first time I read that, I cried. Instead of blaming the vaccine for causing the problem, we blame the children for somehow being defective and the "defect" shows up after we inject them.

Another example of not blaming the vaccine for a reaction comes directly from the National Vaccine Injury compensation table. Only a handful of injuries are covered by this program; if your injury isn't on the table, you don't qualify for compensation. The government says "there is no proof"—no causal association—that the problem that was experienced, the seizure, for example, was caused by the vaccine.

And timing of the injury is important too. For example, the Injury Compensation Table states that if the baby manifests the symptoms of encephalopathy—or brain swelling—within 3 days of being given a DTaP shot, the injury is probably related to the vaccine. If the complication develops on the 4th day—or the 5th, 6th or 7th day—it is not considered to be "causally related" and the parent is ineligible to apply for compensation.

Sort of like saying the black and blue foot you have today had nothing to do with the frozen turkey you dropped on it last week, because the discoloration didn't show up within the time allowed to "prove causation."

Side effects and complications from vaccines are considered inconsequential because their numbers are supposedly "statistically insignificant." This conclusion comes from epidemiological research involving large numbers of participants and has nothing to do with the individual person. Population-based conclusions go against one of the most basic tenants of all of medicine: to treat each person as an individual and believe them when they tell you something went wrong after a vaccine.

A "one in a million" reaction may be rare, but if you are "the one," it is 100% to you.

And even if the one-in-a-million reactions are considered "rare" by the CDC, the health care costs associated with those "rare" reactions are not insignificant. Here's one example.

One recognized complication of the flu shot is a condition called Gullian-Barre Syndrome (GBS). Guillian-Barre is disorder characterized by progressive paralysis, beginning in the feet and advancing up the body, often causing paralysis of the diaphragm and breathing muscles within a matter of hours or days.

Nearly all patients with GBS are hospitalized because of paralysis. The prognosis of GBS varies. Up to 13 percent die and 20 percent more are left significantly disabled, defined, for these purposes, as unable to work for at least a year.

The CDC reports this side effect to be "rare, perhaps 1 or 2 per million flu shots given." Using the numbers determined from a variety of sources—including medical journals and government documents, it can reasonably be assumed that the flu shot may cause 40 cases of GBS per year.

The Healthcare Cost and Utilization Project (HCUP) database reveals that the average hospital charge per person for GBS is nearly $70,000. Add another $40,000 per person for rehabilitation costs after months of paralysis. Therefore the cost to healthcare for this "rare" complication can be approximated to be at least $4.4 million.

This conservative estimate doesn't include lost wages, reduced standards of living for patients who returned to work but had to take a lower paying job because of their illness. And of course, there is no price tag for the "human cost" of being paralyzed and away from your family for months.

The advantageous cost-benefit relationship is one of the main rationalizations given for supporting the national vaccination program at all levels, infants through the elderly. But has anyone seriously analyzed the cost of caring for vaccine complications?

This example of Guillian-Barre represents the cost of just ONE complication. What if the costs for healthcare from all acknowledged side effects were calculated and added to the cost of the National Vaccination programs? What if we add in the parent-observed complications, such as refractory seizures?

Are we getting our money's worth financially? Are we getting our money's worth in terms of a "healthier" nation?

What about other not-so-obvious costs incurred by vaccine mandates—increased taxes and increased health insurance premiums to pay for the shots? Increased administrative costs to track that they have been given? There are many others, but I'll stop there.

There are three things to take away from this introduction:

1. Low infection rates and high vaccination rates should not be the cornerstone of our public health policy. Vaccine reactions should not be discounted, whatever their numbers. Further, the true cost-benefit of the vaccination program must be considered, and what has been presented is barely the tip of the iceberg.

2. Parents, and all adults, must retain their right to refuse vaccines. They are not without risk, and those "rare" complications can result in significant costs, both economic and in terms of human life.

3. Children, and all adults, who refuse to be vaccinated are being discriminated against. They are losing their rights:

    a. Rights and access to a public education.

    b. Rights to access to health care, as doctors discharge them as patients.

    c. Rights to food because often moms on Medicaid are refused food stamps.

These rights—including the right to refuse—must be ensured.

When we give government the power to make medical decisions for us—and force us to vaccinate and medicate our children in the name "health" and "policy" and for "the greater good" we, in essence, accept that the state owns our bodies, and, apparently, our children.

Sherri J. Tenpenny, D.O. is the President and Medical Director of OsteoMed II, a clinic located in the Cleveland area that provides conventional, alternative, and preventive medicine. Dr. Tenpenny has lectured at Cleveland State University and Case Western Reserve Medical School on topics related to alternative health. Nationally, she is a regular guest on many different radio and television talk shows, including "Your Health" aired on the Family Network. She has published articles in magazines, newspapers and internet sites, including, Redflagsdaily.com, Mercola.com and Mothering.com. She has presented at the National Vaccine Information Center's annual meeting and at several international conferences on autism. Dr. Tenpenny is a graduate of the University of Toledo in Toledo, Ohio. She received her medical training at Kirksville College of Osteopathic Medicine in Kirksville, Missouri. Dr. Tenpenny is Board Certified in Emergency Medicine and Osteopathic Manipulative Medicine. Dr. Tenpenny is respected as one of the country's most knowledgeable and outspoken physicians regarding the impact of vaccines on health. Website: www.nmaseminars.com

---

Lorraine Fraser, "Revealed: more evidence to challenge the safety of MMR," *Telegraph,* **June 15, 2002. http://www.telegraph.co.uk/news/main.jhtml?xml=/news/2002/06/16/nmmr16.xml**

Revealed: more evidence to challenge the safety of MMR
by Lorraine Fraser

Scientists have found new evidence to support fears that the MMR vaccine is causing children to develop autism and bowel disease, The Telegraph can reveal today.

Specialists from Trinity College, Dublin, have detected the strain of measles virus used in the MMR jab in tissue samples from the inflamed intestines of 12 children, who each developed autism after receiving the injection.

The results will add further weight to claims that MMR may be responsible for a rapid rise in autism in children over the past decade.

The Department of Health has repeatedly dismissed concerns about its safety, saying epidemiological studies have failed to find a link to autism. It has infuriated worried parents by refusing to allow the alternative of single vaccines to be prescribed on the NHS.

The work was carried out by Prof John O'Leary, a pathologist with a record of important discoveries in the field of virology. Although the finding does not prove that the MRR jab caused autism and bowel disease in the children, it raises urgent questions about the vaccine's role in their condition.

None of the children concerned had shown any sign of disease beforehand. The discovery comes days after the Government seized on a new study to bolster its claims that the MMR vaccine is safe.

The review, from a commercial company which lists the Department of Health as one of its clients, did not, however, consider work published since 1998 by scientists concerned about MMR.

Prof O'Leary's results have been made public in a precis of a scientific presentation released ahead of a meeting of the Pathological Society of Great Britain and Ireland next month. It was greeted with alarm by parents last night.

Jackie Fletcher, of the parents' group JABS, said the findings had profound implications and must be taken seriously. "We have parents shouting that these problems are occurring and what do the Government and health chiefs do—they keep their heads buried in old reports not designed to identify these problems," she said. "No one is listening. Why?"

Ann Hewitt, whose son Thomas, eight, has severe autism and bowel problems, learned earlier this year that Dr. O'Leary had found measles virus in the boy's gut. She and scores of others who received the same news now want to know what is going on.

The new results follow a study by Prof O'Leary and his colleagues, reported in February, in which they found measles virus of unknown origin in gut biopsies from 75 of 91 autistic children with bowel problems.

Measles virus was found in only five of 70 normal youngsters. The team now claims that the new study corroborates their earlier work linking measles virus with the condition and "indicates the origins of the virus to be vaccine strain."

Last night Visceral, a charity set up to fund research into autism and bowel disease, called for MMR to be suspended until studies establish just what the vaccine-strain virus is doing. MMR, which contains live measles mumps and rubella virus, was launched in the UK in 1988 and is given to infants at 12-15 months and four years.

The samples tested in Dublin were from some of nearly 200 youngsters diagnosed with developmental disorder and "new variant inflammatory bowel disease" by doctors at the Royal Free Hospital, in London, where Dr. Andrew Wakefield worked until he was ousted last December.

The controversy over MMR and autism began four years ago when Dr. Wakefield and his colleagues reported in *The Lancet* on 12 children with autistic problems and bowel disease and revealed that the parents of eight of them had said their children regressed developmentally after receiving the MMR jab.

While the genetic code of the strain of measles virus used in MMR differs only minutely from that of the virus responsible for natural infections, Prof O'Leary and his colleagues were able to use a commercially produced molecular probe to distinguish the two.

The probe was designed to detect a single difference in the genetic code of the viruses and to give off a fluorescent signal when it does so. The MMR row became so heated this year that Tony Blair, the Prime Minister—who has refused to say whether his two-year-old son Leo has had the MMR jab—accused Dr. Wakefield and the media of "scaremongering" on the issue.

The chief medical officer, Professor Liam Donaldson, has indicated he would rather resign than abandon official policy on the three-in-one vaccine.

Dr. Wakefield said last night: "Prof O'Leary and colleagues have now provided what may prove to be the most important piece of evidence to date in the case against the MMR vaccine. Parents must at the very least be given a choice of single vaccines.

"Not to do so in the face of these data and all the other evidence we have now published would be negligent in the extreme. It is not acceptable to assume that this vaccine virus is an innocent bystander if your concern is for the safety of the children."

The Department of Health said that it had no plans to review the use of MMR. "This study, if true, does not prove that MMR causes the condition of autism just because the virus is present in the gut. Critical will be independent testing of the teams' samples, which has long been awaited," said a spokesman.

Lorraine Fraser, "Anti-MMR doctor is forced out," *Telegraph*, December 2, 2001. http://www.telegraph.co.uk/news/main.jhtml;jsessionid=U4JZSL0OEVMS BQFIQMFCFFWAVCBQYIV0?xml=/news/2001/12/02/nmmr02.xml

Anti-MMR doctor is forced out
by Lorraine Fraser, Medical Correspondent

The specialist who first raised concerns about the safety of MMR vaccinations has been forced out of his job, *The Telegraph* can reveal.

Andrew Wakefield, a consultant gastroenterologist whose research has linked the vaccine to autism and bowel disease in children, said last night that he had been asked to resign because of his work.

"I have been asked to go because my research results are unpopular," said Dr. Wakefield, an academic at the Royal Free Hospital Medical School in London whose research into the triple measles, mumps and rubella vaccination has caused controversy.

"I did not wish to leave but I have agreed to stand down in the hope that my going will take the political pressure off my colleagues and allow them to get on with the job of looking after the many sick children we have seen.

"They have not sacked me. They cannot; I have not done anything wrong. I have no intention of stopping my investigations."

He has been testing the theory that measles virus from MMR vaccine can colonise the bowel of susceptible children, producing inflammatory bowel disease, which then, via a disruption of the chemical balance in the body and the brain, leads to autism.

Although the specialist admits he has not published proof, he has infuriated ministers by suggesting that the three component vaccines should be given separately.

Dr. Wakefield's departure comes a month after he was made a Fellow of the Royal College of Pathologists in recognition of his research work.

He left his £50,000 job on Friday after 14 years having been told that his ideas were "unwelcome" at University College London, which controls the Royal Free.

The news will please vaccination programme officials in the Public Health Laboratory Service. They have ridiculed his research and still insist that MMR, recommended officially for every child at around 13 months and again at four years, is safe.

He added last night: "I am very concerned that I have been unable to gain any guarantee from the hospital that the children we have already seen, and who need to be seen, will be looked after."

Parents of autistic children involved in his research expressed their anger last night. Some demanded reassurances that the Royal Free Hospital will continue treating their children.

Dr. Wakefield's research has made him a pariah of the medical establishment. As a result, the World Health Organisation felt obliged to announce its support of the MMR vaccine.

The Government has played down concerns since he published a paper in The Lancet in 1998, reporting that he and colleagues had identified a hitherto unknown combination of bowel damage and autism in children whose parents said their previously normal children fell ill after MMR.

The row became a crisis last January when Dr. Wakefield told The Telegraph that he had seen almost 170 children with a similar story and claimed that the Department of Health's contention that MMR had been proven to be safe did not "hold up."

That number, has now reached almost 200. Pressure on the children's gastroenterology unit is so great that it's waiting list risks breaking the NHS's 18-month limit. Parents have appealed to Tony Blair to give it more funds.

The Royal Free Hospital Medical School was unavailable for comment last night.

Lorraine Fraser, "MMR doctor links 170 cases of autism to vaccine," *Telegraph*, June 19, 2001. http://www.telegraph.co.uk/news/main.jhtml?xml=/news/2001/01/21/nmmr21.xml

MMR doctor links 170 cases of autism to vaccine
by Lorraine Fraser, Medical Correspondent

The consultant who first raised concerns about MMR vaccinations has disclosed to The Telegraph that he has identified nearly 170 cases of a new syndrome of autism and bowel disease in children who have had the triple-dose injection.

Andrew Wakefield, a consultant gastroenterologist at the Royal Free Hospital in London, said that in the "majority" of cases parents had documentary evidence that their child's physical and mental decline had followed the vaccination.

Professor Wakefield said: "Last week in our clinic we saw nine or 10 new children with exactly the same story, referred by jobbing paediatricians from around the country who said, 'This child developed normally, had a reaction to MMR and is now autistic.'"

In his first public comments since the row erupted in 1998, when he reported on 12 cases, Professor Wakefield said that he remained seriously concerned by the safety of the vaccine, despite reassurances from the Department of Health.

He said: "The department says that the safety of MMR has been proven. The argument is untenable. It cannot be substantiated by the science. That is not only my opinion but increasingly the view of healthcare professionals and the public.

He said: "Tests have revealed time and time again that we are dealing with a new phenomenon. The Department of Health's contention that MMR has been proven to be safe by study after study after study just doesn't hold up. Frankly, it is not an honest appraisal of the science and it relegates the scientific issues to the bottom of the barrel in favour of winning a propaganda war."

The doctor, who was fiercely attacked by health officials for voicing his doubts three years ago, said in an exclusive interview that he felt driven to break his silence because of the accumulating evidence. His remarks will infuriate the Government and sharpen the dilemma of parents over whether to have children innoculated with MMR.

It emerged last month that a rising number of doctors and nurses were worried about giving second doses of the vaccine, and pressure is growing for its separation into its three component vaccinations, spread over three years. In his 1998 article in *The Lancet*, Professor Wakefield reported finding a devastating combination of bowel disease and autism in 12 children.

His revelation that that figure has reached almost 170 cases will shock parents and doctors and add pressure on the Government to justify its vaccination policy. This month Dr. David Salisbury, the head of the Government's immunisation programme, insisted that MMR was safe.

The vaccine, which contains live measles, mumps and rubella virus, has been given to millions of children in the UK since its introduction in 1988 but the take-up rate has fallen sharply since Dr. Wakefield made his original claims.

Ten days ago health chiefs warned parents that Britain could face a measles outbreak unless more had their children vaccinated with MMR. Professor Wakefield said, however, that if an outbreak were to erupt it would be the fault of the health department, which had "failed to address the safety issues."

The doctor and his colleagues are testing the hypothesis that the measles virus from the vaccine can lodge in the gut of susceptible children, damaging the bowel and causing autism, and that the addition of the mumps virus makes that more likely.

Autism: Abstracts of Recent Scientific Research

Colonic CD8 and gamma delta T-cell infiltration with epithelial damage in children with autism. Furlano RI, Anthony A, Day R, Brown A, McGarvey L, Thomson MA, Davies SE, Berelowitz M, Forbes A, Wakefield AJ, Walker-Smith JA, Murch SH.—University Department of Paediatric Gastroenterology, the Inflammatory Bowel Diseases Study Group, Royal Free and University College School of Medicine, London, United Kingdom. *Journal of Pediatrics*. 2001 Mar;138(3):366–72.

OBJECTIVES: We have reported colitis with ileal lymphoid nodular hyperplasia (LNH) in children with regressive autism. The aims of this study were to characterize this lesion and determine whether LNH is specific for autism. METHODS: Ileo-colonoscopy was performed in 21 consecutively evaluated children with autistic spectrum disorders and bowel symptoms. Blinded comparison was made with 8 children with histologically normal ileum and colon, 10 developmentally normal children with ileal LNH, 15 with Crohn's disease, and 14 with ulcerative colitis. Immunohistochemistry was performed for cell lineage and functional markers, and histochemistry was performed for glycosaminoglycans and basement membrane thickness. RESULTS: Histology demonstrated lymphocytic colitis in the autistic children, less severe than classical inflammatory bowel disease. However, basement membrane thickness and mucosal gamma delta cell density were significantly increased above those of all other groups including patients with inflammatory bowel disease. CD8(+) density and intraepithelial lymphocyte numbers were higher than those in the Crohn's disease, LNH, and normal control groups; and CD3 and plasma cell density and crypt proliferation were higher than those in normal and LNH control groups. Epithelial, but not lamina propria, glycosaminoglycans were disrupted. However, the epithelium was HLA-DR(-), suggesting a predominantly T(H)2 response.

INTERPRETATION: Immunohistochemistry confirms a distinct lymphocytic colitis in autistic spectrum disorders in which the epithelium appears particularly affected. This is consistent with increasing evidence for gut epithelial dysfunction in autism.

Does the MMR vaccine and secretin or its receptor share an antigenic epitope? Mehta BK, Munir KM.—Memorial University of Newfoundland, Newfoundland, Canada. *Medical Hypotheses*. 2003 May;60(5):650–3.

In a subgroup of children with autism-spectrum like conditions symptoms seem to appear as a 'regression' (in normal development). It has been postulated that the onset of such autistic symptoms may involve an autoimmune response against the central nervous system and that the antigenic determinant could possibly be gastrointestinal in origin. It has been suggested that the presence of the measles virus and 'autistic enterocolitis' demonstrates the possibility that the MMR triple vaccine may be mediating the inflammation with possible production of antibodies against the virus containing vaccine. Such an antibody may share antigenic determinant to molecules found in the gut. We propose that this may be secretin or its receptor, found in the gut as well as in the central nervous system. The antibody response to the gut may also conceivably occur in the brain at a critical time in development. The modulation of development by secretin may be a static event possibly occurring at a specific time in early childhood development and if it involves an autoimmune response then a disruption in development may result. These hypothesized events can only occur if the MMR vaccine shares antigenic determinants that resemble secretin or any of its receptor types and remains to be studied.

Abnormal measles-mumps-rubella antibodies and CNS autoimmunity in children with autism. Singh VK, Lin SX, Newell E, Nelson C.—Department of Biology and Biotechnology Center, Utah State University, Logan, Utah 84322, USA. singhvk@cc.usu.edu. *Journal of Biomedical Science.* 2002 Jul–Aug;9(4):359–64.

Autoimmunity to the central nervous system (CNS), especially to myelin basic protein (MBP), may play a causal role in autism, a neurodevelopmental disorder. Because many autistic children harbor elevated levels of measles antibodies, we conducted a serological study of measles-mumps-rubella (MMR) and MBP autoantibodies. Using serum samples of 125 autistic children and 92 control children, antibodies were assayed by ELISA or immunoblotting methods. ELISA analysis showed a significant increase in the level of MMR antibodies in autistic children. Immunoblotting analysis revealed the presence of an unusual MMR antibody in 75 of 125 (60%) autistic sera but not in control sera. This antibody specifically detected a protein of 73-75 kD of MMR. This protein band, as analyzed with monoclonal antibodies, was immunopositive for measles hemagglutinin (HA) protein but not for measles nucleoprotein and rubella or mumps viral proteins. Thus the MMR antibody in autistic sera detected measles HA protein, which is unique to the measles subunit of the vaccine. Furthermore, over 90% of MMR antibody-positive autistic sera were also positive for MBP autoantibodies, suggesting a strong association between MMR and CNS autoimmunity in autism. Stemming from this evidence, we suggest that an inappropriate antibody response to MMR, specifically the measles component thereof, might be related to pathogenesis of autism.

Elevated levels of measles antibodies in children with autism. Singh VK, Jensen RL.—Department of Biology and Biotechnology Center, Utah State University, Logan, Utah, USA. *Pediatric Neurology.* 2003 Apr;28(4):292–4.

Virus-induced autoimmunity may play a causal role in autism. To examine the etiologic link of viruses in this brain disorder, we conducted a serologic study of measles virus, mumps virus, and rubella virus. Viral antibodies were measured by enzyme-linked immunosorbent assay in the serum of autistic children, normal children, and siblings of autistic children. The level of measles antibody, but not mumps or rubella antibodies, was significantly higher in autistic children as compared with normal children (P = 0.003) or siblings of autistic children (P <or= 0.0001). Furthermore, immunoblotting of measles vaccine virus revealed that the antibody was directed against a protein of approximately 74 kd molecular weight. The antibody to this antigen was found in 83% of autistic children but not in normal children or siblings of autistic children. Thus autistic children have a hyperimmune response to measles virus, which in the absence of a wild type of measles infection might be a sign of an abnormal immune reaction to the vaccine strain or virus reactivation.

Association between thimerosal-containing vaccine and autism. Hviid A, Stellfeld M, Wohlfahrt J, Melbye M.—Danish Epidemiology Science Centre, Department of Epidemiology Research, Statens Serum Institut, Copenhagen, Denmark. aii@ssi.dk. *The Journal of the American Medical Association.* 2003 Oct 1;290(13):1763–6.

CONTEXT: Mercuric compounds are nephrotoxic and neurotoxic at high doses. Thimerosal, a preservative used widely in vaccine formulations, contains ethylmercury. Thus it has been suggested that childhood vaccination with thimerosal-containing vaccine could be causally related to neurodevelopmental disorders such as autism. OBJECTIVE: To determine whether vaccination with a thimerosal-containing vaccine is associated with development of autism. DESIGN, SETTING, AND PARTICIPANTS: Population-based cohort study of all children born in Denmark from January 1, 1990, until December 31, 1996 (N = 467 450) comparing children vaccinated with a thimerosal-containing vaccine with children vaccinated with a thimerosal-free formulation of the same vaccine. MAIN OUTCOME MEASURES: Rate ratio (RR) for autism and other autistic-spectrum disorders, including trend with dose of ethylmercury. RESULTS: During 2 986 654 person-years, we identified 440 autism cases and 787 cases of other autistic-spectrum disorders. The risk of autism and other autistic-spectrum disorders did not differ significantly between children vaccinated with thimerosal-containing vaccine and children vaccinated with thimerosal-free vaccine (RR, 0.85 [95% confidence interval [CI], 0.60-1.20] for autism; RR, 1.12 [95% CI, 0.88-1.43] for other autistic-spectrum disorders). Furthermore, we found no evidence of a dose-response association (increase in RR per 25 microg of ethylmercury, 0.98 [95% CI, 0.90-1.06] for autism and 1.03 [95% CI, 0.98-1.09] for other autistic-spectrum disorders). CONCLUSION: The results do not support a causal relationship between childhood vaccination with thimerosal-containing vaccines and development of autistic-spectrum disorders.

MMR vaccine and autism: an update of the scientific evidence. DeStefano F, Thompson WW.—National Immunization Program, Centers for Disease Control and Prevention, 1600 Clifton Road, Mailstop E61, Atlanta, Georgia 30333, USA. fdestefano@cdc.gov. *Expert Review of Vaccines.* **2004 Feb;3(1):19–22.**

An hypothesis published in 1998 suggested that measles-mumps-rubella vaccine may cause autism as a result of persistent measles virus infection of the gastrointestinal tract. Results of early studies were not supportive and in 2001 a review by the Institute of Medicine concluded that the evidence favors the rejection of a causal relationship at the population level between measles-mumps-rubella vaccine and autistic spectrum disorder. Studies published since the Institute of Medicine report have continued not to find an increased risk of autistic spectrum disorder associated with measles-mumps-rubella. The vaccine also has not been found to be associated with a unique syndrome of developmental regression and gastrointestinal disorders. The evidence now is convincing that the measles-mumps-rubella vaccine does not cause autism or any particular subtypes of autistic spectrum disorder.

A comparative evaluation of the effects of MMR immunization and mercury doses from thimerosal-containing childhood vaccines on the population prevalence of autism. Geier DA, Geier MR.—President, MedCon, Inc, Silver Spring, MD, USA. *Medical Science Monitor.* 2004 Mar;10(3):PI33-9. Epub 2004 Mar 1.

BACKGROUND: The purpose of the study was to evaluate the effects of MMR immunization and mercury from thimerosal-containing childhood vaccines on the prevalence of autism. MATERIAL/METHODS: Evaluations of the Biological Surveillance Summaries of the Centers for Disease Control and Prevention (CDC), the U.S. Department of Education datasets, and the CDC's yearly live birth estimates were undertaken RESULTS: It was determined that there was a close correlation between mercury doses from thimerosal—containing childhood vaccines and the prevalence of autism from the late 1980s through the mid-1990s. In contrast, there was a potential correlation between the number of primary pediatric measles-containing vaccines administered and the prevalence of autism during the 1980s. In addition, it was found that there were statistically significant odds ratios for the development of autism following increasing doses of mercury from thimerosal-containing vaccines (birth cohorts: 1985 and 1990-1995) in comparison to a baseline measurement (birth cohort: 1984). The contribution of thimerosal from childhood vaccines (>50% effect) was greater than MMR vaccine on the prevalence of autism observed in this study. CONCLUSIONS: The results of this study agree with a number of previously published studies. These studies have shown that there is biological plausibility and epidemiological evidence showing a direct relationship between increasing doses of mercury from thimerosal-containing vaccines and neurodevelopmental disorders, and measles-containing vaccines and serious neurological disorders. It is recommended that thimerosal be removed from all vaccines, and additional research be undertaken to produce a MMR vaccine with an improved safety profile.

Detection of Measles Virus Genomic RNA in Cerebrospinal Fluid of Children with Regressive Autism: a Report of Three Cases. JJ Bradstreet, M.D.; J El Dahr, M.D.; A Anthony, M.B., Ph.D.; JJ Kartzinel, M.D.; AJ Wakefield, M.B. *Journal of American Physicians and Surgeons*. Volume 9 Number 2 Summer 2004.

In light of encephalopathy presenting as autistic regression (autistic encephalopathy, AE) closely following measles-mumps-rubella (MMR) vaccination, three children underwent cerebrospinal fluid (CSF) assessments including studies for measles virus (MV). All three children had concomitant onset of gastrointestinal (GI) symptoms and had already had MV genomic RNA detected in biopsies of ileal lymphoid nodular hyperplasia (LNH). Presence of MV Fusion (F) gene was examined by TaqMan real-time quantitative polymerase chain reaction (RT-PCR) in cases and control CSF samples. The latter were obtained from three non- autistic MMR-vaccinated children with indwelling shunts for hydrocephalus. None of the cases or controls had a history of measles exposure other than MMR vaccination. Serum and CSF samples were also evaluated for antibodies to MV and myelin basic protein (MBP). MV F gene was present in CSF from all three cases, but not in controls. Genome copy number ranged from 3.7x10 to 2.42x10 per ng of RNA total. Serum anti-MBP autoantibodies were detected in all children with AE. Anti-MBP and MV antibodies were detected in the CSF of two cases, while the third child had neither anti-MBP nor MV antibodies detected in his CSF. Findings are consistent with both an MV etiology for the AE and active viral replication in these children. They further indicate the possibility of a virally driven cerebral immunopathology in some cases of regressive autism.

Thimerosal-containing vaccines and autistic spectrum disorder: a critical review of published original data. Parker SK, Schwartz B, Todd J, Pickering LK.—Department of Pediatrics, Children's Hospital and University of Colorado Health Sciences Center, Denver, Colorado 80262, USA. *Pediatrics*. 2004 Sep;114(3):793–804.

OBJECTIVE: The issue of thimerosal-containing vaccines as a possible cause of autistic spectrum disorders (ASD) and neurodevelopmental disorders (NDDs) has been a controversial topic since 1999. Although most practitioners are familiar with the controversy, many are not familiar with the type or quality of evidence in published articles that have addressed this issue. To assess the quality of evidence assessing a potential association between thimerosal-containing vaccines and autism and evaluate whether that evidence suggests accepting or rejecting the hypothesis, we systematically reviewed published articles that report original data pertinent to the potential association between thimerosal-containing vaccines and ASD/NDDs. METHODS: Articles for analysis were identified in the National Library of Medicine's Medline database using a PubMed search of the English-language literature for articles published between 1966 and 2004, using keywords thimerosal, thiomersal, mercury, methylmercury, or ethylmercury alone and combined with keywords autistic disorder, autistic spectrum disorder, and neurodevelopment. In addition, we used the "related links" option in PubMed and reviewed the reference sections in the identified articles. All original articles that evaluated an association between thimerosal-containing vaccines and ASD/NDDs or pharmacokinetics of ethylmercury in vaccines were included. RESULTS: Twelve publications that met the selection criteria were identified by the literature search: 10 epidemiologic studies and 2 pharmacokinetic studies of ethylmercury. The design and quality of the studies showed significant variation. The preponderance of epidemiologic evidence does not support an association between thimerosal-containing vaccines and ASD. Epidemiologic studies that support an association are of poor quality and cannot be interpreted. Pharmacokinetic studies suggest that the half-life of ethylmercury is significantly shorter when compared with methylmercury. CONCLUSIONS: Studies do not demonstrate a link between thimerosal-containing vaccines and ASD, and the pharmacokinetics of ethylmercury make such an association less likely. Epidemiologic studies that support a link demonstrated significant design flaws that invalidate their conclusions. Evidence does not support a change in the standard of practice with regard to administration of thimerosal-containing vaccines in areas of the world where they are used.

An Investigation of the Association Between MMR Vaccination and Autism in Denmark. GS Goldman, Ph.D., FE Yazbak, M.D., F.A.A.P. *Journal of American Physicians and Surgeons.* Volume 9 Number 3 Fall 2004.

The measles, mumps, rubella (MMR) vaccine was added to the childhood immunization schedule in Denmark in 1987. From 1998 to the present, there has been concern over whether there is an association between MMR vaccination and autism. Prevalence of autism by age category during 1980 to 2002 was investigated, using data from a nationwide computerized registration system, the Danish Psychiatric Central Register, in order to compare the periods preceding and following introduction of MMR vaccine. Prior to a classification change in 1993/1994 and a change in enrollment in 1995, an increase in autism prevalence was noted. Linear regression analysis was performed separately on the trend during 1990 to 1992, the period that preceded the introduction of both effects. The prevalence in 2000 could then be derived excluding the sources of ascertainment bias. Prevalence of autism among children aged 5-9 years increased from a mean of 8.38/100,000 in the pre-licensure era (1980- 1986) to 71.43/100,000 in 2000 and leveled off during 2001-2002. The relative risk (RR) is therefore 8.5 (95% CI, 5.7 to 12.7). After adjusting for greater diagnostic awareness, the RR is 4.7 (95% CI, 3.1 to 7.2). Among individuals less than 15 years old, the adjusted RR is 4.1 (95% CI, 3.5 to 4.9). Longitudinal trends in prevalence data suggest a temporal association between the introduction of MMR vaccine in Denmark and the rise in autism. This contradicts an earlier report. Health authorities should develop safer vaccination strategies and support further investigation of the hypothesized link between the MMR vaccine and autism

Neurodevelopmental disorders following thimerosal-containing childhood immunizations: a follow-up analysis. Geier D, Geier MR.—MedCon, Inc., Maryland, USA. *The International Journal of Toxicology.* 2004 Nov.–Dec.;23(6):369–76.

The authors previously published the first epidemiological study from the

United States associating thimerosal from childhood vaccines with neurodevelopmental disorders (NDs) based upon assessment of the Vaccine Adverse Event Reporting System (VAERS). A number of years have gone by since their previous analysis of the VAERS. The present study was undertaken to determine whether the previously observed effect between thimerosal-containing childhood vaccines and NDs are still apparent in the VAERS as children have had a chance to further mature and potentially be diagnosed with additional NDs. In the present study, a cohort of children receiving thimerosal-containing diphtheria-tetanus-acellular pertussis (DTaP) vaccines in comparison to a cohort of children receiving thimerosal-free DTaP vaccines administered from 1997 through 2000 based upon an assessment of adverse events reported to the VAERS were evaluated. It was determined that there were significantly increased odds ratios (ORs) for autism (OR = 1.8, $p < .05$), mental retardation (OR = 2.6, $p < .002$), speech disorder (OR = 2.1, $p < .02$), personality disorders (OR = 2.6, $p < .01$), and thinking abnormality (OR = 8.2, $p < .01$) adverse events reported to the VAERS following thimerosal-containing DTaP vaccines in comparison to thimerosal-free DTaP vaccines. Potential confounders and reporting biases were found to be minimal in this assessment of the VAERS. It was observed, even though the media has reported a potential association between autism and thimerosal exposure, that the other NDs analyzed in this assessment of the VAERS had significantly higher ORs than autism following thimerosal-containing DTaP vaccines in comparison to thimerosal-free DTaP vaccines. The present study provides additional epidemiological evidence supporting previous epidemiological, clinical and experimental evidence that administration of thimerosal-containing vaccines in the United States resulted in a significant number of children developing NDs.

Thimerosal and autism? A plausible hypothesis that should not be dismissed. Blaxill MF, Redwood L, Bernard S.—Safe Minds (Sensible Action For Ending Mercury-Induced Neurological Disorders), 14 Commerce Drive, PH Cranford, New Jersey 07016, USA. blaxill@comcast.net. *Medical Hypotheses.* 2004;62(5):788–94.

The autism-mercury hypothesis first described by Bernard et al. has generated much interest and controversy. The Institute of Medicine (IOM) reviewed the connection between mercury-containing vaccines and neurodevelopmental disorders, including autism. They concluded that the hypothesis was biologically plausible but that there was insufficient evidence to accept or reject a causal connection and recommended a comprehensive research program. Without citing new experimental evidence, a number of observers have offered opinions on the subject, some of which reject the IOM's conclusions. In a recent review, Nelson and Bauman argue that a link between the preservative thimerosal, the source of the mercury in childhood vaccines, is improbable. In their defense of thimerosal, these authors take a narrow view of the original hypothesis, provide no new evidence, and rely on selective citations and flawed reasoning. We provide evidence here to refute the Nelson and Bauman critique and to defend the autism-mercury hypothesis.

MMR vaccination and autism: what is the evidence for a causal association? Madsen KM, Vestergaard M.—Department of Epidemiology and Social Medicine, The Danish Epidemiology Science Centre, Aarhus, Denmark. KMM@dadlnet.dk. *Drug Safety*. 2004;27(12):831–40.

It has been suggested that vaccination with the measles-mumps-rubella (MMR) vaccine causes autism. The wide-scale use of the MMR vaccine has been reported to coincide with the apparent increase in the incidence of autism. Case reports have described children who developed signs of both developmental regression and gastrointestinal symptoms shortly after MMR vaccination. A review of the literature revealed no convincing scientific evidence to support a causal relationship between the use of MMR vaccines and autism. No primate models exist to support the hypothesis. The biological plausibility remains questionable and there is a sound body of epidemiological evidence to refute the hypothesis. The hypothesis has been subjected to critical evaluation in many different ways, using techniques from molecular biology to population-based epidemiology, and with a vast number of independent researchers involved, none of which has been able to corroborate the hypothesis.

A two-phased population epidemiological study of the safety of thimerosal-containing vaccines: a follow-up analysis. Geier DA, Geier MR.—MedCon, Inc., USA. *Medical Science Monitor.* 2005 Apr;11(4):CR160-70. Epub 2005 Mar 24.

BACKGROUND: Thimerosal is an ethylmercury-containing preservative in vaccines. Toxicokinetic studies have shown children received doses of mercury from thimerosal-containing vaccines (TCVs) that were in excess of safety guidelines. Previously, an ecological study showing a significant association between TCVs and neurodevelopmental disorders (NDs) in the US was published in this journal. MATERIAL/METHODS: A two phased population-based epidemiological study was undertaken. Phase one evaluated reported NDs to the Vaccine Adverse Event Reporting System (VAERS) following thimerosal-containing Diphtheria-Tetanus-acellular-Pertussis (DTaP) vaccines in comparison to thimerosal-free DTaP vaccines administered from 1997 through 2001. Phase two evaluated the automated Vaccine Safety Datalink (VSD) for cumulative exposures to mercury from TCVs at 1-, 2-, 3-, and 6-months-of-age for infants born from 1992 through 1997 and the eventual risk of developing NDs. RESULTS: Phase one showed significantly increased risks for autism, speech disorders, mental retardation, personality disorders, and thinking abnormalities reported to VAERS following thimerosal-containing DTaP vaccines in comparison to thimerosal-free DTaP vaccines. Phase two showed significant associations between cumulative exposures to thimerosal and the following types of NDs: unspecified developmental delay, tics, attention deficit disorder (ADD), language delay, speech delay, and neurodevelopmental delays in general. CONCLUSIONS: This study showed that exposure to mercury from TCVs administered in the US was a consistent significant risk factor for the development of NDs. It is clear from these data and other recent publications linking TCVs with NDs that additional ND research should be undertaken in the context of evaluating mercury-associated exposures and thimerosal-free vaccines should be made available.

An assessment of downward trends in neurodevelopmental disorders in the United States following removal of Thimerosal from childhood vaccines. Geier DA, Geier MR.—Department of Biochemistry, George Washington University, Washington, DC, USA. *Medical Science Monitor.* 2006 Jun;12(6):CR231-9. Epub 2006 May 29.

BACKGROUND: The US is in the midst of an epidemic of neurodevelopmental disorders (NDs). Thimerosal is an ethylmercury-containing compound added to some childhood vaccines. Several previous epidemiological studies conducted in the US have associated Thimerosal-containing vaccine (TCV) administration with NDs. MATERIAL/METHODS: An ecological study was undertaken to evaluate NDs reported to the Vaccine Adverse Event Reporting System (VAERS) from 1991 through 2004 by date of receipt and by date of vaccine administration. The NDs examined included autism, mental retardation, and speech disorders. Statistical trend analysis was employed to evaluate the effects of removal of Thimerosal on the proportion of NDs reported to VAERS. RESULTS: There was a peak in the proportion of ND reports received by VAERS in 2001-2002 and in the proportion of ND reports by date of vaccine administration in 1998. There were significant reductions in the proportion of NDs reported to VAERS as Thimerosal was begun to be removed from childhood vaccines in the US from mid-1999 onwards. CONCLUSIONS: The present study provides the first epidemiological evidence showing that as Thimerosal was removed from childhood vaccines, the number of NDs has decreased in the US. The analysis techniques utilized attempted to minimize chance or bias/confounding. Additional research should be conducted to further evaluate the relationship between TCVs and NDs. This is especially true because the handling of vaccine safety data from the National Immunization Program of the CDC has been called into question by the Institute of Medicine of the National Academy of Sciences in 2005.

A meta-analysis epidemiological assessment of neurodevelopmental disorders following vaccines administered from 1994 through 2000 in the United States. Geier DA, Geier MR.—The Institute for Chronic Illnesses,

Inc., Silver Spring, MD 20905, USA. mgeier@comcast.net. *Neuroen-docrinology Letters*. 2006 Aug;27(4):401–13.

BACKGROUND: Thimerosal is an ethylmercury-containing compound (49.6% mercury by weight) used as at the preservative level in vaccines (0.005% to 0.01%). METHODS: Statistical modeling in a meta-analysis epidemiological assessment of the Vaccine Adverse Event Reporting System (VAERS) for neurodevelopment disorders (NDs) reported following Diphtheria-Tetanus-whole-cell-Pertussis (DTP) vaccines in comparison to Diphtheria-Tetanus-whole-cell-Pertussis-Haemophilus Influenzae Type b (DTPH) vaccines (administered: 1994-1997) and following Thimerosal-containing Diphtheria-Tetanus-acellular-Pertussis (DTaP), vaccines in comparison to Thimerosal-free DTaP vaccines (administered: 1997-2000), was undertaken. RESULTS: Significantly increased adjusted (sex, age, vaccine type, vaccine manufacturer) risks of autism, speech disorders, mental retardation, personality disorders, thinking abnormalities, ataxia, and NDs in general, with minimal systematic error or confounding, were associated with TCV exposure. CONCLUSION: It is clear from the results of the present epidemiological study and other recently published data associating mercury exposure with childhood NDs, additional ND research should be undertaken in the context of evaluating mercury-associated exposures, especially from Thimerosal-containing vaccines.

Update on the National Vaccine Injury Compensation Program. Edlich RF, Olson DM, Olson BM, Greene JA, Gubler KD, Winters KL, Kelley AR, Britt LD, Long WB 3rd.—Distinguished Professor of Plastic Surgery, Biomedical Engineering and Emergency Medicine, University of Virginia Health System, Charlottesville, Virginia; Director of Trauma Prevention, Research and Education, Trauma Specialists, LLP, Legacy Emanuel Hospital, Portland, Oregon. *The Journal of Emergency Medicine*. 2007 Aug;33(2):199–211. Epub 2007 Jun 18.

The National Childhood Vaccine Injury Act of 1986, as amended, established the Vaccine Injury Compensation Program (VICP). The VICP went into effect on

October 1, 1988 and is a Federal "no-fault" system designed to compensate individuals, or families of individuals, who have been injured by covered vaccines. From 1988 until July 2006, a total of 2531 non-autism/thimerosal and 5030 autism/thimerosal claims were made to the VICP. The compensation paid for the non-autism/thimerosal claims from 1988 until 2006 was $902,519,103.37 for 2542 awards. There was no compensation for any of the autism/thimerosal claims. On the basis of the deaths and extensive suffering to patients and families from the adverse reactions to vaccines, all physicians must provide detailed information in the Vaccine Information Statement to the patient or the parent or legal guardian of the child about the potential dangers of vaccines as well as the VICP.

Autism: Facts and Figures

Centers for Disease Control and Prevention, *Measles, Mumps, and Rubella (MMR) Vaccine and Autism Fact Sheet,* July 5, 2007 http://www.cdc.gov/od/science/iso/concerns/ mmr_autism_factsheet.htm

WHAT YOU SHOULD KNOW

■ MMR vaccine protects children against dangerous, even deadly, diseases.

■ Because signs of autism may appear at around the same time children receive the MMR vaccine, some parents may worry that the vaccine causes autism.

■ Carefully performed scientific studies have found no relationship between MMR vaccine and autism.

■ The CDC continues to recommend two doses of MMR vaccine for all children.

ADDITIONAL FACTS

■ MMR is a combination vaccine that protects children from measles, mumps, and rubella (also known as German measles). The first dose of the vaccine is usually given to children 12 to 15 months old. The second dose is usually given between 4 and 6 years of age.

■ In 1998, a study of autistic children raised the question of a connection between MMR vaccine and autism.

■ The 1998 study has a number of limitations. For example, the study was very small, involving only 12 children. This is too few cases to make any generalizations about the causes of autism. In addition, the researchers suggested that MMR vaccination caused bowel problems in the children, which then led to autism. However, in some of the children studied, symptoms of autism appeared *before* symptoms of bowel disease.

■ In 2004, 10 of the 13 authors of the 1998 study retracted the study's interpretation. The authors stated that the data were not able to establish a causal link between MMR vaccine and autism.

■ Other larger studies have found no relationship between MMR vaccine and autism. For example, researchers in the UK studied the records of 498 children with autism born between 1979 and 1998. They found:

  ❑ the percentage of children with autism who received MMR vaccine was the same as the percentage of unaffected children in the region who received MMR vaccine

❑ there was no difference in the age of diagnosis of autism in vaccinated and unvaccinated children

❑ the onset of "regressive" symptoms of autism did not occur within 2, 4, or 6 months of receiving the MMR vaccine.

■ Groups of experts, including the American Academy of Pediatrics, agree that MMR vaccine is not responsible for recent increases in the number of children with autism. In 2004, a report by the Institute of Medicine (IOM) concluded that there is no association between autism and MMR vaccine or vaccines that contain thimerosal as a preservative.

■ There is no published scientific evidence showing that there is any benefit to separating the combination MMR vaccine into three individual shots.

National Center for Immunization and Respiratory Diseases, *Possible Side-effects from Vaccines*, Centers for Disease Control and Prevention, June 12, 2007 http://www.cdc.gov/vaccines/vac-gen/side-effects.htm#mmr

MMR VACCINE SIDE-EFFECTS

What are the risks from MMR vaccine?

A vaccine, like any medicine, is capable of causing serious problems, such as severe allergic reactions. The risk of MMR vaccine causing serious harm, or death, is extremely small.

Getting MMR vaccine is much safer than getting any of these three diseases. Most people who get MMR vaccine do not have any problems with it.

MILD PROBLEMS

■ Fever (up to 1 person out of 6)
■ Mild rash (about 1 person out of 20)
■ Swelling of glands in the cheeks or neck (rare)

If these problems occur, it is usually within 7-12 days after the shot. They occur less often after the second dose.

MODERATE PROBLEMS

■ Seizure (jerking or staring) caused by fever (about 1 out of 3,000 doses)
■ Temporary pain and stiffness in the joints, mostly in teenage or adult women (up to 1 out of 4)
■ Temporary low platelet count, which can cause a bleeding disorder (about 1 out of 30,000 doses)

SEVERE PROBLEMS (VERY RARE)

■ Serious allergic reaction (less than 1 out of a million doses)
■ Several other severe problems have been known to occur after a child gets MMR vaccine. But this happens so rarely, experts cannot be sure whether they are caused by the vaccine or not. These include:
  ❏ Deafness
  ❏ Long-term seizures, coma, or lowered consciousness
  ❏ Permanent brain damage

National Center for Immunization and Respiratory Diseases, *Who Should NOT Get Vaccinated with these Vaccines?* **Centers for Disease Control and Prevention, May 24, 2007 http://www.cdc.gov/vaccines/vpd-vac/should-not-vacc.htm#mmr**

WHO SHOULD NOT GET VACCINATED WITH THESE VACCINES?

MMR (MEASLES, MUMPS, AND RUBELLA) VACCINE

Some people should not get MMR vaccine or should wait.
■ People should not get MMR vaccine who have ever had a life-threatening allergic reaction to gelatin, the antibiotic neomycin, or to a previous dose of MMR vaccine.
■ People who are moderately or severely ill at the time the shot is scheduled should usually wait until they recover before getting MMR vaccine.
■ Pregnant women should wait to get MMR vaccine until after they have given birth. Women should avoid getting pregnant for 4 weeks after getting MMR vaccine.

Some people should check with their doctor about whether they should get MMR vaccine, including anyone who:

■ Has HIV/AIDS, or another disease that affects the immune system

■ Is being treated with drugs that affect the immune system, such as steroids, for 2 weeks or longer.

■ Has any kind of cancer

■ Is taking cancer treatment with x-rays or drugs

■ Has ever had a low platelet count (a blood disorder)

■ People who recently had a transfusion or were given other blood products should ask their doctor when they may get MMR vaccine

Autism Society of America webpage, *Facts and Statistics*, Autism Society of America, 2003, 2006 http://www.autism-society.org/site/PageServer?page-name=FactsStats

FACTS AND STATISTICS, 2003, 2006

AUTISM SOCIETY OF AMERICA

■ 1 in 150 births[1]

■ 1 to 1.5 million Americans[2]

■ Fastest-growing developmental disability

■ 10—17 % annual growth

■ Growth comparison during the 1990s:[3]

   ❑ U.S. population increase: 13%

   ❑ Disabilities increase: 16%

   ❑ Autism increase: 172%

■ $90 billion annual cost[4]

■ 90% of costs are in adult services[4]

■ Cost of lifelong care can be reduced by 2/3 with early diagnosis and intervention[4]

■ In 10 years, the annual cost will be $200-400 billion[5]

NOTES

1. Based on prevalence statistics from the Centers for Disease Control and Prevention (2007).
2. Based on the autism prevalence rate of 2 to 6 per 1,000 (Centers for Disease Control and Prevention, 2001) and 2000 U.S. Census figure of 280 million Americans.

3. U.S. Department of Education's "Twenty-First Annual Report to Congress on the Implementation of the Individuals with Disabilities Education Act" (1999).
4. Jarbrink K, Knapp M, 2001, London School of Economics study: "The economic impact on autism in Britain," 5 (1): 7-22.
5. ASA calculates that the annual cost of autism will increase to $200-400 billion in 10 years. February 2003.

TACAnow.com webpage, *Latest Autism Statistics,* **Talk About Curing Autism, 2007 http://www.tacanow.com/autism/latest_autism_statistics.htm**

LATEST AUTISM STATISTICS, 2007
by TACA (Talk About Curing Autism)

The purposes of this document/web link is to provide the latest in Autism statistics. Statistic information and collection protocols are provided where ever possible. Please see original source as outlined for more details.

AUTISM OCCURRENCE: One in every 150 children born in the US have autism. It is estimated approximately 1 million in the US have this disorder. *NOTE: This number does NOT include: PDD, Asperger's and other spectrum disorders. These statistics are endorsed by the CDC, American Academy of Pediatrics, and other federal organizations.*

U.S. FACTS:

- A new case of autism is diagnosed nearly every 20 minutes
- There are 24,000 new cases diagnosed in the U.S. per year
- The economic impact of autism is more than $90 billion and expected to more
- than double in the next decade.
- Autism receives less than 5% of the research funding of many less prevalent childhood diseases.
- There is no medical detection treatment, or cure for autism.

AUTISM COMPARED TO OTHER DISABILITIES: Autism is the fastest-growing developmental disability in the U.S. today.

AUTISM & CALIFORNIA STATISTICS:

■ EIGHT new cases each day – 7 days a week in California alone!

■ From 1987-1998 there was a 633 % increase in Autism (DSM IV) in the State of California. *(Note: In 1998 mandatory immunizations programs and the MMR vaccine were introduced.)*

■ From 1998–2002 there was an additional 96% increase in Autism (DSM IV) in the State of California.

■ There are 20,277 cases of autism in California as of December 2003.

■ Autism cases represent over 12% of the Regional Center caseload. Annual budget for ASD care is over $171,000,000.

■ In state operated institutions of care there are 3,436 people with autism.

■ Current California Autism diagnosis by quarter:

Quarter	Total # children 3-5 years old	Net gain	Change in net gain
1Q 2003	4228	189	+81
2Q 2003	4466	238	+49
3Q 2003	4558	92	-146
4Q 2003	4611	53	-39
1Q 2004	4793	182	+129
2Q 2004	4894	101	-81
3Q 2004	4997	103	+2
4Q 2004	5156	159	+56
1Q 2005	5307	151	-8
2Q 2005	5446	139	-12
3Q 2005	5539	93	-46

FUNDING RESEARCH: In the late 1990s The National Institutes of Health (NIH) funded just $5 million in Autism Research. Today, the National Institutes of Health funds allocation:

■ $29 billion Total NIH funding

■ $5 billion Funding of relevant NIH departments: Child Health, Mental Health,

■ Environmental Health, Neurological Disorders

■ LESS THAN $100 million* Portion of the $5 billion allocation that directly or indirectly impacts autism research.

*This represents 0.3% of total NIH funding. MUCH MORE FUNDING is needed.

HOW DOES FUNDING FOR AUTISM COMPARE TO OTHER CHILDHOOD DISORDERS & DISEASES?

■ Leukemia 1 in 25,000 Funding: $300 million
■ Muscular Dystrophy 1 in 20,000 Funding: $160 million
■ Cystic Fibrosis 1 in 5,000 Funding: $75 million
■ Juvenile Diabetes 1 in 500 Funding: $140 million
■ Autism 1 in 150 Funding: $15 million (*Dollar amounts reflect approximate annual funds raised by major private advocacy groups.*)

Note: it is important to note that there is no suggestion to place an importance on one disease over another. This funding information above is only to demonstrate the disparity of funding towards autism.

AUTISTICS AGE INFORMATION: In the State of California seven out of ten Autistic individuals are under the age of 13 years.

BETTER DIAGNOSIS? Some have suggested that autism is just being better diagnosed today versus ten years ago and that many cases of mental retardation are now being coded as autism. This would also assume that the experts diagnosing autism before did not know what they were doing. This is NOT TRUE. Autism is the only disorder rising dramatically—mental retardation, Down's syndrome, and cystic fibrosis remain relatively the same.

GIRLS VS. BOYS: Autism often strikes boys more often than girls—roughly four times more common in boys. Statistics being 1 in every 166 children that makes it 1 in every 41 males.

Appendix E

Prozac

■ ■ ■

Prozac: Recent News

FDA Proposes New Warnings About Suicidal Thinking, Behavior in Young Adults Who Take Antidepressant Medications
May 2, 2007 | www.fda.gov

The U.S. Food and Drug Administration (FDA) today proposed that makers of all antidepressant medications update the existing black box warning on their products' labeling to include warnings about increased risks of suicidal thinking and behavior, known as suicidality, in young adults ages 18 to 24 during initial treatment (generally the first one to two months).

The proposed labeling changes also include language stating that scientific data did not show this increased risk in adults older than 24, and that adults ages 65 and older taking antidepressants have a decreased risk of suicidality. The proposed warning statements emphasize that depression and certain other serious psychiatric disorders are themselves the most important causes of suicide.

"Today's actions represent FDA's commitment to a high level of post-marketing evaluation of drug products," said Steven Galson, M.D., MPH, director of FDA's Center for Drug Evaluation and Research. "Depression and other psychiatric disorders can have significant consequences if not appropriately treated. Antidepressant medications benefit many patients, but it is important that doctors and patients are aware of the risks."

People currently prescribed antidepressant medications should not stop taking them. Those who have concerns should notify their health care providers.

The proposed labeling changes apply to the entire category of antidepressants. Results of individual placebo-controlled scientific studies are reasonably consistent in showing a slight increase in suicidality for patients taking antidepressants in early treatment for most of the medications. Available data are not sufficient to exclude any single medication from the increased risk of suicidality.

The proposed labeling update follows similar labeling changes made in 2005 that warned of a suicidality risk in children and adolescents who use antidepressants. At that time, FDA asked manufacturers to add a black box warning to the labeling of all antidepressants to describe this risk and to emphasize the need for appropriate monitoring and close observation, particularly for younger patients taking these medications. In addition, FDA directed manufacturers to develop Medication Guides, FDA-approved user-friendly information for patients, families and caregivers, that could help improve monitoring. Medication Guides are intended to be distributed at the pharmacy with each prescription or refill of a medication.

Also in 2005, FDA began a comprehensive review of 295 individual antidepressant trials that included over 77,000 adult patients with major depressive disorder (MDD) and other psychiatric disorders, to examine the risk of suicidality in adults who are prescribed antidepressants.

In December 2006, FDA's Psychopharmacologic Drugs Advisory Committee agreed that labeling changes were needed to inform health care professionals about the increased risk of suicidality in younger adults using antidepressants. Additionally, the committee noted product labeling needed to reflect the apparent beneficial effect of antidepressants in older adults and to remind health care professionals that the disorders themselves are the most important cause of suicidality.

FDA has been developing language to revise product labeling and update the Patient Medication Guides for these products. Manufacturers of antidepressants will now have 30 days to submit their revised product labels and revised Medication Guides to FDA for review.

BMJ apologizes to Eli Lilly over Prozac
Medical journal retracts allegations made about the drugmaker's disclosure of important Prozac info.
January 27, 2005
http://money.cnn.com/2005/01/27/news/midcaps/bmj_prozac/index.htm

ATLANTA (CNN) - The medical journal BMJ Thursday retracted and apologized for the claim it made early this month that internal industry documents it received from an anonymous source had gone "missing" during a 1994 product liability suit against Eli Lilly and Co., maker of the antidepressant Prozac.

The documents, cited by the journal in a Jan. 1 news article, suggest a link between fluoxetine—the generic name for Prozac—and suicide attempts and violence.

The article said "the missing documents ... include reviews and memos indicating that Eli Lilly officials were aware in the 1980s that fluoxetine had troubling side effects and sought to minimize their likely negative effect on prescribing."

The BMJ said it investigated its "missing" claim after Lilly complained. "That investigation has revealed that all of the documents supplied to the BMJ that were either Eli Lilly (Research) documents or were in the hands of Eli Lilly had in fact been disclosed during the suit," it said in a statement posted on its Web site.

"At the end of the trial, all the documents were preserved by court order or were disclosed by Eli Lilly to the plaintiffs' lawyers in related Prozac claims.

"The BMJ did not intend to suggest that Eli Lilly caused these documents to go missing. As a result of the investigation, it is clear that these documents did not go missing. The BMJ accepts that Eli Lilly acted properly in relation to the disclosure of these documents in these claims. The BMJ is happy to set the record straight and to apologize to Eli Lilly for this statement, which we now retract, but which we published in good faith."

In its original report, CNN reported BMJ's claim and Lilly's denial that the papers had ever been missing.

The London-based BMJ, formerly called the British Medical Journal, did not retract its contention that the documents show the antidepressant is linked to increased risk of suicide or violence.

"All we have retracted is the statement that these documents went missing," wrote acting editor Kamram Abbasi, in an e-mail to CNN.

The BMJ had written that the documents "went missing" during the 1994 lawsuit brought by relatives of victims of Joseph Wesbecker, who five years before shot and killed eight of his co-workers at a Louisville, Ky., printing plant and then killed himself.

Wesbecker, who had a history of depression, had been prescribed Prozac a month before the shootings.

One document cited by the BMJ article was a 1988 report that said 38 percent of depressed patients on Prozac reported such side effects as agitation and nervousness.

That was twice the rate reported by people taking a placebo.

Only recently has the FDA warned that antidepressants can cause "activating" or stimulating symptoms such as agitation, panic attacks, insomnia and aggressiveness.

Plaintiffs in the case tried to show Lilly had withheld key negative data from the FDA and that it was Prozac that pushed Wesbecker over the edge.

Lilly initially won the case, but was later forced to admit that it had made a secret settlement with the plaintiffs during the trial, which meant that the verdict was invalid, the journal said.

Lilly did not immediately respond to a request for comment.

An advisory panel to the Food and Drug Administration in 1991 reviewed the data and concluded that Prozac was safe, though critics point out that several of the panelists had financial ties to Lilly.

They also note that other internal documents show that Lilly excluded 76 of 97 cases of reported suicidality from the data.

Lilly did not immediately respond to that report, though the scientist involved in the reclassification of some of the cases defended doing so, saying that a review of the cases showed they were not suicide attempts.

A critic noted that the reclassifications were made on the basis of record reviews, and that the patients themselves were not interviewed.

The issue has re-emerged on the news media landscape with the upcoming trial of Christopher Pittman, a South Carolina teenager charged with killing his grandparents when he was 12.

His lawyers contend that Zoloft—an antidepressant similar to Prozac—was responsible for his outburst. Trial is scheduled to begin Monday.

In the article, the prestigious medical journal said it had sent the documents to the FDA for review.

The FDA said Thursday it is reviewing them. "Our initial conclusion was that, to date, those materials do not alter the conclusions reached by FDA about Prozac," said spokeswoman Susan Cruzan.

About 54 million people worldwide have taken Prozac, a Lilly spokesman said.

Lilly Settles Prozac Lawsuit
Terms of the deal not disclosed; new litigation in Georgia is targeting metabolization issue.
By Jeff Swiatek November 30, 2002
Indystar.com

A two-year-old Prozac negligence lawsuit, set for trial Tuesday, has been settled out of court by defendant Eli Lilly and Co. and the Pennsylvania plaintiffs.

The case was brought by Diane and Melvin Cassidy, of Monroeville, who in July 2000 picketed outside Lilly's corporate headquarters in Indianapolis, handing out fliers proclaiming, "Lilly, how many people are maimed or dead on your drug today?"

The Cassidys' lawsuit, filed in federal court in Pittsburgh, charged that Diane Cassidy's doctor prescribed the antidepressant Prozac to her for weight loss and that the drug caused suicidal thoughts that led her to slash her wrists and overdose on a painkiller. She suffered intracranial bleeding from the painkiller, which left her paralyzed on one side and mentally impaired, according to the lawsuit, which sought $4.84 million in tangible damages.

The Cassidys were represented by Houston trial lawyer Andy Vickery, who has negotiated settlements of several Prozac cases against Lilly.

Terms of the settlement, reached this week, were not disclosed.

The Indianapolis drugmaker said in a statement that it "made a business decision to settle . . . for factors completely unrelated to the safety and efficacy of Prozac. Such factors included the extensive time demands that litigation would have placed upon our scientists, keeping them away from their primary objective of discovering lifesaving medicines. In no way was our decision to settle in any way motivated by concerns over the safety and efficacy of Prozac."

The settlement comes the same week that a fresh Prozac lawsuit was filed against Lilly, in U.S. District Court in Georgia. It raises a new charge in the more than decade long litigation over Prozac: that Lilly has failed to publicize research showing some people are "poor metabolizers of Prozac" and a test can reveal if a patient might be affected.

The Georgia product-liability and wrongful-death suit, in which Vickery is assisting the plaintiff, was brought by William H. Shell, the widower of LaVerne M. Shell. She shot herself to death at age 63 in November 2000, 11 days after starting on a prescription of Prozac to treat migraine headaches.

The lawsuit charges that a human enzyme dubbed CYP2D6 normally metabolizes or breaks down Prozac and similar drugs in the body, but fails to do so in a minority of people. In their bodies, the active ingredient in Prozac builds up to high levels, putting them at risk of violence and suicide, the lawsuit says.

"Lilly is negligent in failing to make this information public, to convey it to doctors, or otherwise to take reasonable measures to implement appropriate patient screening techniques," the lawsuit says.

Lilly spokesman Blair Austin said that company officials hadn't seen the lawsuit and couldn't comment on the new charge.

The metabolization issue is gaining currency among some activists who publicize side effects from the Prozac class of antidepressants and other drugs.

Self-employed businessman Jim Harper of Glendale, Calif., who runs a Web site called Prozactruth.com, said he hopes to soon offer a DNA test through his site that can tell if a person is a poor metabolizer of Prozac and related drugs.

"I should not have to be the one" to publicize the test, Harper said Friday. "I'd rather be doing other things on my nights and weekends." But drug companies and doctors aren't doing enough to warn users of serious side effects from antidepressants, said Harper, who noted he receives hundreds of e-mails a week from people who read his Web site.

Harper said he hopes to arrange to sell the test for about $245 through Genelex Corp. of Redmond, Wash., a direct-to-consumer DNA testing firm.

Prozac: Abstracts of Recent Scientific Research

Fluoxetine dose-increment related akathisia in depression: implications for clinical care, recognition and management of selective serotonin reuptake inhibitor-induced akathisia. Hansen L.- Department of Psychiatry, Royal South Hants, Southampton, UK. lh4@soton.ac.uk *J Psychopharmacol.* 2003 Dec;17(4):451–2.

We report the case of a 22-year-old woman presenting major depressive episode with severe akathisia after an increase in fluoxetine. The patient developed severe restlessness and de novo suicidal ideation approximately 1 week after the dosage of fluoxetine was doubled, 1 year on from when the drug was first introduced. This case illustrates the importance of being alert to movement disorders in patients treated with selective serotonin reuptake inhibitors. The clinical implications are discussed. A management strategy based on the evidence in the existing literature is suggested.

Serotonin transporter polymorphisms and adverse effects with fluoxetine treatment. Perlis RH, Mischoulon D, Smoller JW, Wan YJ, Lamon-Fava S, Lin KM, Rosenbaum JF, Fava M. - Department of Psychiatry, Massachusetts General Hospital, Boston 02114, USA. *Biol Psychiatry.* 2003 Nov 1;54(9):879–83

BACKGROUND: The short (S) allele of the serotonin transporter gene-linked polymorphic region (5HTTLPR) has been associated with poorer antidepressant response in major depressive disorder (MDD) and with antidepressant-induced mania. This study investigated a possible association with treatment-emergent insomnia or agitation. METHODS: Thirty-six outpatients with MDD were genotyped at 5HTTLPR and treated with open-label fluoxetine up to 60 mg/day. Treatment-emergent adverse effects were assessed at each study visit. RESULTS: Of nine subjects homozygous for the "S" allele, seven (78%) developed new or worsening insomnia, versus 6 of 27 (22%) non-"S"-homozygous subjects (Fisher's exact p =.005). Similarly, six of nine subjects homozygous for the "S" allele (67%) developed agitation, versus 2 of 27 (7%) of non-"S"-homozygous subjects

(Fisher's exact p =.001). CONCLUSIONS: The "S" allele of the 5HTTLPR may identify patients at risk for developing insomnia or agitation with fluoxetine treatment. This preliminary result requires confirmation in larger samples.

Inhibition of risperidone metabolism by fluoxetine in patients with schizophrenia: a clinically relevant pharmacokinetic drug interaction. Spina E, Avenoso A, Scordo MG, Ancione M, Madia A, Gatti G, Perucca E.- Department of Clinical and Experimental Medicine and Pharmacology, Section of Pharmacology, University of Messina, Messina, Italy. espina@unime.it *J Clin Psychopharmacol.* 2002 Aug;22(4):419–23

The effect of fluoxetine on the steady-state plasma concentrations of risperidone and its active metabolite 9-hydroxyrisperidone (9-OH-risperidone) was evaluated in 10 patients with schizophrenia or schizoaffective disorder. Patients stabilized on risperidone (4-6 mg/day) received additional fluoxetine (20 mg/day) to treat concomitant depression. One patient dropped out after 1 week due to the occurrence of akathisia associated with markedly increased plasma risperidone concentrations. In the other subjects, mean plasma concentrations of risperidone increased during fluoxetine administration from 12 +/- 9 ng/mL at baseline to 56 +/- 31 at week 4 (p < 0.001), while the levels of 9-OH-risperidone were not significantly affected. After 4 weeks of combined treatment, the levels of the active moiety (sum of the concentrations of risperidone and 9-OH-risperidone) increased by 75% (range, 9-204%, p < 0.01) compared with baseline. The mean plasma risperidone/9-OH-risperidone ratio also increased significantly. During the second week of adjunctive therapy, two patients developed Parkinsonian symptoms, which were controlled with anticholinergic medication. These findings indicate that fluoxetine, a potent inhibitor of the cytochrome P450 enzyme CYP2D6 and a less potent inhibitor of CYP3A4, reduces the clearance of risperidone by inhibiting its 9-hydroxylation or alternative metabolic pathways. This interaction may lead to toxic plasma risperidone concentrations. In addition to careful clinical observation, monitoring plasma risperidone levels may be of value in patients given adjunctive therapy with fluoxetine.

Manic behaviors associated with fluoxetine in three 12- to 18-year-olds with obsessive-compulsive disorder. Go FS, Malley EE, Birmaher B, Rosenberg DR. - Department of Psychiatry at the University of Pittsburgh Medical Center, Pennsylvania, USA. *J Child Adolesc Psychopharmacol.* 1998;8(1):73–80.

In a sample of 40 youths (ages 11-17) with obsessive-compulsive disorder (OCD) and mood disorders who were treated with behavior therapy, 20 patients received serotonin reuptake inhibitors (SRIs) and 20 did not. In open-label clinical treatment, 30% of the patients (6/20) treated with SRIs developed manic or hypomanic symptoms (5/15 on fluoxetine, 1/1 on sertraline). Symptoms included impulsivity, grandiosity, pressured speech, and disinhibition and did not resemble akathisia or "behavioral activation." These behaviors emerged despite gradual dose elevation (2-5 mg/wk), conservative dosing (maximum 40 mg daily), and careful weekly outpatient monitoring of each patient. Fluoxetine-induced mania occurred at doses as low as 10 mg daily. It is unclear whether mania/hypomania would appear in OCD children without comorbid mood disorders or, alternatively, whether OCD is a stronger risk factor than mood disorder for manic switch in SRI-treated youths. Clinicians are advised to be aware of the risk and to be vigilant in monitoring manic and hypomanic behaviors when using SRIs to treat OCD in youth, even with low doses and gradual dose elevation.

Open fluoxetine treatment of mixed anxiety disorders in children and adolescents. Fairbanks JM, Pine DS, Tancer NK, Dummit ES 3rd, Kentgen LM, Martin J, Asche BK, Klein RG. - Department of Child Psychiatry, College of Physicians and Surgeons, Columbia University, New York, New York, USA. *J Child Adolesc Psychopharmacol.* 1997 Spring;7(1):17–29.

An open-label pilot study examined fluoxetine treatment in 16 outpatients (9-18 years old) with mixed anxiety disorders. Following nonresponse to psychotherapy, fluoxetine monotherapy was started at 5 mg daily and was increased weekly by 5 or 10 mg daily for 6-9 weeks until improvement occurred or to a maximum of 40 mg (children under 12) or 80 mg (adolescents). Among patients on fluoxetine, severity of illness ratings were "much improved" (mean final Clinical Global Impression scale score 2.8 +/- 0.7). Clinical improvement occurred in 10 of 10 patients with current separation anxiety disorder, 8 of 10 with social phobia, 4 of 6 with specific phobia, 3 of 5 with panic disorder, and 1 of 7 with generalized anxiety disorder. Mean time to improvement was 5 weeks. Mean doses were 24 mg (0.7 mg/kg) for children and 40 mg (0.71 mg/kg) for adolescents. Side effects were transient and included drowsiness (31% of patients), sleep problems (19%), decreased appetite (13%), nausea (13%), abdominal pain (13%), and excitement (13%). No patient developed disinhibition, akathisia, or suicidality. These preliminary findings suggest fluoxetine effectiveness in separation anxiety disorder and social phobia. Youths with only one anxiety disorder appeared to respond to lower doses of fluoxetine than patients with multiple anxiety disorders (0.49 +/- 0.14 versus 0.80 +/- 0.28 mg/kg, p < 0.05).

Movement disorders associated with the serotonin selective reuptake inhibitors. Leo RJ. - Department of Psychiatry, School of Medicine, State University of New York at Buffalo 14215, USA. *J Clin Psychiatry*. 1996 Oct;57(10):449–54.

BACKGROUND: To review the case reports and case series of movement disorders ascribed to the use of serotonin selective reuptake inhibitors (SSRIs). METHOD: Reports of SSRI-induced extrapyramidal symptoms (EPS) in the literature were located using a MEDLINE search and review of bibliographies. RESULTS: Among the 71 cases of SSRI-induced EPS reported in the literature, the most common side effect was akathisia (45.1%), followed by dystonia (28.2%), parkinsonism (14.1%), and tardive dyskinesia-like states (11.3%). Among patients with Parkinson's disease treated with SSRIs, there were 16 cases of worsening parkinsonism. Patients who developed dystonia, parkinsonism, or tardive dyskinesia were older on average than patients with akathisia; 67.6% of affected patients were females. Fluoxetine, the most commonly prescribed SSRI to date, was implicated in 53 (74.6%) of cases of SSRI-induced EPS. Several reports (57.7%) were confounded by the concomitant use of other medications that can contribute to the development of EPS. CONCLUSION: SSRI-induced EPS are probably related to agonism of serotonergic input to dopaminergic pathways within the CNS. Several patient-dependent and pharmacokinetic variables may determine the likelihood that EPS will emerge. Although these side effects are infrequent, clinicians should be alert to the possibility of their occurrence.

Efficacy, adverse events, and treatment discontinuations in fluoxetine clinical studies of major depression: a meta-analysis of the 20-mg/day dose. Beasley CM Jr, Nilsson ME, Koke SC, Gonzales JS. - Eli Lilly and Company, Lilly Corporate Center, Indianapolis, Ind 46285, USA. *J Clin Psychiatry*. 2000 Oct;61(10):722–8.

BACKGROUND: The efficacy and safety of fluoxetine in adults with moderate-to-severe major depression are well established. However, most analyses combined dosages (20-80 mg/day) of the compound. We hypothesized that in patients taking 20 mg/day, efficacy would be maintained but the incidence of adverse events would be lower. We present a meta-analysis of efficacy and safety data for fluoxetine, 20 mg/day. METHOD: Data were from 3 double-blind studies (N = 417) that included patients with moderate-to-severe major depression (DSM-III or DSM-III-R criteria) who received placebo or fixed-dose 20-mg/day treatment with fluoxetine. Efficacy was assessed using the Hamilton Rating Scale for Depression (HAM-D; HAM-D-17 total score and anxiety/somatization, retardation, sleep disturbance, and cognitive disturbance factors) and response and remission rates. Safety assessments included treatment-emergent adverse events, reasons for discontinuation, and adverse events leading to discontinuation. Adverse events were evaluated to determine the emergence of activation and/or sedation. RESULTS: At 20 mg/day, fluoxetine-treated patients demonstrated significantly greater remission and response rates and mean changes on HAM-D-17 total score and anxiety/somatization, retardation, and cognitive disturbance factor scores than placebo-treated patients (p < .001). The incidence of specific adverse events leading to discontinuation and the frequency of study discontinuations due to adverse events were similar among fluoxetine-treated and placebo-treated patients (6.1% vs. 5.8%, p = .879). Several adverse events (insomnia, asthenia, somnolence, gastroenteritis, decreased libido, chills, and confusion) occurred significantly more frequently among fluoxetine-treated patients. A significant change in sedation, but not activation, occurred in patients in the fluoxetine 20-mg/day group compared with the placebo group. CONCLUSION: These data affirm that fluoxetine at 20 mg/day is efficacious, safe, and of similar activation potential when compared with placebo in patients with major depression.

Extrapyramidal reactions and the selective serotonin-reuptake inhibitors.

Caley CF. - School of Pharmacy, University of Connecticut, Hartford, USA.
Ann Pharmacother. 1997 Dec;31(12):1481–9.

OBJECTIVE: To review the known published reports of extrapyramidal reactions (EPRs) associated with the use of selective serotonin-reuptake inhibitors (SSRIs). DATA SOURCES: Information was selected from a MEDLINE search (January 1990 to January 1996) of English-language medical literature. Manual searches of pertinent journal article bibliographies were also performed. DATA EXTRACTION: Appropriate information from all reports obtained was included, with specific attention directed toward patient age, gender, primary psychiatric diagnosis, total daily SSRI dosage, dosage escalation strategy, and concurrent psychotropic medications. DATA SYNTHESIS: Reports of EPRs associated with SSRI use have been accumulating in the medical literature for several years. More commonly associated with high-potency antipsychotics, EPRs can have an adverse impact on medication compliance and hospital read-missions. The proposed hypothesis for EPRs occurring with SSRI use involves serotonin's inhibitory actions on extrapyramidal dopamine activity. Other possible contributing factors include pharmacokinetic interactions or drug-disease interactions. EPRs may include dystonias, dyskinesias, akathisia, parkinsonism, exacerbations of Parkinson's disease, and possibly the neuroleptic malignant syndrome. The majority of SSRI-related reactions appear to occur within the first month of treatment. Information from available case reports does not strongly support any consistent risk factor, although some worth considering may include total SSRI daily dose, rapid dose escalation strategies, increased age, female gender, concurrent psychotropics known to also precipitate EPRs, and concurrent disease states such as Parkinson's disease. Since SSRI-related EPRs have occurred in different situations with different possible contributing factors, clinical pharmacy practitioners and other healthcare providers should remain aware of these reactions and carefully consider educating and monitoring their patients accordingly. CONCLUSIONS: The use of SSRIs may be associated with the development of EPRs; therefore, appropriate monitoring should be considered for patients so that optimal pharmaceutical care may be provided.

Recognition and management of acute neuroleptic-induced extrapyramidal motor and mental syndromes.Dose M. - BKH Taufkirchen, Germany.

Pharmacopsychiatry. 2000 Sep;33 Suppl 1:3–13.

After nearly 50 years of therapeutic application of neuroleptics, diagnosis and classification of neuroleptic-induced extrapyramidal syndromes still concentrate on their "neurological" (motor) aspects. Psychiatric (mental) aspects are in general—if at all—regarded as "secondary" to motor symptoms. Psychiatric side effects of neuroleptics (including psychotic exacerbations during neuroleptic treatment) have, however, anecdotally been reported since 1954 but never developed into a systematic classification. Accordingly, psychiatric manifestations of extrapyramidal side effects frequently are overlooked, misdiagnosed as psychotic deteriorations and treated by increased dosing of neuroleptics instead anticholinergics, which in addition are falsely suspected of bearing a high addictive potential and the risk of development of tardive dyskinesia. It is suggested that neuroleptic-induced basal ganglia dysfunction results in motor as well as mental extrapyramidal side effects, whose recognition and management is essential to achieve better tolerability of and thereby compliance with neuroleptic treatment.

Fluoxetine-related death in a child with cytochrome P-450 2D6 genetic deficiency.Sallee FR, DeVane CL, Ferrell RE.- Department of Psychiatry, University of Cincinnati, Ohio 45267, USA. salleefr@email.uc.edu *J Child Adolesc Psychopharmacol* 2000 Spring;10(1):27–34

The clinical course of a 9-year-old diagnosed with attention-deficit hyperactivity disorder, obsessive-compulsive disorder, and Tourette's disorder and treated with a combination of methylphenidate, clonidine, and fluoxetine is described. The patient experienced over a 10-month period, signs and symptoms suggestive of metabolic toxicity marked by bouts of gastrointestinal distress, low-grade fever, incoordination, and disorientation. Generalized seizures were observed, and the patient lapsed into status epilepticus followed by cardiac arrest and subsequently expired. At autopsy, blood, brain, and other tissue concentrations of fluoxetine and norfluoxetine were several-fold higher than expected based on literature reports for overdose situations. The medical examiner's report indicated death caused by fluoxetine toxicity. As the child's adoptive parents controlled medication access, they were investigated by social welfare agencies. Further genetic testing of autopsy tissue revealed the presence of a gene defect at the cytochrome P450

CYP2D locus, which results in poor metabolism of fluoxetine. As a result of this and other evidence, the investigation of the adoptive parents was terminated. This is the first report of a fluoxetine-related death in a child with a confirmed genetic polymorphism of the CYP2D6 gene that results in impaired drug metabolism. Issues relevant to child and adolescent psychopharmacology arising from this case are discussed.

Fluoxetine and violent death in Maryland. Frankenfield DL, Baker SP, Lange WR, Caplan YH, Smialek JE. - Johns Hopkins University, School of Public Health, Baltimore, MD *Forensic Sci Int.* **1994 Feb;64(2-3):107–17.**

A retrospective Medical Examiner case review of all deaths in Maryland where either fluoxetine or tricyclic antidepressant (TCA) use was forensically detected was conducted for the time period January 1987-July 1991. Case records and toxicology reports from the Office of the Chief Medical Examiner were reviewed to determine cause and manner of death, circumstances of death, demographic information on the decedent, prior medical history of the decedent, and presence and level of either fluoxetine or TCA in various body fluids/tissues. Suicide was the manner of death most frequently associated with TCA and fluoxetine detection. Violent methods were more often associated with fluoxetine suicides than with TCA suicides (65% v. 23%, P < 0.001). Demographic characteristics of antidepressant-related deaths in Maryland were similar to those of the entire USA. Possible explanations for the results obtained include the inherent lower lethality of fluoxetine compared to the TCAs, necessitating the use of additional means to complete the act of suicide; that physicians may have switched more impulsive, high risk patients to this new agent as it became available, thus creating a selection bias for more violence-prone individuals in the fluoxetine group; or that fluoxetine may be associated with induction of violence and/or suicidal ideation. Further research examining the possible association of these agents with violent acts is warranted.

Unexpected deaths in depressed medical inpatients treated with fluoxetine. Spier SA, Frontera MA. - Psychiatric Consultation Service, Mercy Medical Center, Baltimore, MD 21202. *J Clin Psychiatry*. 1991 Sep;52(9):377–82.

BACKGROUND: Depression in the medically ill is underdiagnosed and undertreated. Fluoxetine would appear promising in this population because of its efficacy and benign side effect profile, but it has not been systematically studied in the medically ill. METHOD: The authors report the cases of three seriously medically ill patients, seen in psychiatric consultation while patients on a general medical service, who were treated with fluoxetine for depression. Each was an elderly white female with pulmonary disease and atrial arrhythmias, including atrial fibrillation, and each was prescribed diuretics, nitrates, and other cardiac and/or pulmonary agents. RESULTS: Each patient died within 10 days of beginning fluoxetine treatment, from unexplained causes. CONCLUSIONS: The authors hypothesize that direct cardiac effects mediated by fluoxetine, or other factors, may have been contributory. The effects of fluoxetine on electrolytes, fluoxetine's possible effects on drug levels, and serotonin's effect on the pulmonary system are examined. Other antidepressant agents should be considered in this particular population until further data are available.

Memory loss in a patient treated with fluoxetine. Joss JD, Burton RM, Keller CA. - Ambulatory Services, Good Samaritan Regional Medical Center, Corvallis, OR, USA. jjoss@samhealth.org *Ann Pharmacother.* 2003 Dec;37(12):1800–3.

OBJECTIVE: To report a case of severe memory loss in an elderly patient after initiation of fluoxetine. CASE SUMMARY: An 87-year-old white woman was started on fluoxetine for depression, and the dose was titrated to 20 mg/d. She developed progressive memory loss over the next 6 weeks for which she ultimately was hospitalized. Other potential causes for her memory loss were ruled out. After fluoxetine was discontinued, the patient's memory improved significantly over the next 2 months. An objective causality assessment indicated a possible relationship between the memory loss and fluoxetine in this patient. DISCUSSION: Our report documents a case of severe reversible memory deterioration after initiating fluoxetine. Fluoxetine has a favorable adverse effect profile when compared with older classes of antidepressants. Postmarketing studies and isolated case reports, however, suggest that fluoxetine may harm memory in some patients. Some selective serotonin-reuptake inhibitors (SSRIs) appear to cause memory loss more frequently than others. CONCLUSIONS: Clinicians should be aware of the possible effects of fluoxetine (and possibly other SSRIs) on memory.

Fluoxetine-induced extrapyramidal symptoms in an adolescent: a case report. Diler RS, Yolga A, Avci A. *Swiss Med Wkly* 2002;132:125–126.

We present a 15-year-old girl with depression, an obsessive compulsive disorder and conduct disorder, who developed EPS (torticollis, bradykinesia and cogwheel rigidity) while on fluoxetine. No other cause of EPS was present. The patient responded well to benztropine but re-experienced EPS when benztropine was stopped. Fluoxetine and benztropine were used concomitantly for 21.2 months and the patient has been off medication for 2 months without EPS. This case report shows that EPS can and does occur in youth with SSRI. Clinicians should be aware of the SSRIs as a potential causative factor for EPS.

Fluoxetine-induced tremor: clinical features in 21 patients. M. Serrano-Dueñas - Servicio de Neurología del Hospital Carlos Andrade Marín, Instituto Ecuatoriano de Seguridad Social, Facultad de Medicina de la Pontificia, Universidad Católica del Ecuador, Quito, Ecuador. *Parkinsonism & Related Disorders* Volume 8, Issue 5, June 2002, Pages 325–327

We report a cohort of 21 patients (12 females and nine males), with a mean age of 42.4 years, who developed tremor after receiving fluoxetine at a mean dose of 25.7 mg per day. The mean latency period for tremor appearance was 54.3 days. Severity was found to be mild. In all patients, tremor was postural, with $P<0.0005$, compared to patients with rest tremor and $P<0.05$ compared to action/intention-tremor patients. The frequency range was 6–12 Hz/s. After fluoxetine was discontinued, tremor disappeared in 10 patients after a mean latency period of 35.5 days. In the remaining 11 patients, tremor persisted up to the end of the observation period (a mean of 449 days). We believe that this tremor phenomenon is due to the involvement of the red nucleus and the inferior olivary nucleus through their projections to the thalamus and the spinal cord.

Fluoxetine-induced Exacerbation of Chorea in Huntington's Disease? A Case Report. S. Chari,[1] S. H. Quraishi,[1] A. K. Jainer.[1] The Caludon Centre, Clifford Bridge Road, Coventry CV2 2TE, UK

INTRODUCTION

Huntington's chorea continues to pose challenges in the management of both psychiatric and neurological symptoms. The disorder, which was first described in 1872, is widely acknowledged to be due to a gene mutation that lies in the short arm of Chromosome 4. The pathology mainly affects the basal ganglia, in particular the caudate nucleus and the putamen. Wanker [10] recently wrote about the accumulation of highly insoluble intracellular protein aggregates in neuronal inclusions as a hallmark of Huntington's disease (HD), Parkinson's disease (PD), and several other late-onset neurodegenerative disorders. The aggregates formed generally have a fibrillar morphology, consist of individual beta-strands, and are resistant to proteolytic degradation. Myrianthopolous estimated the prevalence to be in the range of 4 to 7 per 100,000 population in the UK [6]. The inheritance is autosomal dominant, with 50 % of the offspring being affected and virtually all manifesting the disease.

Heathfield [3] concluded that the symptoms were almost equally divided between neurological and psychiatric symptoms. The neurological symptoms of chorea - hemichorea, dysarthria, ataxia, disturbance in fine motor task completion, and a conspicuous slowness of movement - are well recognized. The psychiatric symptoms of cognitive impairment giving rise to a subcortical dementia, pervasive apathy, self-neglect, marked depression, persecutory delusions, and suicide are also well known [5].

THE CASE

We write about the case of a 46-year-old Caucasian gentleman, with a diagnosis of Huntington's disease confirmed in 1995 by the West Midlands Regional Genetic Services in the UK. His mother had died at the age of 47 from the same illness. He was referred to the psychiatric services by a neurologist, who had been seeing him since 1995. The reason for the referral was for the management of excessive hand washing, which had reached a disabling degree and met the criteria for an ICD-10 [11] diagnosis of an obsessive-compulsive disorder (OCD).

Unfortunately, the degree of OCD was not quantified using standardized scales. Prior to this referral, he had never been in contact with psychiatric services and had not suffered from symptoms of OCD.

The neurologist treated the patient's chorea with tetrabenazine, which depletes dopamine at the nerve endings, at a dose of 25 mg three times daily orally, but this appeared to cause a deterioration in his symptoms. He was then started on haloperidol at a dose of 5 mg twice daily orally, which seemed to reduce his symptoms of chorea, but, unfortunately, no scales were used to quantify the difference. Following psychiatric assessment in November 1999, he was started on 20 mg of fluoxetine orally, a selective serotonin reuptake inhibitor (SSRI) to control his OCD symptoms. He was considered for cognitive behavioral therapy but was felt to be an unsuitable candidate because of the severity of his chorea.

Within a couple of days, he noticed a marked exacerbation of his chorea, and this continued over the two weeks that he was taking fluoxetine. This exacerbation of the chorea was corroborated by the patient, his wife, and the neurologist.

On review at the psychiatric clinic, the fluoxetine was stopped and he was switched to clomipramine, a tricyclic antidepressant that is known to be effective in the treatment of OCD, but he continued on haloperidol at a dose of 5 mg twice daily orally. The clomipramine was initiated at a dose of 25 mg per day and titrated upwards to achieve a dose of 100 mg per day.

In July 2000, he was seen by a neuropsychiatrist with a special interest in movement disorders, who felt that risperidone 1 mg four times per day instead of the haloperidol would be more suitable. This did not change his physical situation significantly, but his depression became more pronounced, with a pervasive low mood, tearfulness, low energy, and no motivation. His sleep became more erratic, with early morning wakening and a poor appetite. However, the depression and the OCD were brought under control by increasing the clomipramine to 200 mg per day.

Though the management of OCD is often difficult and has periodic relapses, we are pleased to report that to date there has been no relapse of his psychiatric symptoms, and he continues to be seen on a monthly basis. Unfortunately, his gait and chorea are getting worse and he and his family are aware of the prognosis of his illness.

CONCLUSION

We highlight two learning points in this case report. The first point is the occurrence of OCD as a psychiatric manifestation of Huntington's chorea. Second is the possibility of an exacerbation of chorea or other movement disorders when treated with SSRIs in general and fluoxetine in particular.

Given that fluoxetine is now generically available at a low cost, there will be greater prescribing and consequently a greater potential for such side effects, which may not be easily recognized or managed.

REFERENCES

1. Bharucha KJ, Sethi KD. Complex movements disorders induced by fluoxetine. *Movement Disorders* 1996; 11 (3): 324–326. This article in: PubMed.
2. Bird ED, Iverson LL. Huntington's chorea - postmortem measurement of glutamic acid decarboxylase, choline acetyltransferase and dopamine in basal ganglia. *Brain* 1974; 97: 457–472 This article in: PubMed.
3. Heathfield KWG. Huntington's chorea. *Brain* 1967; 90: 203–232 This article in: PubMed.
4. Jimenez-Jimenez FJ, Molina JA. Extrapyramidal symptoms associated with selective serotonin reuptake inhibitors, epidemiology, mechanisms and management. *CNS Drugs* 2000; 14 (5): 367–379. This article in: PubMed.
5. Lishman WA. Organic Psychiatry. Oxford Blackwell Science 1998 , p. 469–470.
6. Myrianthopolous NC. Huntington's chorea. *J Med Gen* 1966; 3: 298–314 This article in: PubMed.
7. Saxena S Brody AL, Schwart JM, Baxter LR. Neuroimaging and frontal-subcortical circuitry in obsessive-compulsive disorder. *B J Psych* 1998; 173 (suppl 35): 26–37. This article in: PubMed.
8. Scicutella A. Late-life obsessive-compulsive disorder and Huntington's disease. *J Neuropsy Clin Neurosci* 2000; 12: 228–289. This article in: PubMed.
9. Spokes EGS. Neurochemical alterations in Huntington's chorea: a study of post-mortem brain tissue. *Brain* 1980; 103: 179–210. This article in: PubMed.
10. Wanker EE. Protein aggregation in Huntington's and Parkinson's disease: implications for therapy. *Mol Med Today* 2000; 6 (10): 387–391. This article in: PubMed.
11. World Health Organisation (eds). The ICD - 10 classification of mental and behavioural disorders. Geneva WHO 1995

Mania and Tramadol-Fluoxetine Combination. Ana Gonzalez-Pinto, M.D., Harkaitz Imaz, M.D., Jose Luis Pérez De Heredia, M.D., Miguel Gutierrez, M.D., And Juan Antonio Micó, M.D. Vitoria, Spain. *Am J Psychiatry* 158:964–965, June 2001 Letter to the Editor.

To the Editor: Tramadol is a centrally acting analgesic that actives the muopioid receptor and enhances the action of serotonin and noradrenaline by interference with their uptake and release mechanisms. It has been suggested (1) that tramadol could be useful in the treatment of obsessive-compulsive disorder associated with the use of selective serotonin reuptake inhibitors (SSRIs). Discussion has included possible pharmacological interaction, leading to side effects such as serotonin syndrome. Also, tramadol-induced mania in a patient with bipolar disorder has been reported (2), but to our knowledge, there are no reports of tramadol-induced mania in patients with unipolar disorder. We present a report of a patient with serotonin syndrome and mania who had no previous history of manic episodes and was being treated with fluoxetine and tramadol.

Ms. A was a 72-year-old woman who had been treated with fluoxetine, 20 mg/day, for the last 10 years. She had had no cognitive deficits, had never been hospitalized, and had had only one previous major depressive episode, occurring 10 years before. She had been taking acetaminophen for the last year for articular pain. She was planning to take a trip, so her doctor prescribed tramadol to relieve the pain. After 18 days of taking tramadol, 150 mg/day, and fluoxetine, 20 mg/day, Ms. A began to feel nervous, had a temperature of 37.2°C, piloerection, and muscular contractions.

She stopped taking tramadol, and her physical symptoms disappeared by day 21. Nevertheless, she was agitated, euphoric, and hyperactive, slept less than 3 hours a day, and demonstrated rapid speech and paranoid ideation. She was conscious and oriented at all times. Ms. A was hospitalized for 3 days and stopped taking fluoxetine; haloperidol treatment was initiated at 5 mg/day. The results of a physical examination were normal. After discharge, her symptoms continued, so by day 31 she was hospitalized again. She then began treatment with olanzapine, 10 mg/day. Two weeks later she was euthymic and was discharged from the hospital while taking olanzapine, 10 mg/day.

This case of serotonin syndrome and mania in the same patient could be due to the fluoxetine-tramadol treatment combination. Tramadol contains a mono-O-desmethyl metabolite that has less serotonergic activity than tramadol. The rate of production of this metabolite is influenced by the CYP2D6 system. Fluoxetine could previously have inhibited CYP2D6 production, and, consequently, tramadol would have accumulated in serum, conveying a greater risk of adverse effects.

Also, preclinical reports have suggested an antidepressant effect with tramadol therapy (3). If this is the case, tramadol could induce mania itself in a manner similar to that of antidepressants, although the present episode probably was precipitated by coadministration of two compounds with similar mechanisms of action. In conclusion, it is important to consider the potential risk of inducing mania and serotonergic syndrome when using tramadol combined with SSRIs.

REFERENCES

1. Goldsmith TB, Shapira NA, Keck PE Jr: Rapid remission of OCD with tramadol hydrochloride (letter). *Am J Psychiatry* 1999; 156:660–661.
2. Watts BV, Grady TA: Tramadol-induced mania (letter). *Am J Psychiatry* 1997; 154:1624.
3. Rojas-Corrales MO, Gibert-Rahola J, Mico JA: Tramadol induces antidepressant-type effects in mice. *Life Sci* 1998; 63:175–180.

Antisocial violent offenders with attention deficit hyperactivity disorder demonstrate akathisia-like hyperactivity in three-channel actometry. Tuisku K, Virkkunen M, Holi M, Lauerma H, Naukkarinen H, Rimon R, Wahlbeck K. - Helsinki University Central Hospital, Department of Psychiatry, Helsinki, Finland. katinka.tuisku@hus.fi. *J Neuropsychiatry Clin Neurosci.* 2003 Spring;15(2):194–9.

Actometry enables quantitative and qualitative analysis of various hyperactivity disorders. Antisocial violent offenders have demonstrated diurnal increases in motor activity that may be related to attention deficit hyperactivity disorder (ADHD) that often precedes antisocial development. Motor restlessness in ADHD has common features with neuroleptic-induced akathisia. In this study, three-channel actometry was used to compare 15 antisocial violent offenders who had a history of ADHD with 15 healthy control subjects and 10 akathisia patients. The Barnes Akathisia Rating Scale (BARS) was used for clinical evaluation of akathisia symptoms. Ankle movement indices and the ankle-waist ratio differentiated the antisocial patients from the healthy controls significantly, with no overlap, and the same parameters expectedly differentiated the akathisia patients from the healthy controls. The repetitive, rhythmic pattern of akathisia was found in 13 of the 15 antisocial patients. Nine of the antisocial patients scored 2 or 3 (mild to moderate akathisia) on the BARS. Thus, the motor hyperactivity of antisocial ADHD patients has common features with mild akathisia. This may be due to a common hypodopaminergic etiology of ADHD and akathisia.

The relationship of akathisia with suicidality and depersonalization among patients with schizophrenia. Cem Atbasoglu E, Schultz SK, Andreasen NC. - Department of Psychiatry, Ankara University, Ankara, Turkey. atbasoglu@superonline.com. *J Neuropsychiatry Clin Neurosci.* **2001 Summer;13(3):336–41.**

An association of suicidality and depersonalization with akathisia has been reported, but it is not clear whether these phenomena are specific to akathisia or are nonspecific manifestations of distress. The authors used the Barnes Akathisia Rating Scale, Brief Psychiatric Rating Scale, and Hamilton Rating Scale for Depression (Ham-D) to examine the relationships between suicidality, depersonalization, dysphoria, and akathisia in 68 patients with schizophrenia or schizophreniform disorder. Akathisia was associated with higher scores on the Ham-D ratings of suicidality, depersonalization, and agitation. In a logistic regression model, depressive mood and subjective awareness of akathisia appeared to be the only predictors of suicidality and depersonalization, respectively. These findings support the association between akathisia and both suicidality and depersonalization. However, these symptoms appear to be nonspecific responses to accompanying depressive mood and the subjective awareness of the akathisia syndrome, respectively.

Fluoxetine-induced anaesthesia of vagina and nipples. A. Michael and C. Mayer - Department of Psychiatry, West Suffolk Hospital, Bury St Edmunds IP33 2QZ. *The British Journal of Psychiatry* **(2000) 176: 299**

Antidepressant drugs cause a variety of sexual side-effects. However, antidepressant-induced changes in sexual sensations are rare. We report a case of fluoxetine-induced loss of sensation of vagina and nipples.

A 48-year-old married woman with recurrent depression had good antidepressant response to fluoxetine 20 mg. However, her compliance with the medication was poor resulting in recurrences. While euthymic and on no antidepressants, her sexual function was normal. When depressed she has moderate decrease in libido. With fluoxetine 20 mg her depression remitted and her libido returned to normal. However, she developed a complete loss of sexual sensation of her nipples and vagina. Touch and pain sensations were also impaired, but only to a lesser extent. This lead to decreased satisfaction with sexual life and consequently poor compliance with the medication. Even when she became briefly hypomanic on fluoxetine, the lack of sensation persisted. We substituted her fluoxetine with trazodone 400 mg. She remained euthymic. By the fifth week her vaginal and nipple sensations returned to normal. The frequency of sexual inter-course and satisfaction improved to premorbid levels.

This is the first report of fluoxetine-induced loss of sensation of vagina and nipples. Fluoxetine-induced anaesthesia of penis (Neill, 1991; Measom, 1992) and vagina (King & Horowitz, 1993), which did not improve with dosage reduction or addition of cyproheptadine, but did with discontinuation of fluoxetine, have been reported. Ellison & DeLuca (1998) reported a case of genital anaesthesia caused by fluoxetine that did not improve with addition of cyproheptadine or yohimbine but responded to Ginkgo biloba. Ginkgo biloba is a Chinese herbal remedy for a variety of disorders and has diverse neurochemical effects. The mechanism of antidepressant-induced sexual anaesthesia remains elusive. The fact that the anaesthesia persisted even during the fluoxetine-induced hypomanic state confirms that this was not part of the depressive syndrome.

Sexual side-effects of antidepressant drugs cause distress, strain relationships, impair quality of life and reduce compliance with treatment. Enquiring routinely about side-effects, especially sexual side-effects of antidepressants, would help to improve compliance with treatment.

REFERENCES

Ellison, J. M. & DeLuca, P. (1998) Fluoxetine-induced genital anaesthesia relieved by Ginkgo biloba extract. *Journal of Clinical Psychiatry*, 59, 199–200.

King, V. L. & Horowitz, I. R. (1993) Vaginal anesthesia associated with fluoxetine use. *American Journal of Psychiatry*, 150, 984–985.

Measom, M. O. (1992) Penile anaesthesia and fluoxetine. *American Journal of Psychiatry*, 149, 709.

Neill, J. R. (1991) Penile anaesthesia associated with fluoxetine. *American Journal of Psychiatry*, 148, 1603.

Reversible galactorrhea and prolactin elevation related to fluoxetine use. Peterson MC. - Division of General Internal Medicine, University of Utah School of Medicine, Salt Lake City, USA. mike.peterson@utahtele-health.net. *Mayo Clin Proc.* **2001 Feb;76(2):215–6.**

Fluoxetine, an antidepressant of the selective serotonin reuptake inhibitor class, may stimulate prolactin release by pituitary lactotrophs. A 71-year-old woman taking estrogen replacement therapy developed galactorrhea after initiation of flu-oxetine for depression and was found to have an elevated prolactin level. Fluox-etine was discontinued with resolution of the patient's galactorrhea and normalization of her prolactin level.

Hyponatremia associated with sertraline and fluoxetine: a case report. Raphael K, Tokeshi J. - University of Hawaii, John A. Burns School of Med-icine, USA. *Hawaii Med J.* **2002 Mar;61(3):46–7.**

The syndrome of inappropriate antidiuretic hormone secretion (SIADH) is a rare but serious adverse effect of the selective serotonin reuptake inhibitors (SSRIs). Although many case reports describe this association, few report the effect of rechallenge with another SSRI. We present a case of an elderly patient who developed hyponatremia with sertraline and SIADH when rechallenged with fluoxetine.

Muscle changes in the neuroleptic malignant syndrome. Behan WM, Madigan M, Clark BJ, Goldberg J, McLellan DR. - University Department of Pathology, Western Infirmary, Glasgow, UK. wmb1q@clin-med.gla.ac.uk. *J Clin Pathol.* **2000 Mar;53(3):223–7.**

AIMS: To characterise the skeletal muscle changes in the neuroleptic malignant syndrome (NMS). METHODS: Detailed light and ultrastructural examination was carried out on skeletal muscle from three cases of NMS, two associated with recreational drugs (3,4-methlenedioxymethylamphetamine (MDMA, Ecstasy) and lysergic acid diethylamide (LSD)) and one with antipsychotic drugs (fluox-etine (Prozac) and remoxipride hydrochloride monohydrate (Roxiam)). RESULTS: The muscles were grossly swollen and oedematous in all cases, in one with such severe local involvement that the diagnosis of sarcoma was con-sidered. On microscopy, there was conspicuous oedema. In some fascicles less than 10% of fibres were affected whereas in others more than 50% were pale and enlarged. There was a spectrum of changes: tiny to large vacuoles replaced most of the sarcoplasm and were associated with necrosis. A striking feature in some fibres was the presence of contraction bands separating segments of oede-matous myofibrils. Severe endomysial oedema was also detectable. There was a scanty mononuclear infiltrate but no evidence of regeneration. CONCLU-SIONS: The muscle changes associated with NMS are characteristic and may be helpful in differential diagnosis.

Prozac: Safety Statement

PROZAC Safety Information, 2006 Eli Lilly and Company
http://www.prozac.com/common_pages/safety_information.jsp

IMPORTANT INFORMATION ABOUT PROZAC (FLUOXETINE HYDROCHLORIDE)

WHAT IS PROZAC?

PROZAC is a medicine approved by the FDA for the treatment of Major Depressive Disorder, Obsessive-Compulsive Disorder, Bulimia Nervosa and Panic Disorder in adults.

PROZAC is also approved for the treatment of Major Depressive Disorder and Obsessive-Compulsive Disorder in pediatric patients (children and adolescents).

PROZAC is available by prescription only.

WHAT IS THE ACTIVE INGREDIENT IN PROZAC?

PROZAC contains fluoxetine hydrochloride, the same ingredient as found in Prozac® Weekly™, Sarafem®, and generic versions of PROZAC.

WHO SHOULD NOT TAKE PROZAC?

You should not take PROZAC if you:
■ are allergic to PROZAC, or any of its components, or have had a bad reaction to PROZAC or generic fluoxetine previously.
■ are taking a type of antidepressant medicine known as a monoamine oxidase inhibitor (MAOI), such as Nardil® (phenelzine sulfate) or Parnate® (tranylcypromine sulfate). Using an MAOI together with many prescription medicines, including PROZAC, can cause serious or even life-threatening reactions. You must wait at least 14 days after you have stopped taking an MAOI before you can

take PROZAC. Also, you need to wait at least 5 weeks after you stop taking PROZAC before you take an MAOI.

■ are taking a type of antipsychotic medicine known as Mellaril® (thioridazine). Also, you need to wait at least 5 weeks after you stop taking PROZAC before you take Mellaril.

■ are taking a type of antipsychotic medicine known as Orap® (pimozide).

In clinical studies, antidepressants increased the risk of suicidal thinking and behavior in children, adolescents, and young adults with depression and other psychiatric disorders. Anyone considering the use of PROZAC or any other antidepressant in a child, adolescent, or young adult must balance this risk with the clinical need. Short-term studies did not show an increase in the risk of suicidality with antidepressants compared to placebo in adults beyond age 24; there was a reduction in risk with antidepressants compared to placebo in adults aged 65 and older. Depression and certain other psychiatric disorders are themselves associated with increases in the risk of suicide. Patients of all ages who are started on antidepressant therapy should be monitored appropriately and observed closely. Families and caregivers should discuss with the doctor any observation of worsening of depression symptoms, suicidal thinking and behavior, or unusual changes in behavior. PROZAC is approved for use in pediatric patients (children and adolescents) with MDD or obsessive compulsive disorder (OCD).

WHAT SHOULD I TALK TO MY DOCTOR OR PHARMACIST ABOUT?

Patients on antidepressants and their families or caregivers should watch for worsening depression symptoms, unusual changes in behavior and thoughts of suicide, as well as for anxiety, agitation, panic attacks, difficulty sleeping, irritability, hostility, aggressiveness, impulsivity, restlessness, or extreme hyperactivity. Call the doctor if you have thoughts of suicide or if any of these symptoms are severe or occur suddenly. Be especially observant at the beginning of treatment or whenever there is a change in dose. You should not stop taking PROZAC abruptly. Talk to your doctor before you stop taking PROZAC.

If you get a rash or hives while taking PROZAC, call your doctor right away because this can be a sign of a serious medical condition.

Be sure to tell your doctor if you are taking SARAFEM, PROZAC Weekly, or generic versions of PROZAC since these contain fluoxetine hydrochloride, the same active ingredient found in PROZAC.

Tell your doctor about all the nonprescription and prescription medicines you are taking, including those for migraine to avoid a potentially life-threatening condition. Also, tell your doctor if you are taking or plan to take any vitamins, herbal supplements or alcohol.

Be sure to tell your doctor if you are taking PROZAC and are taking or plan to take non-steroidal anti-inflammatory drugs or aspirin since combined use of these drug products have been associated with an increased risk of bleeding.

You should tell your doctor if you are pregnant, plan to become pregnant, or are breast-feeding while you are taking PROZAC.

Tell your doctor if you have diabetes. The dose of diabetes medicine may change when you start or stop taking PROZAC.

Tell your doctor about any other medical conditions you may have especially liver disease or seizures.

Tell your doctor if you have ever been told you had Bipolar Disorder ("Manic Depression") or have had a "manic" or "psychotic" episode.

WHAT ARE POSSIBLE SIDE EFFECTS OF PROZAC?

Some people experience side effects like nausea, difficulty sleeping, drowsiness, anxiety, nervousness, weakness, loss of appetite, tremors, dry mouth, sweating, decreased sex drive, impotence, or yawning. Most of these tend to go away within a few weeks of starting treatment and, in most cases, aren't serious enough to cause people to stop taking PROZAC.

PROZAC can cause changes in sexual desire or satisfaction.

Do not drive a car or operate dangerous machinery until you know what effects PROZAC may have on you.

Contact your doctor or healthcare professional if you get a rash or hives, or other side effects that concern you while taking PROZAC.

Index

❖ ❖ ❖

T

About Gary Null, Ph.D.

Time magazine called him *"The New Mr. Natural." My Generation* magazine dubbed him one of the top health gurus in the United States. For over three decades, Gary Null has been one of the foremost advocates of alternative medicine and natural healing.

A multi award-winning journalist and *New York Times* bestselling author, Dr. Null has written over seventy books on nutrition, self-empowerment, and public health issues, including his most recent, *Power Aging*. His syndicated public radio show, *Natural Living with Gary Null*, earned twenty-one *Silver Microphone Awards* and is the longest-running, continuously aired health program in America at twenty-seven years. Currently, *The Gary Null Show* can be heard on the Internet at www.garynull.com, from 12:00 noon to 1:00 p.m. EST. Null also broadcasts on Mondays, Tuesdays, and Wednesdays on WPFW (89.3 FM), from 3:00 p.m. to 4:00 p.m. EST, in Washington DC. In addition, he can be heard in Los Angeles on *Something's Happening with Roy of Hollywood* on KPFK (90.7 FM), from 12:00 a.m. to 5:30 a.m. PST. Lastly, Dr. Null can be heard on Sunday evenings on the Health Radio Network at 8:00 p.m. EST, broadcast over a growing national network of radio stations.

The Gary Null Show is not a "chit-chat" show but, rather, an on-air health forum featuring knowledgeable guests and well-researched scientific information that is presented objectively and in layperson's terms. The program's combination of provocative interviews, controversial commentary, and listener call-ins motivates listeners to change their lives for the better.

Gary Null holds a Ph.D. in human nutrition and public health science. He has been a consistent voice on how to live a longer, more vital life through work that embraces the body, mind and spirit. Gary believes that much of what our society accepts as inevitable markers of aging are actually manifestations of a preventable disease process. Gary's philosophy has influenced countless Americans to achieve a healthier, more fulfilling lifestyle. He is also the author of the *New York Times* bestsellers, *Get Healthy Now!* and *The Encyclopedia of Natural Healing*.

As the senior editor and lead investigator for the *Caveat Emptor*, plus host of ABC Radio Network and WABC radio, Gary Null captured the attention of hundreds of thousands of people who saw that he was unafraid to address controversial issues involving public health and alternative health practices in this country. As a reporter, Gary conducted more than one hundred major investigations into issues such as AIDS, chronic fatigue, heart disease, cancer, diet and exercise, stress management, arthritis, vaccines, and allergies. Television programs such as *20/20* and *60 Minutes* have used his material.

As a documentary filmmaker, Gary has achieved critical acclaim. He's produced over twenty films and videos on health and nutrition topics, including the following award-winning productions: *Age Is Only A Number*; *Overcoming Depression and Anxiety Disorders Naturally* (for which he received a coveted Gold CINDY [Cinema In Industry] Award); *Deconstructing The Myth of AIDS* (winner of the Audience Award for Best Documentary at both the New York and Los Angeles International Independent Film and Video Festivals); *Fatal Fallout* (winner of both Best Director and Best Documentary awards at the New York International Independent Film and Video Festival), and *Drugging of Our Children* (Winner of 2005 Best Documentary at World Houston International Film Festival and Key West Indy Fest).

Additionally, Gary Null's special programs, such as *Kiss Your Fat Goodbye—Get Fit Now* and *Seven Steps to Perfect Health*, are regularly featured during public television fundraising drives, spurring strong viewer contributions whenever broadcast.

Gary Null was a founder and director of health and nutrition certificate programs at Pratt Institute and the School of Visual Arts. He was the founder of the National Health Resources Council and the Nutrition Institute of America, where he has also served as a Director of Nutrition. As an athlete, Gary has trained thousands of marathon runners and walkers through his Natural Living Walking and Running Club. He is a TAC Master Champion athlete and was twice the MAC Track and Field Masters Athlete of the Year.

Gary Null has been featured in numerous publications, including *The Daily News*, *Time*, *People*, *Fitness*, *Time Out*, and *Vegetarian Times*. Throughout the years, he has garnered much recognition for his dedication, advocacy, and in-depth coverage of vital health issues, receiving the Truth in Journalism Award for Investigative Reporting and the Human Rights Award from the Citizens Commission on Human Rights. His scholarly and academic papers have been published in such journals as *The Townsend Letter for Doctors*, *The Journal of Orthomolecular Medicine*, and *The Journal of Applied Nutrition*.

Gary Null lives in New York City and Florida.

Achievement Awards

EDUCATIONAL

The Consumer Education Award: Health Resources Council - 1991
NY Regional Alumni Award for Exceptional Public Service: Union Institute - 1995

ENVIRONMENTAL

Environmental Lifetime Achievement Award: Earth First Foundation

JOURNALISM

Truth in Journalism Award: American Chiropractic Association Investigative Reporting - 1995
Truth in Journalism Award: Health Education AIDS Liaison - 1991
Health Journalism Award, Investigative Reporting: American Chiropractic Association - 1981, 1985

HUMAN RIGHTS

Human Rights Award: Citizens Commission on Human Rights - 1995
Special Investigations Award: Mental Health Patients' Rights
International Human Rights in Broadcast Journalism: American Chiropractic Association - 1994

SELECT DOCUMENTARY FILM AND RADIO AWARDS

2007 TEMECULA VALLEY INTERNATIONAL FILM FESTIVAL
Special Jury Prize: *Gulf War Syndrome—Killing Our Own*

ACTION ON FILM INTERNATIONAL FILM FESTIVAL
Best Documentary: *Gulf War Syndrome—Killing Our Own*

LONG ISLAND INTERNATIONAL FILM EXPO
Alan Fortunoff Humanitarian Film Award: *AIDS Inc.*

INDIE GATHERING
Best Documentary - First Place: *Gulf War Syndrome—Killing Our Own*
Best Documentary - Third Place: *AIDS Inc.*

WORLDFEST HOUSTON INTERNATIONAL FILM FESTIVAL
Best Documentary - Platinum Award: *Gulf War Syndrome—Killing Our Own*
Best Documentary - Silver Award: *AIDS Inc.*

THE HOBOKEN INTERNATIONAL FILM FESTIVAL
Winner Best Documentary and Best of the Festival Chariman's Award: *AIDS Inc.*

THE ACCOLADE COMPETITION
Award of Excellence: *AIDS Inc.*

2006 SANTA CLARITA VALLEY FILM FESTIVAL
Winner Best Documentary: *Friendly Fire—Exposing Gulf War Syndrome*

INDIE GATHERING
Best Documentary - Second Place: *Friendly Fire – Exposing Gulf War Syndrome*
Best Documentary - Third Place: *The Drugging of Our Children*
Best Documentary - Fourth Place: *Prescription for Disaster*

WORLDFEST HOUSTON INTERNATIONAL FILM FESTIVAL
Best Documentary - Platinum Award: *Prescription for Disaster*

RED BANK INTERNATIONAL FILM FESTIVAL
Best Documentary: *Prescription for Disaster*

SEDONA INTERNATIONAL FILM FESTIVAL
Finalist, Best Documentary: *The Drugging of Our Children*

KENT FILM FESTIVAL
Official selection: *Prescription for Disaster*

RED BANK INTERNATIONAL FILM FESTIVAL, SECRET CITY
FILM FESTIVAL, CACKALACKY FILM FESTIVAL, AUSTRALIAN
INTERNATIONAL FILM FESTIVAL, SANTA CLARITA VALLEY
FILM FESTIVAL
Official selection: *Friendly Fire – Exposing Gulf War Syndrome*

AUSTRALIAN INTERNATIONAL FILM FESTIVAL
Official selection: *Prescription for Disaster*

AUSTRALIAN INTERNATIONAL FILM FESTIVAL AND TACOMA
FILM FESTIVAL
Official selection: *The Drugging of Our Children*

2005 WORLDFEST HOUSTON INTERNATIONAL FILM FESTIVAL
Best Documentary - Platinum Award: *The Drugging of Our Children*

KEY WEST INDIEFEST
Best Documentary: *The Drugging of Our Children*

NEW YORK FILM FESTIVAL
Finalist Best Documentary: *The Drugging of Our Children*

WINNIPEG INTERNATIONAL FILM FESTIVAL
Finalist Best Documentary: *The Drugging of Our Children*

PALM BEACH INTERNATIONAL FILM FESTIVAL
Finalist Best Documentary: *The Drugging of Our Children*

GOLDEN FILM FESTIVAL
Finalist: *The Drugging of Our Children*

MARCH OF DIMES ACHIEVEMENT IN RADIO (AIR)
Awards Finalist: *Best News Series; Aids in Africa, Women's Health Issues*

SAN FRANCISCO WORLD FILM FESTIVAL
Finalist Best Documentary: *The Drugging Of Our Children*

ARPA INTERNATIONAL FILM FESTIVAL
Finalist Best Documentary: *The Drugging Of Our Children*

BLACK BEAR FILM FESTIVAL
Official Selection: *The Drugging Of Our Children*

SILVER MICROPHONE AWARD
National Finalist: *The Hidden Side of Psychiatry*

SILVER MICROPHONE AWARD
National Finalist: *Psychiatry's Bias Against Blacks*

SILVER MICROPHONE AWARD
National Finalist: *Sugar, Sweet Suicide*

SILVER MICROPHONE AWARD
National Finalist: *Pain, Profit & Politics of AIDS*

SILVER MICROPHONE AWARD
National Finalist: *Rediscovering The Legacy Of Women's Health*

SILVER MICROPHONE AWARD
National Finalist: *The Popes*

SILVER MICROPHONE AWARD
National Finalist: *Death By Medicine*

SILVER MICROPHONE AWARD
National Finalist: *Fluoride Toxicity*

SILVER MICROPHONE AWARD
National Finalist: *Causes of Cancer*

SILVER MICROPHONE AWARD
National Finalist: *The Overmedicating Of Our Children*

SILVER MICROPHONE AWARD
National Finalist: *Thyroid Health*

2004 NEW YORK FESTIVALS
Certificate of Distinction, Finalist Winner: *Deconstructing the Myth of AIDS*

MARCH OF DIMES ACHIEVEMENT IN RADIO (AIR)
Awards Finalist: *Anti Depressants, Are they Safe?*

ZOIE FILM FESTIVAL
Second Place Award for Best Documentary: *Gulf War Syndrome: A Deadly Legacy*

2003 SARASOTA FILM FESTIVAL
Cultural Impressions Documentary Film Award: *Deconstructing the Myth of AIDS*

NEW YORK INTERNATIONAL INDEPENDENT FILM & VIDEO FESTIVAL, LOS ANGELES SCREENING
Grand Jury Prize, Best Director of a Documentary: *Fatal Fallout*

WORLD MEDIA FESTIVAL HAMBURG
Intermedia Globe Gold Lifestyle Documentary: *Supercharge Your Immune System*

HONOLULU INTERNATIONAL FESTIVAL
Jury Category of Integral Realization: *Deconstructing the Myth of AIDS*
Honorable Mention: *Fatal Fallout*

MARCH OF DIMES ACHIEVEMENT IN RADIO (AIR)
Awards Finalist, Best Non-Music show: *Natural Living With Gary Null*
Awards Finalist, Best Syndicated Show Originating in New York: *ECT: A Second Opinion*

HEALTH AND SCIENCE COMMUNICATIONS ASSOCIATION (HeSCA)
Leadership in Health & Science Communication: *Deconstructing the Myth of AIDS*

WORLDFEST HOUSTON
Gold Award: *Deconstructing the Myth of AIDS*

ZOIE FILM FESTIVAL
Awards Finalist: *Deconstructing the Myth of AIDS*

COLUMBUS INTERNATIONAL FILM & VIDEO FESTIVAL *THE CHRIS AWARDS*
Bronze Plaque: *Supercharge Your Immune System*
Honorable Mention: *Fatal Fallout, Deconstructing the Myth of AIDS*
Certificate of Participation: *Power Aging*

ANNAPOLIS FILM FESTIVAL
Awards Finalist: *Fatal Fallout*

NEW YORK FESTIVALS
Awards Finalist: *Deconstructing the Myth of AIDS*

2002 US INTERNATIONAL FILM & VIDEO FESTIVAL
Certificate for Creative Excellence: *Deconstructing the Myth of AIDS*

2001 COLUMBUS INTERNATIONAL FILM & VIDEO FESTIVAL, *THE CHRIS AWARDS*
Honorable Mention: *De-Stress Now!*

SILVER MICROPHONE AWARDS
National Finalist: *Women's Health Issues*

WORLDFEST HOUSTON
Special Jury Gold Award: *It's Not Your Fault You're Fat*

NEW YORK INTERNATIONAL INDEPENDENT FILM & VIDEO
FESTIVAL
Best Documentary, Current Issues, Medicine & Health: *Deconstructing the Myth of AIDS*

LOS ANGELES INTERNATIONAL INDEPENDENT FILM & VIDEO
FESTIVAL
Best Documentary, Medicine & Health Research: *Deconstructing the Myth of AIDS*

1999   CINDY INTERNATIONAL
Silver Award: *Gulf War Syndrome: A Deadly Legacy*

Mature Media
Bronze Award: *Staying Young Forever*

1998   NEW YORK INTERNATIONAL INDEPENDENT FILM & VIDEO
FESTIVAL
Bronze Award: *AIDS: A Second Opinion*
Gold Award, Investigative Documentary: *Gulf War Syndrome: A Deadly Legacy*

ATHLETIC AWARDS

Silver Medal: Summer World Games, Spain, 20K team championship - 2005
Silver Medal: Summer World Games, Puerto Rico - 2003
Outstanding Male Racewalker: Florida - 1996
Track and Field Masters Athlete of the Year: Metropolitan Athletic Congress - 1995
Outstanding Achievement Award: Metropolitan Athletic Congress - 1994
Master Championship Track and Field Athlete of the Year: Metropolitan Athletic Congress - 1992
Grand Prix Indoor Champion: Metropolitan Athletic Congress - 1992

Books by Gary Null

7 Steps to Overcoming Cardiovascular Disease
7 Steps to Overcoming Anxiety and Depression
7 Steps to Overcoming Arthritis and Back Pain
90's Healthy Body Book
AIDS: A Second Opinion
Baby Boomer's Guide to Getting it Right the Second Time Around
Be Kind to Yourself
Biofeedback, Fasting and Meditation
Black Hollywood
Black Hollywood: 1970–Today
Change Your Life Now
Clearer, Cleaner, Safer, Greener
Encyclopedia of Natural Healing
For Women Only
Gary Null's Guide to Joyful, Healthy Life
Gary Null's Perfect Health System
Gary Null's Ultimate AntiAging Program
Gary Null's Ultimate Lifetime Diet
Germs, Biological Warfare, Vaccinations
Get Healthy Now!
Healing with Magnets
Healing Your Body Naturally
Herbs for the Seventies
How to Get Rid of the Poisons in Your Body
How to Keep Your Feet and Legs Healthy for a Lifetime
How to Turn Your Ideas into Dollars
Joy of Juicing Recipe Guide
Man and His Whole Earth
Mind Power
Natural Organic Beauty Book
Natural Pet Care
New Vegetarian Cookbook
No More Allergies
Nutrition Source Book for the 80's

Power Foods

Power Aging

Profitable PartTime Home Based Businesses

✓ *Protein for Vegetarians*

Reverse the Aging Process Naturally

Secrets of the Sacred White Buffalo

Successful Pregnancy

Supercharge Your Heath!

The Clinician's Handbook of Natural Healing

The Complete Handbook of Nutrition

The Complete Guide to Health and Nutrition

The Complete Question and Answer Book of General Nutrition

✓ *The Egg Project*

The Vegetarian Handbook

The Vegetarian Handbook

Vegetarian Cooking for Good Health

Who Are Your Really?

Whole body Health and Sex Book

Why Your Stomach Hurts

Women's Health Solutions

7 Steps to Perfect Health

A Little Bit of Everything Good

Choosing Joy

Complete Guide to Healing Your Body Naturally

Complete Handbook of Nutrition

Food Combining Handbook

Food Mood Body Connection

Gary Null's International Vegetarian Cookbook

Gary Null's Power Aging

Gary Null's Ultimate Lifetime Diet

Good Food, Good Mood

Handbook of Skin and Hair

Nutrition and the Mind

The Complete Guide to Sensible Eating

Ultimate Training

Gary Null Video Documentaries

AIDS Inc.

Deconstructing the Myth of AIDS

The Drugging of our Children

Fatal Fallout

Friendly Fire

Gulf War Syndrome – Killing Our Own

Prescription For Disaster

7 Steps to Perfect Health

Age is Only a Number

Art of Health - 4-Part Box Set

Art of Health - Living a Dynamic Life

Art of Health - Cooking Up Good Health

Art of Health - Natural Healing Part 1

Art of Health - Natural Healing Part 2

De-Stress Now

For Women Only

Get Healthy Now

How To Live Forever

It's Not Your Fault You're Fat

Kiss Your Fat Goodbye—Get Fit Now

Mind Power

Natural Pet Care

Power Aging

Supercharge Your Immune System

7 Steps to Total Health

AIDS: A Second Opinion

AIDS: The Untold Story

Allergies: A Natural Approach

Alternative Approach to Disease

Dental Care: A Natural Approach

Detoxification: A Natural Approach

Diet for Lifetime

Eye Care: A Natural Approach

Guilt Free Vegetarian Desserts

Hair Care: A Natural Approach
Healing Your Body Naturally
Nice & Easy
Overcoming Cardiovascular Disease Naturally
Overcoming Depression & Anxiety Disorders
Overcoming Fatigue: A Natural Approach
Pain A Natural Approach
Preparing Live Foods with Gary Null & Roberta Atti
Sexual Healing
Shopping Healthy with Gary Null
Total Health Step 5 (Update) Shopping Healthy with Gary Null
Sick, Twisted & Living the American Dream Part 1
Sick, Twisted and Living the American Dream Part 2
Sick, Twisted and Living the American Dream Part 3
Sick, Twisted and Living the American Dream Part 4
Staying Young Forever
Stress Management: A Natural Approach
Anger: Taming the Beast Within
Change Your Life
Choosing Your Essential Needs
Embracing Our Bliss
Embracing Passion
Enhancing Self Esteem
Expanding Into Consciousness
Honor Your Self
How To Manifest A Beautiful Life
I'm Not Finished Yet
Letting Go of Fear
Life Energies
Rebalance Your Life
The 13th Step
Vaccine-Nation
Wake Up and Get Healthy
You're Smarter Than You Think

Other Titles by Gary Null, Ph.D. from Seven Stories Press

Get Healthy Now!: A Complete Guide to Prevention, Treatment and Healthy Living (2006)

The fully revised and updated edition to the national bestseller *Get Healthy Now!* includes new research and nutritional advice for treating allergies, diabetes, PMS, andropause, and everything in-between. From healthy skin and hair to foot and leg care, and featuring an up-to-date Alternative Practitioners Guide, *Get Healthy Now!* is your one-stop guide to becoming healthier from top to bottom, inside and out.

Let "the new Mr. Natural" (*Time* magazine) show you the best alternatives to drugs, surgical intervention, and other standard Western techniques. Drawing from methods that have been supported by thousands of years of use in other societies, as well as more recent discoveries in modern medicine, this comprehensive guide to healthy living offers a wide range of alternative approaches to help you stay healthy.

Germs, Biological Warfare, Vaccinations: What You Need to Know (2002)
with James Feast

In response to deepening concerns of the threat of germ warfare and bioterrorism, *Germs, Biological Warfare, Vaccinations: What You Need to Know* is the first book to discuss traditional methods of combating germ warfare while also offering simple, natural alternative approaches to preventing and treating diseases caused by biological agents.

Germs, Biological Warfare, Vaccinations includes

➤ a historical review of the use of biological weapons from 400 BC to the present day;

➤ a list of bacteria, viruses, fungi, and toxins considered to be biological weapons, including Anthrax, Botulism, and Ebola viruses—along with definitions and descriptions of the various agents, symptoms, and treatment options;

➤ information on how to detoxify, de-acidify, and de-stress;

➤ natural ways to boost your immune system, including the use of herbs, vitamins, minerals, and nutrients;

➤ and a discussion of traditional versus alternative approaches, focusing on the safety and effectiveness of each.

➤ Also included is a resource guide listing key organizations—including Web sites and support groups—that offer information about natural prevention and treatment of infectious diseases.

Women's Health Solutions (2002)

For the legions of women turning to alternative health practices today, *Women's Health Solutions* is a compendium founded in holistic principles, and featuring the most up-to-date clinical experiences and published research. *Women's Health Solutions* covers general physical and mental issues, as well as those particular to women, including

➤ anemia

➤ birth control

➤ breast cancer

➤ chronic fatigue syndrome

➤ diabetes

➤ endometriosis

➤ infertility

➤ lupus

➤ menopause

➤ multiple sclerosis

➤ occupational disorders

➤ premenstrual syndrome

- sexual dysfunction
- sexually transmitted diseases
- stroke
- urinary incontinence
- varicose veins
- vulvar disorders
- and much more.

In each of its thirty-eight chapters, this encyclopedia includes a thorough discussion of each health problem and the recommended preventions and treatments, emphasizing tried and proven alternative approaches from acupuncture and Ayurveda to Chinese medicine and Hellerwork, to Reiki and yoga techniques.

Complemented by a resource guide and tips on how to select an alternative health practitioner, the unconventional approaches found in *Women's Health Solutions* are bound to empower women to take their health into their own hands.

AIDS:
A Second Opinion (2001)

In this first book to bring both establishment and dissenting views of the AIDS crisis into one volume, Gary Null unravels the half-truths that many argue have marred the study of this disease from the start. In clear, jargon-free prose, the book offers an unbiased, unflinching discussion of all sides of each issue.

AIDS: A Second Opinion argues that the AIDS drama has exposed problematic issues having to do with the functioning of US medical institutions. Null explores a new type of health care, grounded in patients' own choices and dispositions, that poses a challenge to the top-down, expert-controlled medical systems favored by the establishment.

Drawing from Null's many years of study of alternative, traditional, and orthodox medicine as well as from interviews with many long-term survivors, the book dissects the claims of the AZT and drug-cocktail approach to treating AIDS and offers a trilogy of treatment strategies based on wide views of how to enhance the immune system and improve overall functioning.

Natural Pet Care:
Your Spectacular Pet (2000)
with James Feast

Right now, there are more pets in America than people, and many count their pets among the most beloved members of their family. However, a surprising number of pet owners are not aware that the lifestyle they provide their companions may not be a healthy one.

Gary Null has helped countless Americans improve their diets and their health with his natural approach to healthy living and skepticism of the healthcare and pharmaceutical industries. Now, with *Natural Pet Care*, he carefully and compassionately lays out the ways we can improve our pets' health and lives. *Natural Pet Care* includes

> ➤ "Animals on the Move," which explains the importance of proper exercise;

> ➤ "Everybody in the Tub!" which covers natural bathing and grooming products and techniques;

> ➤ "The Impetuous Pet," which helps in understanding your animal's behavior;

> ➤ and appendices for those seeking holistic veterinary care, pet friendly lodgings and animal friendly organizations.

Natural Pet Care also provides sources for natural pet foods and products, while scrutinizing the pet food industry. He describes, for instance, that almost any dog owner would be horrified to learn what really goes into most commercial dog foods—even some of the more expensive brands—including "slaughterhouse throwaways" and diseased animal parts. As an alternative, Null offers "The Tao of Chow," in which he recommends countless natural alternatives that can easily be made at home—recipes included—and which can prolong and improve your pet's life. With this book on your reference shelf, you and your spectacular pet will be ready to tackle anything naturally!

Natural Pet Care deals extensively with the health of dogs and cats, but also is devoted to other common pets, including birds, rabbits, ferrets, fish, horses, rodents, and snakes. Long overdue, Gary Null's *Natural Pet Care* will help pet owners provide their furry, feathered, and scaled companions with the healthy lifestyle they need and deserve.

For Women Only!:
Your Guide to Health Empowerment
(1999, 2001)
with Barbara Seaman

Both a reference work and a health guide, *For Women Only!* joins together hands-on advice from the country's leading health practicioners with essays, interviews, and commentary by leading thinkers, activists, writers, doctors, and sociologists. Contributors include the Boston Women's Health Book Collective, Susan Brownmiller, Phyllis Chesler, Angela Davis, Charlotte Perkins Gilman, Germaine Greer, Shere Hite, Erica Jong, the National Black Women's Health Project, Gloria Steinem, Sojourner Truth, and Naomi Wolf, among many others.

How To Keep Your Feet and Legs Healthy
For a Lifetime:
The Complete Guide to Foot and Leg Care
(1999)
with Howard Robins

Written by Dr. Gary Null and Dr. Howard Robins, a foot specialist, *How to Keep Your Feet and Legs Healthy for a Lifetime* tells you everything you always wanted to know about your most active body parts. It includes chapters on the true course of athlete's foot and how to prevent it, a complete manual of foot massage, a guide to proper foot wear, advice on how to treat common foot ailments and deformities, optimum performance exercises for walkers, joggers and runners, pointers for athletes to help them avoid sports injuries, and much more.

The Complete Guide to Sensible Eating
(1998)

The bestselling comprehensive guide for anyone interested in starting or maintaining a holistic approach to their health, *The Complete Guide to Sensible Eating* features new chapters including "Holistic Dentistry," "Pain Management Techniques," "Phytochemicals," and "Reversing the Aging Process." It also contains chapters on detoxification, homeopathy, herbs, and healing. Null offers a hands-on, alternative approach to nutrition and health, integrating exercise and other weight management techniques with individual nutritional needs.

The book contains over fifty original recipes and advice on how to rotate foods in the diet, as well as chapters that demonstrate how to handle food allergies and how to find an alternative practitioner to best suit your health needs.

Nutrition and the Mind (1996)

Renowned nutritionist Gary Null interviews twenty-five distinguished physicians about the origins and treatments for alcoholism, depression, food allergies, chronic fatigue, Alzheimer's, hypoglycemia, PMS, and behavioral problems in children, among other conditions. In case after case, the doctors found that certain mental and physical conditions can be caused by vitamin deficiencies, environmental toxins, hormonal imbalances, food allergies, or the inability of the body to absorb certain nutrients.

The doctors show that frequently these conditions respond to nutritional treatments, especially when conventional approaches have failed. "Calcium and magnesium deficiencies can produce anxiety attacks in some people," explains Michael Schacter, M.D., a New York psychiatrist and graduate of Columbia University's College of Physicians and Surgeons. "By correcting some of these nutrient imbalances, we can reduce tremendously the chances of a person having panic attacks."

Null also cites studies which show a link between low thyroid conditions and depression, and other studies which reveal chronic underlying vitamin and mineral deficiencies in alcoholics. In both types of cases, nutrient supplements are used to treat the underlying physical condition and can relieve psychological and emotional distress.

Other topics covered in *Nutrition and the Mind* include

➤ the connection between toxins in the environment and mental disorders,

➤ nutritional treatments that can be used with Prozac for treating mood disorders,

➤ a special section on mental disorders in children, and

➤ the benefits of the "wonder drug" Tryptophan, which was banned by the FDA.

Nutrition and the Mind also includes groundbreaking case studies; a history of orthomolecular medicine ("the right amount of the right nutrients"), which began with the work of Nobel prizewinner Dr. Linus Pauling; and a list of recent scientific articles that describe the link between nutrition and illness.

About the Editor

AMY McDONALD has worked in the medical publishing field for nearly twenty years. She has edited many articles and several books, including *Women's Health Solutions* and the national bestseller *Get Healthy Now!*, both by Gary Null.